SQUAMOUS CELL CARCINOMA

Edited by **Xiaoming Li**

Squamous Cell Carcinoma
Edited by Xiaoming Li

Published by InTech
Janeza Trdine 9, 51000 Rijeka, Croatia

Publishing Process Manager Vedran Greblo

Technical Editor Teodora Smiljanic

Cover Designer InTech Design Team

Additional hard copies can be obtained from orders@intechopen.com

Squamous Cell Carcinoma, Edited by Xiaoming Li
p. cm.
ISBN 978-953-51-0024-9

For EU product safety concerns:
IN TECH d.o.o., Prolaz Marije Krucifikse Kozulić 3, 51000 Rijeka, Croatia,
info@intechopen.com or visit our website at intechopen.com.

Meet the editor

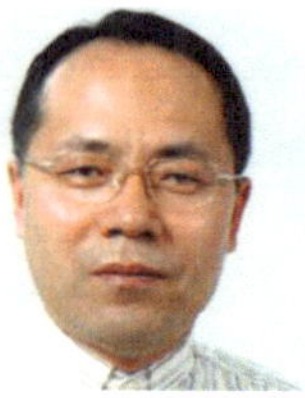

Xiaoming Li, MD, PhD is now Professor and Director of Department of Otolaryngology Head & Neck Surgery, Bethune International Peace Hospital, China. He is now the Head of Surgical Head and Neck Oncology Section, Chinese Otolaryngology Head and Neck Surgery Society. His special interest in clinic is surgical management of head and neck cancers including tumor resection and one-stage reconstruction. His expertise in surgical salvage for advanced recurrent head and squamous cell carcinomas (HNSCC) is recognized in that he gave two special talks in round table session on reconstructive surgery for HNSCC and one keynote lecture on salvage surgery of recurrent HNSCC in recent two IFOS world congresses. Over the years, he conducted a series of studies on the clino-pathologic features of HNSCC, defining some important factors for predicting metastasis and recurrence. He also devotes himself to in-depth investigation on molecular aspects of tumor invasion and progression, and therapeutic resistance of HNSCC. He was a research scientist from 1999 to 2002 in the National Cancer Institute (NCI), NIH, USA. He was visiting professor of several universities in the world. He published a paper in Nature in 2003 for definition of a new pathway on TNF receptor signaling. His research work is now focusing on genetic manipulations of resistance of HNSCC to chemoradiation by targeting some genes and cell populations such as cancer stem cells.

Contents

Preface

Squamous cell carcinoma (SCC) represents a common malignancy of mankind. It originates in the squamous epithelia covering the external surface of the body or lining the inner surface of lumen of different body systems. Because of the diversity in the location of the primary tumors, patients may present with distinct clinicopathologic manifestations, making it necessary to manage them individually and multidisciplinarily. Even with marked advances in the understanding of the disease and treatment modalities, there are still many difficult problems to solve and unclear questions to address.

This book is unique in that it supplies an in-depth discussion of a series of interesting topics on SCC. Firstly, the features and management of some specific SCC is discussed to give the readers the general principles in dealing with these uncommon and sophisticated conditions. Some new concepts in adjuvant therapy including neoadjuvant therapy and gold nanoparticle-based photo dynamic therapy are introduced, the latter of which shows a great promise in the treatment of SCC. Secondly, a detailed discussion of molecular aspects of tumor invasion and progression in SCC is provided with the emphasis on the roles of some important factors. The role of tumor microenvironment in head and neck SCC is specifically discussed, which is comprised of cellular and non-cellular components. Thirdly, as a relatively new concept, the roles of cancer stem cells (CSC) in cancer therapy of SCC are described. Molecular mechanisms involving therapeutic resistance and new therapeutic strategies targeting CSC are discussed in detail. Finally, other aspects concerning SCC are also included, which involve the assessment, genetic manipulation and its possible clinical implications for the treatment of SCC. It is really our hope that the book can point to some new areas deserved for further investigation on SCC, and much progress in the understanding and treatment of the disease be made in the near future.

To be frank, it is really such an extensive topic to discuss about SCC. Moreover, within a book containing limited chapters, we are definitely unable to cover nearly all related issues on SCC. Our intent in writing the book "Squamous Cell Carcinoma" is to provide the readers with not very comprehensive but exclusive presentations on some special issues in the recent advances in the study of SCC. Perhaps, many important parts concerning diagnosis and treatment of SCC have been missed, which seems to be our regret for this book.

I wish to give special thanks to all contributors of the book around the world. Without the great efforts and excellent work they made, the publication of the book would not have been realized. I finally express my love and thanks to my wife and other family members for their constant understanding, support, love and patience in helping such a project to a final success.

Professor and Director Xiaoming Li
Department of Otolaryngology Head Neck Surgery,
Bethune International Peace Hospital
China

Part 1

Features and Managment of Some Specific Squamous Cell Carcinomas

1

Metastasis of Head and Neck Squamous Cell Carcinoma

Xiaoming Li, Yupeng Shen, Bin Di and Qi Song
Bethune International Peace Hospital
China

1. Introduction

Head and neck squamous cell carcinoma (HNSCC) is the sixth most common cancer worldwide and accounts for approximately 650,000 new diagnoses and 350,000 cancer deaths every year (Parkin, et al., 2005). In the United States, HNSCC accounts for approximately 5% of all cancer cases diagnosed per year. Even with significant advances in operative skills such as reconstructive microvascular free tissue transfer, and in adjuvant therapies such as hyperfractioned radiotherapy and concomitant chemoradiation, the 5-year survival of the HNSCC has not been markedly improved in the past three decades. The number of annually diagnosed cases amounts to over 42,000 individuals and results in more than 12,000 deaths per year in the United States. As is known, HNSCC is a locoregional disease notoriously for regional and distant metastases, representing the leading cause of death in HNSCC patients. Although surgical resection of isolated metastases is beneficial for some patients, the overall efficacy of surgery, chemotherapy or radiotherapy is still limited. The main reason for the poor 5-year survival may be that the most important prognostic factors for these patients are not only local control, but regional and distant metastases as well.

2. Development of metastasis

Metastasis is defined as the spread of disease from one organ or part to another not directly connected with it through the blood, lymph, or serosal surfaces. Recent investigations disclose the mysterious aspects of the cancer metastasis. The development of metastasis of tumor is a multi-step process, in which multiple genes participate in and play different roles. With regard to the regional lymph node metastasis, several important gene proteins related to mirovascular angiogenesis and lymphogenesis function as promoters of regional lymph node metastasis. For the regional metastasis to occur, it is necessary for tumor cells to enter the microvessels to gain the pathway to the lymphatic channels. After entering the tumor-draining lymphatic channels, the tumor cells migrate to the regional lymph nodes in the neck, in which they settle and form the foci of micrometastasis. In the event of distant metastasis, several processes determine the tumor spreading to other organ systems, including angiogenesis, tumor invasion into local stroma and vascular system, circulation of tumor cells, arrest of tumor cells at distant site, and colony formation at secondary site. It is obvious that tumor invasion into stroma and vascular system is a prerequisite to the development of distant metastasis, which involves attachment of tumor to the basement membrane, degradation of extracellular matrix components, migration of malignant cells to the stroma and ultimate invasion to the surrounding blood vessels or lymphatic channels. Recently, results from several studies indicate that the disseminated cancer cells alter their adjacent stroma into a "metastatic" microenvironment that is similar to the primary tumor microenvironment in which they can survive and proliferate. A better understanding of the gene expression pattern and molecular biologic mechanisms of metastasis in HNSCC may be beneficial for exploration of new effective therapies to prevent the development of metastasis and to improve the survival of these patients.

2.1 Genes involved in metastasis

Development of metastatic carcinoma is associated with masses of molecules involved in cell adhesion, migration, and invasion in HNSCC. Further insight into the molecular basis of metastasis in HNSCC could lead to advances in screening, diagnosis, and treatment with improved clinical outcome. Multiple gene products are involved in angiogenesis, all of which have been demonstrated to be critical for regulating angiogenic phenotype. This has raised the need for comprehensive analysis of the angiogenic phenotype using microarray analysis and global proteomic approaches. Complex interplay between positive and negative regulators determines the degree of neovascularization in and around the tumor. And now emerging evidence suggests that the lymphangiogenic factors may also play important roles in lymph node metastasis in many cancers.

2.1.1 Vascular endothelial growth factor (VEGF)

As a key regulator of angiogenesis, the role of VEGF has been extensively studied. Tumor cells enter the circulation by penetration through proliferating capillaries that have fragmented basement membrane. Further progress in this multi-step cascade is controlled by the positive and negative regulators of angiogenesis. Recent studies have shown that VEGF receptor-expressing cells from the bone marrow arrive at a specific site of future metastasis even prior to arrival of metastatic cells (Ellis, 2008). First and foremost, VEGF is a highly potent angiogenic agent that acts to increase vessel permeability and enhance endothelial cell growth, proliferation, migration and differentiation (Johnstone & Logan, 2007). In addition, VEGF promotes angiogenesis in many different tumor types. VEGF levels may affect tumor growth, metastatic potential, and response to radiotherapy. VEGF expression may prove to be an important prognostic factor in head and neck cancer (Smith, et al., 2000); VEGF positivity is the most significant predictor of poor prognosis. Accordingly, the potent role of VEGF in angiogenesis has spurred interest in using this molecule as a therapeutic target in antiangiogenetic therapy.

2.1.2 Matrix metalloproteinases (MMP)

As is known, MMP has the ability to degrade connective tissues such as the basement membrane, which is a crucial step in the initiation of metastatic process, thus serving as a positive regulator of metastasis. Expression levels of molecules involved in tissue remodeling and extracellular matrix (ECM) adhesion, especially *MMP-1* and *integrin-3,* can provide an accurate biomarker system for predicting the risk of cervical lymph node metastasis in oral squamous cell carcinoma (Nagata, et al., 2003). In order to breech the basement membrane and invade the connective tissue stroma, HNSSC must produce enzymes capable of degrading the extracellular matrix. General classes of these proteolytic molecules include MMPs, named for their dependence on Zn^{2+} as a catalyst, and the plasminogen activators. The MMPs are a large group of secreted proteinases that require zinc for catalytic activity. MMP-2 and MMP-9 are the largest members of this gene family. They are able to degrade connective tissue, among other substrates, the basement membrane collagen, which appears to be very crucial in tumor cell invasion and in the process of metastasis.

The association of the expression of MMP-9 and MMP-2 with mode of tumor invasion and nodal involvement has previously been found in squamous cell carcinoma, and recently its utility has been proven in oral cancers (Miyajima, et al., 1995, Patel, et al., 2007). However, some studies have shown that the activation of MMP-2 was more prominent as compared with MMP-9 in malignant oral SCCs. Elevated activation ratio of MMP-2 has also correlated significantly with lymph node metastasis in oral SCCs. Accordingly, MMP-2 was considered by some investigators as more selective molecular marker for prediction of metastatic potentials of oral SCCs (Patel, et al., 2007). Certain other studies have shown results favoring the use of MMP-9 as a prognostic indicator (Ruokolainen, et al., 2004). Association between MMP-9 and vascular endothelial growth factor expression or micro vessel density has been found in head and neck carcinoma (Riedel, et al., 2000). The summary of MMPs produeced by HNSCC is illustrated in table 1.

MMP	Name	Substrate
Collagenases		
MMP-1	Interstitial	Collagens I, II, III, V, IX
	collagenase	Collagens I, II, III, V, IX
MMP-8	Neutrophil	Elastin
MMP-12	collagenase	Collagen III
MMP-13	Metalloelastase	
	Collagenase3	
Stromelysins		
MMP-3	Stromelysin 1	Proteoglycans, collagen IV, gelatins
MMP-7	Matrilysin	Fibronectin, collagen IV
MMP-10	Stromelysin 2	Proteoglycans, collagen IV, gelatins
MMP-11	Stromelysin 3	Laminin and fibronectin
Gelatinases		
MMP-2	Gelatinase A	Gelatin, collagens IV and V
MMP-9	Gelatinase B	Gelatin, collagens IV and V

Table 1. MMP produced by HNSCC

2.1.3 Endostatin

Endostain exhibits specific inhibitory action on the proliferating endothelial cells of newly formed blood vessels, representing one of the better defined and most potent negative regulators of angiogenesis (O'Reilly, et al., 1997). Earlier studies have shown that plasma levels of endostatin in patients with HNSCC have been associated with histologic grade, recurrence, and survival rate (Homer, et al., 2002). However, the immunohistochemical expression of endostatin and collagen XVIII in SCC tissues and their significance for the growth and metastatic potential of these tumors have not been widely studied. In a recent study, the levels of endostatin were lower in the primary tumors of cases with multiple metastatic lymph nodes compared with non metastatic tumors. The differences in endostatin expression between these tumors corresponded well with the levels of collagen XVIII, suggesting that the reduction in endostatin expression in the node positive group is because of decreases in the production of the precursor molecule collagen XVIII. On the other hand, these results contradict with those of Homer *et al* (Homer, et al., 2002), who observed a positive trend between higher levels of endostatin and nodal metastasis and an association between increased endostatin expression and higher tumor grade, recurrence, and death in patients with HNSCC. The authors attributed this discrepancy to differences in methods used, as these investigators measured the circulating levels of endostatin, whereas this study assessed the levels in tissue samples (Nikitakis, et al., 2003).

2.1.4 Others

E-cadherin is an important molecule that promotes cell to cell adhesion which serves as a positive regulator of metastasis. Low expression of E-cadherin should be considered as a high-risk group for late cervical metastasis when a wait-and-see policy for the neck is adopted (Lim, et al., 2004). The plasminogen activators (PAs) are another class of proteases that have been confirmed to play important parts in invasion and metastasis of HNSCC. PAs are neutral serine proteases which catalyze the synthesis of plasmin from plasminogen. Plasmin is a fibrinolytic enzyme, also active in degrading type IV collagen and laminin.

2.2 Molecular pathologic changes during development of metastasis

HNSCC will progress from carcinoma in situ, to microinvasive carcinoma, to an invasive tumor with stromal invasion, and to a deeply invasive tumor with lymphatic metastasis. The essential element in the transition from carcinoma in situ or preinvasive to invasive carcinoma is the destruction of the underlying basement membrane.A reasonable interpretation of these studies is that increased degradation of basement membrane correlates with increased invasion and metastasis. Adherence to the basement membrane and extracellular matrix components is another method by which tumor cells can facilitate local invasion and metastasis. Alterations in tumor cell adherence and the expression of these cell surface ligands may facilitate invasion, metastasis, and neovascularization.

2.2.1 Detachemnt and migration of tumor cells

Essential characteristics of cancer are the ability to invade surrounding tissues and metastasize to regional and distant sites. The events attendant to local invasion by an epithelial tumor include loss of adhesion to surrounding tumor cells and basement membrane, production of enzymes and mediators which facilitate the incursion of malignant cells into the subjacent connective tissue. Therefore, the late stages of cancer involve progressive tumor invasion and metastasis, which are the stages that ultimately affect vital functions and cause death in patients. Many important histopathologic and molecular events associated with tumor progression and metastasis. Development of invasive carcinoma is associated with focal dissolution of the basement membrane and extracellular matrix (ECM), detachment, and migration of cells into the submucosal tissue. HNSCCs that exhibit a streaming pattern of small clusters of cells through the ECM are associated with more aggressive behavior and poor prognosis. HNSCCs exhibit alterations in expression of a repertoire of cell adhesion molecules and ECM substances that function in attachment and migration.

2.2.2 Angiogenesis

In 1972, Folkman first articulated the hypothesis that tumor growth was angiogenesis-dependent. Characteristics of prevascular tumors include a linear growth phase, absence of intratumoral vessels, and size limited to < 1 mm^3. Once tumors become vascularized, obtaining nutrients and exchanging metabolic waste products with the host become more efficient and the growth properties of the tumor change. Characteristics of tumors in the 'vascular phase' are histological demonstration of intratumor capillary networks, size> 1 mm^3, and an exponential growth phase (Folkman, 1990, 1992). Tumor progression to a size that becomes visible and has an effect on adjacent structures requires an increase in supply of oxygen and nutrients and removal of waste, which implies that new blood vessel formation is critical in cancer progression (Folkman, 1996). Enlargement of tumors to a size beyond 0.5 cm exceeds the range for diffusion of oxygen from existing vessels and necessitates new blood vessel formation, called neoangiogenesis. Angiogenesis is increased in various human cancers, including HNSCCs, and correlates with tumor progression and metastasis. Vascular endothelial growth factor (VEGF) has been shown to be a key regulator of angiogenesis.

The ability to stimulate new blood vessel growth (neovascularization or angiogenesis) is an integral part of organogenesis, reproduction, and wound healing and repair, and in this context it is short term and self-limiting. Pathologic angiogenesis is not autoregulated and results from alterations in growth control, which are parts of particular disease processes. However, the ability of a tumor to stimulate an angiogenic response should directly determine the capability of a tumor to metastasize and ultimately kill the host. The evidence regarding microvessel density as a predictor of nodal metastasis, or response to treatment in HNSCC remains conflicting, furthermore initially good correlations between microvessel density and outcome recently being challenged. Tumors invade local connective tissues by the production of proteinases and the expression of cell surface markers which facilitate attachment to components of the extracellular matrix. Tumor size is limited by the diffusion of nutrients from adjacent blood vessels, however, tumors circumvent this limitation by recruiting host capillaries to form an intratumor blood supply.

2.2.3 Lymphoangiogenesis

Lymphangiogenesis is associated with locoregional disease recurrence in early-stage oral carcinoma (Munoz-Guerra, et al., 2004). The presence of intratumoral lymphangiogenesis is a useful discriminator in predicting the outcome of patients with absence of lymph node metastasis. Various studies has stressed on the impact of tumor thickness as a significant factor that had predictive value for local disease recurrence, survival and neck metastasis. The rationale was that the depth of invasion would determine proximity to blood and lymphatic vessels and facilitate the ability of the tumor to expand. In most cases, metastasis in squamous cell carcinoma occurs via the lymphatic vessels and dilation of lymphatic vessels is frequently found in oral tumors with lymph node involvement. However, the influence of intratumoral or peritumoral lymphangiogenesis on squamous cell carcinoma of the oral cavity is still controversial.

Several markers have been utilized in the study of lymphangiogenesis. The main disadvantage of this method is that it relies on quantitative rather than qualitative differences between lymphatic and blood vessels and therefore requires a certain amount of subjective interpretation. In addition, most antibodies used react with both blood vessels and lymph vessels (Hannen & Riediger, 2004). Some of these studies have correlated the presence of VEGF-C in the tumor cells with an increased likelihood of lymph node metastasis in oral SCC, which seems promising (Kishimoto, et al., 2003, Shintani, et al., 2004, Warburton, et al., 2007). An association between lymphangiogenic growth factors, intralymphatic growth and tumor metastasis has been suggested. However, the role of intratumoral lymphangiogenesis in the progression of squamous cell carcinomas has not been studied. Tumor invasion of capillaries and lymphatics leads to dissemination of tumors and the establishment of histologically identical tumors at secondary sites.

2.2.4 Cellular components of tumor microenvironment

It has been shown that during progression, squamous cell carcinomas undergo additional changes needed for growth and metastasis that depend on the host (Chen, et al., 1997). Inflammatory cells infiltrating squamous cell carcinomas are one of the host components that promote growth and metastasis. New vessel formation is commonly associated with an increase in inflammatory cells. Growth of the tumor epithelia and angiogenesis is also accompanied by increased infiltration of inflammatory cells and proliferation of fibrous stroma. These inflammatory cells bear a stem cell marker called CD34 and appear to differentiate into granulocytes and endothelial cells that form new blood vessels. Granulocytes have been found to promote growth and metastasis. Granulocytes from the host can release growth factors and proteases that stimulate growth and invasion of tumor cells. Several studies have suggested that tumor cells capable of inducing host inflammatory and stromal cell responses grow, invade, and metastasize more rapidly.

Squamous cell carcinomas also induce proliferation of stromal fibroblasts. Fibroblasts also secrete factors and ECM substances that can promote growth. The establishment of metastases requires cell arrest and vessel formation in a new location. HNSCC shows a predilection for metastases to the lymphatics, lungs, liver, and bone marrow, suggesting that the cells and substrate of the reticuloendothelial system provide a favorable environment for arrest and formation of squamous cell carcinoma metastases. Non-malignant cells within the tumor microenvironment also play important roles in modulating tumor progression and metastases. Functional studies have identified several tumor-promoting functions for macrophages in primary tumors. These include promotion of angiogenesis, tumor cell invasion, migration and intravasation.

Local tissue invasion and migration into the subjacent connective tissue matrix by HNSCC are dependent of the production of cell surface molecules, enzymes and motility factors. In addition to the production of these locally active molecules, HNSCC produces growth factors or cytokines which target other cell types. Cytokines are low molecular-weight proteins which affect cell-cell communication and signal cellular proliferation, differentiation, activation, and migration.

3. Biological processes of the metastatic cascade

Tumor metastasis is ultimately the result of an imbalance between forces favoring and opposing the development of secondary tumors. The first steps in the development of distant metastases involve (1) the initiation of the primary tumor in a genetically susceptible host, (2) the promotion and progression of malignant cell gene mutations favoring clone expansion, and (3) uncontrolled proliferation of these malignant clones of cells due to the actions of autocrine growth factors and growth factor receptors.

The risk of distant spread is related to primary tumor site, its local and regional extension, and the phenotype (Li, et al. 2009). Distant metastases are particularly important in supraglottic laryngeal and pharyngeal cancers (Buckley, 2000). Factors which favor the development of metastases include the primary tumor's ability to activate oncogenes, downregulate tumor suppressor genes, express cell-surface adhesion molecules, synthesize and respond to autocrine and paracrine growth and motility factors, secrete proteases, and produce angiogenic and immunosuppressive cytokines. Factors opposing the development of metastases include activated tumor suppressor and antimetastasis genes, enhanced host immune responses, synthesis of protease and angiogenesis inhibitors by both the tumor and the host, and anatomic and structural barriers. All of these phenomena are the result of multiple gene mutations culminating in the development of secondary tumors at distant sites.

Fidler and colleagues (Fidler & Hart, 1982) articulated the principal of tumor heterogeneity, which is now widely accepted. The development of local-regional and distant metastases begins with the initiation of the primary tumor and ends with the establishment of metastatic clones throughout the host. Several processes including the differential expression of cell adhesion molecules, release of metalloproteinases, and angiogenesis occur at multiple points in the metastatic cascade. This cascade involves an sequential process including tumor invasion into local stroma and vascular system, circulation of tumor cell and arrest at the distant site, and clonal formation at secondary site.

3.1 Invasion into local stroma and vascular system

The process of tumor invasion involves attachment of the tumor to the basement membrane, degradation of extracellular matrix components, and migration of the malignant cells into the surrounding stroma. We will refer again the process when we consider the establishment of the tumor at a secondary (distant) site.

3.2 Circulation of the tumor and arrest at the distant site

Metastatic tumors, regardless of how they exist in the circulation, will establish distant metastases either by mechanical impaction or attachment to the endothelial cell surfaces. Mechanical impaction of the tumor/lymphocyte/platelet emboli will occur when the diameter of the embolus approaches that of the vessel. The tumor will then adhere to the lumen surface of endothelial cells and begin to grow. The second mechanism is the attachment of single tumor cells to the exposed basement membrane on the subendothelial side of the capillary lumen.

3.3 Colony formation at the secondary site

The common theoretical mechanisms exist for determining the locations of distant metastases were first articulated by Fidler as the 'seed and soil hypothesis' of tumor metastasis. These mechanisms include: (1) tumor metastasis equally to all organs, but preferentially only grow in locations which provide appropriate growth factors (soil); (2) circulating tumor cells have receptors specific for the endothelial cells of only certain target organs (seed), and (3) circulating tumors have receptors for specific chemotactic factors produced by the target organ. These factors result in the preferential attraction of the tumors to the target organ (seed soil) (Markus, 1988).

4. Lymph node metastasis of HNSCC

The status of the regional lymphatics is one of the most important prognostic indicators in patients with head and neck cancer. HNSCCs that are localized to the primary site without regional lymph node metastasis have excellent cure rates with either surgery or radiation therapy. The presence of regional metastases results in cure rates that are approximately half of those obtainable if metastasis to the regional lymphatics is not present. Thus the treatment of the neck has become one of the most actively debated topics in the field of head and neck oncology.

4.1 Patterns

The primary sites for HNSCC are mainly in the oral cavity, oropharynx, hypopharynx and larynx. In 1972, Lindberg published the location of nodal metastases in patients with squamous carcinoma of the upper aerodigestive tract as determined by clinical examination (Lindberg, 1972). This review consisted of 2,044 previously untreated patients with HNSCC. The presence of nodal metastasis and its location was assessed and correlated with the location and stage of the tumor at the primary site. Primary sites were divided into oral tongue, floor of mouth, retromolar trigone/anterior faucial pillar, soft palate, tonsillar fossa, base of tongue, oropharyngeal walls, supraglottic larynx, hypopharynx and nasopharynx. Fifty-seven percent of patients presented with clinical evidence of metastasis in the cervical nodes. Lindberg showed that for lesions of the oral tongue, floor of mouth, retromolar trigone/anterior faucial arch and soft palate, the incidence of cervical nodal metastasis increased with the size of the primary tumor. However, the incidence of nodal metastasis did not correlate with the size of the primary in tumors of the tonsillar fossa, base of tongue, supraglottic larynx, and hypopharynx.

Clinicopathological studies on the specimens from surgical removal of primary tumors and the associated treatment neck dissection tissues revealed patterns and impacting factors of cervical lymph node metastasis in HNSCC (Li, et al., 1996). For oral cavity cancers, the most common neck regions for neck node metastasis are level I to level III. Whereas, cervical lymph node metastasis from the cancers of oropharynx, hypopharynx and larynx are most frequently found in level II to level IV. Lindberg demonstrated that squamous cell carcinomas of the upper aerodigestive tract tend to metastasize to the neck in a predictable pattern. By far, the most common site of metastasis by all tumors is to the ipsilateral level II nodes. Tumors that lie within the oral cavity anterior to the circumvallate papillae have a propensity to metastasize to levels I through III, with levels IV and V seldom involved. Tumors of the oropharynx have a low propensity to metastasize to level I; metastasis is most common to level II with decreasing incidence of metastasis in levels III and IV. These tumors have a higher rate of metastases to level V than oral cavity tumors but the rate is still low. Tumors of the supraglottic larynx and hypopharynx rarely metastasize to level I, again metastases were most common to level II with a decreasing incidence in levels III and IV and metastases to level V were infrequent. Contralateral metastases were uncommon in cancers of the floor of mouth, oral tongue, hypopharynx, and retromolar trigone/anterior faucial arch. In contrast, tumors of base of tongue, oropharyngeal walls, soft palate, supraglottic larynx, and tonsil have substantial rates of contralateral metastases.

Lindberg's data clearly showed that in cases of squamous cell carcinoma of the upper aerodigestive tract, with the exception of nasopharyngeal carcinoma, nodal metastasis occurs in a predictable pattern and it may, in certain instances, be sound to exclude dissection of the level V lymph nodes. However, this study provides only information on clinically positive nodal metastasis—it provides no information on the incidence and location of occult nodal metastasis. Such information on microscopic metastasis can only be obtained from a surgical specimen. Byers and colleagues published one such study (Byers, et al., 1988) in 1988. They examined the specimens of 428 patients undergoing 648 modified neck dissections and correlated the location of the pathologically positive lymph nodes with the primary site. The majority of these neck dissections were selective neck dissections and therefore not all of the lymph node levels at risk were examined in each patient. This study essentially confirms the clinical data of Lindberg (Lindberg, 1972) that lesions anterior to the circumvallate papillae are most likely to metastasize to lymph nodes levels I through III and lesions within the hypopharynx and larynx to levels II through IV. It must be pointed out, however, that the majority of these dissections were less than comprehensive and therefore the low incidence of metastasis to certain nodal levels may simply reflect the lack of sampling of those levels.

In order to fully assess all the lymph node levels at risk for a particular primary site, surgical specimens should include all lymph node levels (comprehensive neck dissection). Just such information is provided in a series of studies by Shah and colleagues, (Candela, et al., 1990, Candela, et al., 1990, Shah, et al., 1990) which involved 1,081 previously untreated patients who underwent 1,119 classic RNDs for squamous carcinoma of the upper aerodigestive tract. The operations consisted of 343 elective RND in the clinically N0 setting and 776 therapeutic RND in the clinically N+ setting. In patients with primary tumors of the oral cavity undergoing therapeutic RND, the majority of metastatic nodes were located in levels I to III; level IV was involved in 20 percent of specimens and level V in only 4 percent. In those with primary oropharyngeal tumors, the majority of metastases were located in levels II to IV; levels I and V were involved in 17 percent and 11 percent of the specimens respectively. Therapeutic neck dissection in hypopharyngeal tumors showed that the majority of metastases were located in levels II to IV, while levels I and V were involved in 10 percent and 11 percent of the specimens, respectively. Primary tumors of the larynx metastasized to levels II through IV with levels I and V being involved in 8 percent and 5 percent of the specimens, respectively.

In the setting of elective RND in patients with primary tumors of the oral cavity, the majority of metastases were located in levels I to III; levels IV and V were involved in 9 percent and 2 percent of the specimens, respectively. In patients with primary tumors located in the oropharynx, the majority of metastases were located in levels II to IV; levels I and V were involved in 7 percent of the specimens. Patients with tumors of the hypopharynx undergoing elective RND had the majority of metastases in levels II to IV, while levels I and V were not involved in any of the specimens. Primary tumors of the larynx metastasized primarily to levels II through IV, while levels I and V were involved in 14 percent and 7 percent of the specimens, respectively. O'Brien et al.(O'Brien, et al., 2000) found occult metastatic disease in 30% of patients, and Lim et al (Lim, et al., 2006, Lim, et al., 2006) found it in 28%.

The question of metastasis to level V was addressed by another study by Davidson and colleagues. (Davidson, et al., 1993) They examined the specimens of 1,123 patients undergoing 1,277 RNDs and found metastases to level V in only 3 percent of patients. Level V metastases were highest in patients with hypopharyngeal and oropharyngeal primary sites (7% and 6% respectively). Only 3 of the 40 patients with level V metastases had these in the face of a clinical N0 stage. They concluded that the incidence of metastases to level V was small in general, and extremely unlikely in the clinically N0 patient.

4.2 Risk factors

Clinicopathologic factors associated with the development of cervical lymph node metastasis have been well studied for other locations like tongue, mouth floor, and cheek, in particular concerning tumor size (in tongue carcinoma≥3 mm), tumor depth (≥4 mm in tongue carcinoma), differentiation, mode of invasion, microvascular invasion, and histologic grade of malignancy (Kurokawa, et al., 2002, Sparano, et al., 2004, Wallwork, et al., 2007). The presence or absence of lymph node metastasis is a major prognostic factor for survival in patients with negative cervical lymph nodes (Hiratsuka, et al., 1997). A high incidence (20–30%) of cervical metastasis of cancer in the tongue/mouth floor has been well studied (Kurokawa, et al., 2002, Sparano, et al., 2004, Wallwork, et al., 2007). But very few studies have been performed concerning squamous cell carcinoma of the maxilla (Simental, et al., 2006). Sparamo et al(Sparano, et al., 2004) and Kruse et al (Kruse & Gratz, 2009) reveal that the higher the grading, the higher the risk of cervical metastasis. Therefore, regarding the proportion of late cervical metastasis, the question arises whether an elective neck dissection should be provided in early-stage squamous cell carcinoma. Capote et al. (Capote, et al., 2007) reported that in pT1N0 and pT2N0 oral squamous cell carcinoma, neck dissection therapy was a significant prognostic factor for recurrence and survival. Therefore, tumor size, tumor depth, and differentiation should be taken into consideration for the planning of neck dissection for squamous cell carcinoma of the upper jaw. Also the mode of invasion plays an important role in therapy planning because in certain localizations like the palate, the tumor does not need to invade very deeply before reaching the bone.

4.3 Prognostic factors

As an independent prognostic factor, cervical lymph node metastasis has a great impact on disease-free and overall survival of patients with HNSCC. Among various clinicopathological factors, the most important prognostic factors are pN+, numbers of positive node (more than 3 positive nodes), lower level of invasion, and especially the extracapsular nodal spread (ECS) (Di, et al., 2009). A review of literature reveals the impacts of clinicopathological factors on neck recurrence. For example, if residual disease after neck dissection, 2 or more pathologic lymph nodes, extracapsular spread (ECS), more than 3 cm-diameter pathologic lymph node and invasion of soft tissue are found in neck dissection specimens, the risk of neck recurrence is considered to be high (Li, et al., 2009). Since treatment neck dissections for HNSCC vary from selective neck dissection (SND) to radical neck dissection (RND), it is necessary to analyze the clinicopathologic risk factors for regional recurrence in a group of positive-node patients treated with such neck dissections and postoperative radiotherapy (PORT) in order to determine which patients need further adjuvant therapy and further short-interval follow-up. However, the majority of the literatures draw these conclusions in the absence of adjuvant radiotherapy. Furthermore, some reports show that these factors have no statistical significance in predicting regional failure following neck dissection and adjuvant PORT. It is now well established that the development of cervical metastases, in particular those with extranodal extension of tumor, negatively impacts both regional control and survival of patients with laryngeal carcinoma (Myers & Fagan, 1999).

4.4 Modern concepts in management of cervical lymph node metastasis in HNSCC

The lymphatic system of the head and neck is complicated (Fisch, 1964). An extensive analysis of 2044 medical records of patients with HNSCC who had not received prior treatment led Lindberg to divide nine lymph node regions on each side and, additionally, the parited lymph nodes (Lindberg, 1972). The lymph fluid of the upper aerodigestive tract is drained via about 300 regional cervical lymph nodes, which are divided according to the current classification established by Robbins (Robbins, et al., 2002) into nine lymph node levels (level I–VI). It is well understood that an incomplete surgical resection margin is the most important single factor for tumor recurrence, which is determined not only by the experience of the surgeon but also by the limitation of surgical excision. For example, if multiple nodes or ECS of neck diseases are present, it may be difficult to obtain adequate surgical resection margins or to resect all metastatic lymph nodes in the neck. Recurrence in the neck is more likely to occur in patients with these neck situations. For this reason, it is widely accepted that ECS is a marker for biologically aggressive disease and patients with HNSCC who have evidence of ECS need aggressive multimodality therapies including surgery, PORT and, even chemotherapy.

4.4.1 Detection of lymph node metastasis

Most tumors of the head and neck initially metastasize to the regional lymph nodes. The presence of cervical metastases is the most significant oncological factor in the prognosis of HNSCC (SCC) because early detection and treatment may prevent distant metastases (Gray, et al., 2000). The assessment of cervical lymph nodes is known to be extremely difficult clinically. Despite recent advances in the fields of radio diagnosis, its utility to detect occult neck metastasis still lacks considerable power. Owing to the high number of undersized lymph node metastases, the non-invasive neck staging methods are limited to a maximum accuracy of 76% (Stuckensen, et al., 2000). Pre-surgical staging of the neck has become more complex over the years. Clinical assessment of the neck by palpation, while providing critical information, is inadequate in its sensitivity for detecting metastatic disease to the cervical nodes. Error rates as high as 40 percent have been reported when physical examination alone is used to evaluate the neck (Teichgraeber & Clairmont, 1984). Patient factors such as a short, obese neck, as well as prior irradiation play a role in decreasing the accuracy of this technique. Clearly, radiologic assessment of the neck adds to the sensitivity and specificity of preoperative neck evaluation.

4.4.1.1 Comouterized tomography (CT) and magnetic resonance imaging (MRI)

Computerized tomography (CT) and magnetic resonance imaging (MRI) have become the workhorses of imaging modalities in HNSCC. Size criteria are frequently used as indicators of metastatic involvement. Other features such as central necrosis or ring-enhancement aid in specificity but are relatively infrequent findings. Generally, a subdigastric node measuring > 15 mm, a submandibular node > 12 mm, and other nodes > 10 mm are suspicious for involvement. Using criteria such as these, the accuracy of detecting neck disease approaches 90 percent (John, et al., 1993). Size, however, is certainly not pathognomonic for cancerous involvement of lymph nodes. Even in the patient with an identified squamous cell carcinoma of the upper aerodigestive tract, a myriad of alternative causes of enlarged lymph nodes exist. Further, microscopic foci of disease may exist in nodes of normal size. As CT or MRI is often employed to evaluate the primary lesion, inclusion of the neck in the area of study incurs nominal additional expense and no morbidity. Although CT and MRI provide excellent anatomic detail and are the current modalities of choice, they provide little information on the biology of the lymph node.

4.4.1.2 Positron emssion tomography (PET)

Several studies have evaluated fluorodeoxyglucose (FDG) PET in this setting, attempting to identify the patients who need neck dissection. In 3 studies totaling 48 patients, in which a sentinel node biopsy with immunohistochemistry was used as the gold standard, the detection rate of PET was between 0% and 30%, making PET an unreliable modality in this clinical setting (Civantos, et al., 2003, Stoeckli, et al., 2002). This is not unexpected, given that 40% of cervical nodal metastases are less than 1 cm in size and PET detection rate for nodes less than 1 cm is reported at 71% (Menda & Graham, 2005). Numerous promising pilot studies have evaluated sentinel node biopsy (SNB), up to 16% patients required additional immunohistochemistry (IHC) on the sentinel nodes to detect metastasis (Civantos, et al., 2006). Owing to these inadequacies in detection of occult nodal metastasis, surgical dissection and serial histologic examination are the currently accepted "yardsticks".

Another problem that should be considered seems to be the detection of micrometastasis. The assessment of the status of cervical lymph nodes is difficult, and therefore a treatment of patients with a clinical stage N0 neck is controversial. In most studies, the use of CT has an error rate ranging from 7.5 to 19%(van den Brekel, et al., 1990). In the late 1990s, the PET using F-18 FDG, a functional imaging methodology that provides information about tissue glucose metabolism, was applied. Consequently, a high FDG accumulation is manifested on PET images, but inflammation also reveals an increased FDG uptake and can lead to false-positive results. On the other hand, low tumor metabolic activity, the presence of small lesions, and hypoglycemia can lead to false-negative results (Murakami, et al., 2007). Concerning cervical lymph nodes, Ng et al. (Ng, et al., 2005) reported that sensitivity and specificity of PET images were 75% and 93%, respectively. Sigg et al. (Sigg, et al., 2003) reported a sensitivity of 93% and a specificity of 100%. PET together with CT images showed a 15% increase in the accurate identification of nodal staging over using the PET images alone (Jeong, et al., 2007). PET/CT seems to have a higher sensitivity and specificity for detecting lymph node metastasis (Leong, et al., 2006, Wild, et al., 2006).

4.4.1.3 Ultrasound

Due to its non-invasiveness and affordability, ultrasound (US) has been investigated as a potential tool in evaluating neck disease. Factors such as size, irregular margins, and echo characteristics of lymph nodes have been shown to have predictive value in assessing involved nodes. The overall sensitivity of this approach, however, is limited due to the operator-dependant nature of ultrasound.(John, et al., 1993) Some authors have proposed ultrasound in combination with ultrasound-guided fine needle aspiration as an approach to diagnosis. Takes and colleagues (Takes, et al., 1998) examined, with ultrasonography, 64 necks staged N0 based on physical examination. Those with nodes greater than 5 mm in size underwent ultrasound-guided needle biopsy. Results were further verified with histopathologic examination and the findings compared with CT of the neck for detection of involved nodes. They found a 48 percent sensitivity, 100 percent specificity, and 79 percent accuracy for ultrasound versus 54, 92, and 77 percent respectively for CT. These results demonstrate that, in experienced hands, ultrasound can be a useful tool. Its widespread application, however, is limited by the technical expertise required for accurate interpretation.

4.4.2 Management

4.4.2.1 General principles

The type, grade, site and stage of the primary tumor determine the risk of cervical metastases and hence the type of treatment modality. Treatment of the neck in patients with clinical evidence of nodal metastasis has traditionally been surgical. In recent decades, this has been extended to include a combination of surgery and radiation therapy. The role of chemotherapy in the management of neck disease remains controversial and is currently being actively investigated. In oral tongue carcinoma, the risk of neck metastasis is significantly associated also with the depth of tumor invasion (Pentenero, et al., 2005). The patterns of spread of cancer to cervical lymph nodes are predictable, based on the anatomical location of the primary tumor. Therefore, in the absence of clinical evidence of neck disease, the pathological features of the primary tumor along with its site of origin and clinical T stage are used to stratify the risk of positive neck metastases and, consequently, the need for a neck dissection. When the risk for positive neck lymph nodes exceeds 15-20%, elective neck dissection is indicated - not only as treatment but also to evaluate the need for adjuvant therapy. A selective neck dissection, directed to the basins at risk for lymphatic spread, is commonly used for this purpose. The presence of palpable neck disease mandates comprehensive clearance of the lymphatic basins in the neck. Radical neck dissection was considered the primary modality for treatment of HNSCC with clinical evidence of cervical metastases. However, sacrificing vital structures during radical neck dissection causes severe disabilities in patients and a markedly reduced quality of life. Advances in the anatomic elucidation of the neck, enhanced understanding of the biological behavior of tumors, and improved surgical methods have contributed to the emergence of the functional neck dissection technique, resulting in excellent survival and functional outcome(Shah & Gil, 2009). Exact knowledge of the anatomy of the neck and its adjacent structures and the risk and location of common cervical metastases is essential for the operative treatment of HNSCC.

Although primary tumor control is achievable in early tumors with minimally invasive surgery, such as transoral or robot-assisted procedures, the management of the neck is still an important consideration in the treatment of HNSCC. Surgical management of the neck in patients with pharyngeal cancers does not usually involve a dissection of the retropharyngeal lymph node (RPLNs). Neck dissections do not routinely address RPLNs, creating a potential for recurrence in the retropharynx and the need to address this nodal basin with radiotherapy (Tauzin, et al., 2010). Treatment of the neck in patients with clinical evidence of nodal metastasis has traditionally been surgical. In recent decades this has been extended to include a combination of surgery and radiation therapy. The role of chemotherapy in the management of neck disease remains controversial and is currently being actively investigated.

4.4.2.2 Adjuvant therapy

Although the practical value of postoperative radiotherapy (PORT) for improving survival in HNSCC is well acknowledged, it remains controversial whether this postoperative radiotherapy, an adjuvant treatment, could prevent recurrence in the neck in patients having ECS. Smeele et al. found that PORT dose of 62.5 Gy and more could increase neck control rates in patients with ECS treated with surgery and PORT for HNSCC. Peters et al. demonstrated that metastatic lymph nodes with ECS were adequately controlled by PORT at dosage of 63 Gy or more (Peters, et al., 1993). However, Prim et al. reported that the 3-year recurrence rates in the neck were 10.7% in patients without ECS and 49.6% with ECS in squamous cell carcinoma of the larynx with pathologically proven lymph node metastasis, and PORT did not appear to improve the outcome (Prim, et al., 1999). Shingaki et al. found that PORT did not decrease the rate of neck recurrence in patients of oral cavity carcinomas with ECS (Shingaki, et al., 2003). These findings suggest that the exact value of PORT in controlling neck recurrence needs to be further documented and recommended for adjuvant chemotherapy. Our findings suggest that the presence of ECS remains a determined risk factor for neck recurrence after surgery and adjuvant PORT in N^+ patients with HNSCC. There were no significant risk factors associated with regional failure in ECS^- group. Except for PORT, no additional adjuvant therapy is required for N^+ patients without ECS. However, more adjuvant therapies are to be considered after PORT in patients with ECS for the purpose of a more effective neck control.

4.4.2.3 Scenario in the management of an N0 neck

Due to the fact that the prognosis of patients suffering from squamous cell carcinoma of the upper aerodigestive tract depends significantly on the presence or absence of lymph node metastasis, the question of detecting clinically occult lymph node metastases is still important concerning the management of the clinical N0 neck. The published rate of lymph node metastasis depends on the location of the primary tumor, with values from 12% to over 50% (median, 33%) (Hosal, et al., 2000). Numerous authors favor elective treatment of the lymphatic region (neck dissection) if the presence of occult lymph node metastasis can be expected with a probability of 20% or more. However, other authors prefer to adopt a "wait and see" strategy, although this requires both great compliance from the patient and great expertise on the part of the responsible physician to identify metastasis early. Another argument in favor of elective neck dissection versus a "wait-and-see" strategy is the significant deterioration of the survival rate when neck disscetion is due after clinical disease is detected (Godden, et al., 2002).

Regarding the current scenario in the management of an N0 neck, there are presently three policies advocated, which include elective neck irradiation, prophylactic neck dissection or close observation. The choice of therapy often takes into consideration T stage, site of primary, grade, compliance for follow-up, or the probability for occult metastasis [>20%]. Treatment of the neck, even when included with the primary treatment, often confers additional costs, morbidity and prolonged treatment time to the patient. Most often, a single modality treatment is used to treat the primary site and neck. The choice of which is dictated by the treatment of the primary site. There is no conclusive evidence to show if this elective neck treatment approaches contribute to improved overall survival for the patients with HNSCC and clinically negative neck.

4.4.2.4 Sentinel node and elective neck dissection

The elective treatment of the regional lymphatic drainage can generally be performed either surgically or radiotherapeutically. The choice of one of these procedures generally depends on the therapy of the primary tumor. An advantage of elective neck dissection over radiotherapy is that the histological examination of the neck dissection specimen can give important information for deciding therapy, as well as about the prognosis. Thus, the sentinel node concept for squamous cell carcinomas of the upper aerodigestive tract is quite appealing. Furthermore, limits and pitfalls of SLNs for HNSCC discussed elsewhere illustrate that an advanced intranodal tumor growth with extracapsular metastatic spread, leads to a significant reduction of the radiotracer uptake (Dunne, et al., 2001). Even small, clinically unsuspected lymph nodes may reveal extracapsular tumor growth with resulting lack of radiopharmacon accumulation (Coatesworth & MacLennan, 2002). The dominating metastatic region of pharyngeal and laryngeal carcinomas is mainly level II and less commonly, level III. Carcinomas of the anterior oral cavity drain mostly into level I and less commonly into level II. Accordingly, neck dissection of these lymph node levels can be expected to include the majority of clinically occult metastases. With this background, it must still be clarified whether the intraoperative identification of the radiolabeled SLN is appropriate to reduce the extent of selective neck dissection in the suspected N0 neck, or whether neck dissection can be completely avoided in the case of histologically-proven tumor-free SLN. Opponents of such a procedure argue that selective neck dissection already has a morbidity that must be considered. Supporters of sentinel lymphadenectomy stress both protecting the intact, i.e. non-metastatic, cervical lymph node systems and reducing the extent of surgery. Scarring contractures, paresthesia, and persisting lymph edemas can be reduced by a selective SLN dissection. Current research aims to optimize surgical access to the SLNs. The first results on endoscopically performed selective lymphadenectomy led to the assumption that this method of lymph node dissection could achieve some significance in the therapy of the clinical N0 neck, provided that it is based on the SLN concept (Werner, et al., 2004).

However, the techniques would have to be optimized. Furthermore, prospectively collected data should be gathered and analyzed. Within such an investigation, it would make sense to examine frozen sections of the excised lymph node. Depending on the histopathological result, a surgical resection of the lymphatic drainage in the form of a selective neck dissection could then be indicated. At present, the technical diversity and importance of endoscopic lymphadenectomy in the neck shows scientific and clinical potential. The question about the significance of the procedure, however, can not yet be answered conclusively.

5. Distant metastasis

Generally, distant metastasis is defined as tumor spread to other organ systems from its primary site. As a relatively rare but clinically relevant event, the development of distant metastasis is usually difficult to predict in clinic, especially when initial treatment planning is made.

5.1 Clinicopathlological features of distant metastasis in HNSCC

5.1.1 The incidence and common sites of distant metastasis in NHSCC

Alavi et al. (Alavi, et al., 1999) reviewed 342 patients with mucosal HNSCC, and 47 (13.7%) had distant metastases. Five patients (1.5%) had metastases to infraclavicular lymph nodes (axilla, inguinal and presternal). The clinical detection of metastatic foci occurs in 10% to 30% of cases, whereas autopsy studies yield an incidence of about 50% of cases with metastases below the clavicle (Amer, et al., 1979, Dennington, et al., 1980). Clinical data in recently reported studies indicates an incidence of 4% to 23.8%, whereas autopsy data documents that 12% to 57% of cases had disseminated disease(Dennington, et al., 1980). Merino and associates (Merino, et al., 1977) in an analysis of 546 of 5019 untreated patients with squamous carcinoma of the upper respiratory tract who completed curative treatments, found clinically manifested metastases below the clavicle in 10.9% of the cases. The risk of subpathological distant metastases has also to be considered. New and highly sensitive investigations (immunohistochemistry, molecular analysis and FDG-PET/CT) and serial sectioning of nonregional lymph nodes and at risk organs may increase the detection of distant micrometastases in head and neck cancer patients. Probably the different reported incidence depends on the selection criteria of screening for distant metastases and the characteristics of the patients included (Leon, et al., 2000).

The lungs, bones (especially the vertebrae, ribs, and skull) and the liver are the most common sites of hematogenous distant metastases from HNSCC (Gowen & Desuto-Nagy, 1963). During the follow-up period after the initial treatment, 6.2% of the patients were diagnosed of having distant metastasis. The most common sites of distant metastasis were the lungs (58%) and the bones (22%). The lung is clearly the most common site of distant spread. The incidence of pulmonary metastases is also high in patients who present with extensive soft tissue extension of the primary or metastatic regional nodal disease. Holsinger et al, from the Anderson Cancer Center in Houston, provided a panel of clinical and histopathological predictors that may identify patients at the greatest risk for development of distant metastases in HNSCC (Holsinger, et al., 2000). In their study, the 5-year incidence of distant metastasis was 15.1 % (94/622). Pulmonary metastases were most commonly found: 65.9% to the lung, 4.2% to the mediastinum, 2.1 % to the pleura. Metastases to bone (22.3%) and to the liver (9.5%) were the next most commonly encountered. Thirty (31.9%) patients with distant metastases presented with more than one metastatic site. Lung was the most common site for solitary metastasis. The most common site for bony metastasis was the spine (12.7%), followed by skull (4.2%), rib (3.1 %), and axial bones (femur, humerus; 2.1 %). More than half of patients with osseous metastases presented with multiple sites. The patients who present with jugular vein invasion or extensive soft tissue disease in the neck clearly have a high incidence of pulmonary metastases. Other less common sites of metastases include the mediastinum, adrenal gland, brain, pericardium, kidney, and thyroid gland (Troell & Terris, 1995).

5.1.2 Risk factors

Taken into consideration to be relatively important factors in clinic, clinical T stage, N stage, tumor site, tumor thickness, differentiation, pattern of invasion, vascular and/or lymphatic invasion, bone and/or cartilage invasion, perineural invasion, and lymph nodal status have been reported to be associated with distant metastasis in HNSCC. However, the conclusions concerning the role of each independent factor differ among the various authors. In a recent study, we successfully demonstrated that primary tumor site, level of tumor invasion and numbers of levels with positive lymph node are closely related to the occurrence of distant metastasis in HNSCC (Li, et al., 2009).

The incidence of metastases is influenced by T and N stage, as well as control of the primary lesion. As local and regional control of head and neck cancer has improved, distant metastases have become an increasingly common cause of death. (Vikram, et al., 1984) The disturbance of the lymphatic system in the cervical region resulting from radiotherapy or neck dissection can result in alternative pathways of lymphatic drainage. These newly formed pathways of drainage can ultimately result in lymphatic dissemination of head and neck cancers to sites below the clavicles. Metastasis from head and neck carcinomas to infraclavicular lymph nodes has been reported very infrequently in the literature (Nelson & Sisk, 1994). Recognition of this phenomenon is crucial in the evaluation of patients with recurrent head and neck cancer, especially when salvage surgery is entertained.

The incidence of distant metastases is directly related to the clinical stage of the tumor, with high incidence of distant metastases in stage IV tumors, particularly in patients who present with advanced nodal disease. The distant metastasis ratio was much higher in patients with T3 to T4, N2 to N3 lesions who received postoperative radiotherapy. It is reported that locally extensive lesions T3 and T4 are most likely to metastasize and that nodal involvement is also associated with increased risk of distant spread. Lesions arising in the larynx and hypopharynx have a greater predilection to metastasize than oral lesions, although true vocal cord lesions infrequently metastasize as demonstrated by Snow and coworkers(Snow, et al., 1980). In data of Merino (Merino, et al., 1977), 8% of all patients who had local control developed metastases, while 23% of those with T3 to T4 lesions had local control and developed distant spread.

The incidence of pulmonary metastases is extremely high in patients who present with bilateral N3 disease. Disease stage showed a striking correlation with the risk for distant metastases (as follows): stage I, 1 %; stage II, 14%; stage III, 15%; stage IV, 20% ($p < 0.0003$).

Advanced disease (T stage> 3 and N stage> 2a) was significantly correlated statistically with the development of distant metastases ($p < 0.003$). The authors found that certain clinical features (extent of cervical metastasis or N stage) and histopathologic data (evidence of lymphatic or vascular invasion and extension beyond the confines of the lymph node) are associated with significantly increased rates of distant metastases.

Spector (Spector, 2001) report a retrospective tumor registry analysis of patients with HNSCC of the larynx and hypopharynx who were treated with curative intent between January 1971 and December 1991. In 2,550 patients, the mean age, sex and tumor differentiation did not affect the incidence of distant metastases. The overall incidence of distant metastases was 8.5% (217/2,550 patients) with the following distribution: glottis 4.4%, supraglottis 3.6%, subglottis 14%, aryepiglottic fold 16%, pyriform sinus 17% and posterior hypopharynx 17.6%. The overall 5-year disease-specific survival for distant metastases was 6.4%. Distant metastases were related to advanced local disease (T3 + T4), lymph node metastases at presentation (N+), tumor location (hypopharynx) and locoregional tumor recurrence ($p = 0.028$). A meta-analysis of variables which predispose to a higher incidence of distant metastases indicate that tumor location (hypopharynx> larynx), advanced primary disease (T3 + T4), regional disease (N+), locoregional recurrences, and advanced regional metastases (N2 + N3) are statistically significant. The salvage rate for distant metastases was poor (6.4%) and significantly worse than the salvage rate for delayed regional node metastases (42%) or second primary malignancies (38%) ($p = 0.001$). The onset period of distant metastases was greatest between 1.5 and 6 years post initial treatment with a mean of≤3.2 years.

Research for clinicopathlological features of distant metastasis in HNSCC is of clinical implications in the diagnosis and treatment of the disease. Strong prognostic indicators that predict development of distant metastases are the presence and number of lymph node metastases in the neck, and extranodal spread. Once distant metastases are detected, patients have a very poor prognosis. The time interval between the diagnosis of distant metastasis and death is less than 2 years in greater than 90% of such cases.

5.1.3 Retrograde dissemination

Alvarez reported a retrospective study of 633 patients with HNSCC to describe the clinical characteristics of the distant metastasis. During the follow-up period after the initial treatment, 6.2% of the patients were diagnosed of having distant metastasis (Alvarez Marcos, et al., 2006). The site of primary tumor was hypopharynx in 14.4%, unknown origin in 11.8% and oropharynx in 8.5%. Three year overall survival in patients with distant metastasis was 2.5% (versus 49,5% in the control group).

Nonregional lymph node dissemination should be classified as distant metastasis but axillary and mediastinal metastases can be part of a regional dissemination of HNSCC. Metastases to lymph nodes of the upper mediastinum are very common among patients with subglottic, hypopharynx and thyroid carcinomas. Axillary metastases are found at autopsy in 2-9% of the patients who died of HNSCC and are frequently associated with skin implantation in aggressive recurrent head and neck carcinomas. The possible explanations for this location of metastasis were retrograde dissemination due to lymph system blockage, further tumor dissemination after a parastomal recurrence, hematogenous dissemination, and metastasis from a second primary tumor (Kowalski, 2001).

5.2 Diagnose of distant metastasis in HNSCC

5.2.1 Schemes for screening

Because distant metastasis has an important impact on survival, early detection of this unfavorable status in HNSCC is substaintial for therapeutic strategy regulation. The metastatic workup for patients with head and neck cancer frequently includes examination of the cervical lymph nodes as well as chest radiography, liver function tests, and a serum calcium level determination. This evaluation may fail to detect metastases to distant lymph nodes in patients who present with recurrent or second primary cancers after previous therapy that has affected the cervical lymphatics. A predictable pattern of lymphatic metastasis based on tumor histology and site of origin has also been well documented for most cancers that arise in the head and neck region.

The diagnostic and screening procedures used for distant metastasis in HNSCCs are sometimes equivalent and sometimes complementary. The available methods for the assessment of tumor status include: (1) conventional radiographs (X-rays); (2) sectional imaging - CT, magnetic resonance imaging (MRI), positron emission tomography (PET); (3) ultrasound and ultrasound-guided fine needle biopsy; (4) radionuclide scanning; (5) endoscopic examination and (6) histological and cytological investigations - conventional histology, semiserial sections, immunohistochemistry, molecular analysis and techniques of cell culture.

As the lungs, bones and the liver are the most common sites of distant metastases from HNSCC, routine examination about these organs should be performed for high risk patients of metastasis in HNSCC. The prevalence of metastases at autopsy (37-57%) is much higher than in clinical studies (4-26%) (Leon, et al., 2000). This suggests that distant metastases in head and neck cancer are often asymptomatic, which raises the question of screening. Any investigations used for screening need to be sensitive, highly specific, inexpensive, noninvasive and readily available (Troell & Terris, 1995). In the absence of useful screening tests, metastases are usually detected by specific investigation of suspicious symptoms. Plain X-rays, computed tomography (CT) and bone scanning are the most frequently used investigations.

Chest CT is recommended for high-risk patients, especially during the follow-up period. Intensified evaluation and management are mandatory for indeterminate small solitary pulmonary nodules because of the high rate of malignant neoplasms (Hsu, et al., 2008). Otherwise, cross-sectional imaging with CT and MR imaging is commonly used for tumor metastasis detection.

Recently, PET using the radiotracer 18F FDG is widely used to evaluate patients with HNSCC. The combinated technique, PET/CT, provides anatomic and functional information and is useful for identification of an unknown primary tumor, detection of distant metastasis, establishing radiation-therapy planning, assessing therapy response, and long-term surveillance for recurrence. Positron emission tomography-computed tomography with fluorodeoxyglucose F18 (FDG-PET/CT) is widely used to evaluate patients with HNSCC. PET/CT can provide early, accurate detection of bone metastases from HNSCC and to determine the impact of detecting occult bone metastases on patient care. Use of FDG-PET/CT in restaging HNSCC allows for detection of occult lung, liver and bone metastases, and this early detection frequently influences therapeutic decision making (Basu, et al., 2007).

5.2.2 Confirmation of miscellaneous distant metastases

5.2.2.1 Pulmonary metastasis

Chest computed tomography (CT) scan is clearly more sensitive in identifying and localizing pulmonary metastasis than plain chest radiography, which can serve as a useful screening tool.

Treatment of pulmonary metastases requires some evaluations concerning control of the primary site and regional lymph nodes, and the general physiological and mental condition of the patients as well as the patient's willingness to be treated. In addition, to determine the optimal treatment, especially when considering surgical treatment, it is necessary to exclude other metastases and to precisely define the sequence after the surgery. Surgical excision is indicated as the optimal treatment for a solitary metastasis tumor of the lung when chemoimmunotherapy is ineffective. The patients who have jugular vein invasion or extensive soft tissue encroach in the neck clearly have a high incidence of pulmonary metastases.

5.2.2.2 Bone metastasis

Because metastasis to osseous tissue is the second most common presentation of distant metastases, bone scan is an important and sensitive test. However, because of its non specificity, CT-directed needle biopsies may be necessary to establish diagnosis.

5.2.2.3 Liver metastasis

Hematogenous spread to liver rarely occurs without evidence of pulmonary and bone disease. Although liver function tests may detect abnormality, elevation in liver enzymes ordinarily carries low sensitivity or specificity for liver involvement. Confirmation most often requires a diagnostic CT scan followed by ultrasound-guided needle biopsy.

5.2.2.4 Brain metastasis

Brain metastasis is a rare occurrence from head and neck cancer, it is particularly more probable in tumor involving the temporal bone simply because of its proximity to the cranial vault. CT scan and magnetic resonance imaging (MRI) provide the highest sensitivity of screening for intracranial disease well before neurological manifestations become apparent.

5.3 Management of distant metastasis in HNSCC

5.3.1 Prevention

It has been noted that, with the modern therapeutic regimens, the outcome of patients with distant metastasis from HNSCC remains dismal. Salvage therapy of metasesectomy or ionizing radiation is not sufficient to obtain a higher cure rate, when distant metastasis is at presence. It seems that optimal therapeutic strategies for distant metastasis may be adjuvant chemotherapy after surgery and postoperative radiotherapy at target groups of patients who are at high risk of developing distant metastasis. According to findings in our previous study (Li, et al., 2009), we propose that patients with multilevel nodal involvement in the neck, primary tumor localization at oropharynx, hypoparynx and larynx, and primary tumor invasion into muscle, bone or cartilage are at highest risk of developing distant metastasis in HNSCC. Therefore, these subsets of patients with high risk factors should be considered for a more through evaluation for detecting distant metastasis and a more increasing utilization of adjuvant chemotherapy for preventing distant metastasis. However, it must be mentioned that screening for distant metastasis in the follow-up doses little help in improving the outcome, since there is mostly no possibility of a curative intervention.

5.3.2 Surgery

Treatment of metastases is generally difficult. The difficulty seems to be caused by the low sensitivity of metastatic tumor cells to anticancer drugs and radiation. Surgery and radiotherapy are the main treatment modality of morning metastases for HNSCC. Metastasized regional lymph nodes are usually controlled by surgical removal (Shah & Andersen, 1994). However, surgical removal of distant metastatic tumors is usually not easy, especially in patients with multiple organ metastases. Because of these difficulties in conservative and surgical treatments, distant metastases are lethal in most patients.

Treatment planning for cases with axillary metastasis must take in consideration the likelihood of other regional recurrences and/or distant metastasis. Also, the presence of a second primary tumor must be ruled out. Whenever axilla is the only site of cancer recurrence, a standard axillary dissection must be considered. Upper mediastinal metastases from subglottic and hypopharyngeal cancer are managed by paratracheal and mediastinal dissection through the neck and postoperative radiotherapy (Kowalski, 2001).

Surgery is sometimes useful in the treatment of bone metastases. For example, pulmonary metastasectomy of isolated metastasis has been shown to be of benefit in selected patients (Wedman, et al., 1996). Surgery is sometimes useful in the treatment of bone metastases, although radiotherapy is the standard first-line treatment. In metastatic brain tumor, surgical resection should also be considered for patients with solitary brain metastasis and no extracranial disease or controlled extracranial disease. Whole-brain radiotherapy is routinely administered postoperatively (Hoegler, 1997). Although surgical removal of isolated solid metastatic tumors in liver is sometime carried out, adjuvant chemoradiation is the mainstream in the treatment modalities.

Occasionally, surgical resection of metastases is useful for metastases that do not respond to radiotherapy and in weight-bearing or high-stress areas (subtrochanteric region of the hip, mid-femoral diaphysis, mid-humeral metaphysis). Surgical stabilization can improve the remaining quality of life in these patients if it is carried out early enough (Sim, et al., 1992). A brief, fractionated course of radiotherapy is usually given postoperatively (Hoegler, 1997).

5.3.3 Chemotherapy

Head and neck cancer metastases are responsive to chemotherapy and the use of multiple agents may increase response rate. Unfortunately, neither single agent nor combinations of drugs have any significant impact on survival (de Mulder, 1999). The exception may be nasopharyngeal carcinoma, where platinum-based chemotherapy may increase survival even in the presence of distant metastases (Gebbia, et al., 1993). Chemotherapy also acting as a radiosensitizer, increases survival in advanced metastasis in HNSCC.

Neoadjuvant chemotherapy with the cisplatin and fluororacil (PF) regimen in HNSCC patients has no effect on locoregional relapse. However, it shows a small but significant benefit in reducing distant metastasis and improving the overall survival (Su, et al., 2008). Many new chemotherapy ways are attempted in a broader sense of targeted therapy.

Multi-modality treatment or targeted therapy-containing management does not significantly improve overall survival.

Systemic chemotherapy management of extensive metastasis in HNSCC patients is a major concern. The drugs most commonly used clinically are the platin compounds (cisplatin and carboplatin), taxanes (docetaxel and paclitaxel), 5-FU, methotrexate, and ifosfamide. In an effort to improve response rates and, hopefully, survival time, combination chemotherapy needs to be developed.

5.3.4 Radiotherapy

Radiotherapy is the standard first-line treatment of bone metastases in HNSCC. Radiotherapy also has a role in the infrequent patients with brain metastases, especially for solitary brain metastasis with no extracranial diseases or have been controlled. It relieves clinical symptoms in 70-90% of patients (Hoegler, 1997). The use of stereotactic radiosurgical treatment remains to be defined. It is most often used to treat solitary metastases in previously irradiated patients.

Radiotherapy is unlikely to cure even solitary lung metastases. However, it may have a palliative role and increase survival when there are a limited number of foci, small metastases and locoregional control (Sugawara & Kaneta, 1983). Approximately 50% of patients with cancer develop bone metastases, although they are relatively unusual in head and neck cancer. They can cause pain and affect weight-bearing areas and consequently have a significant impact on quality of life. The role of radiotherapy in the palliation of bone metastases is well supported in the literature, with reported response rates of around 70-90% (Arcangeli, et al., 1998, Hoegler, 1997). The pain relief is complete in nearly half of the responders (Uppelschoten, et al., 1995) (Steenland, et al., 1999). If patients fail to respond to the first treatment, then they may respond to re-treatment.

5.3.5 Associated targeting therapy

Recently, molecular targeting biologicals with a different toxicity profile and hopefully less late damage to functionally important tissues may open new strategies in primary and adjuvant treatment of HNSCC. The principal strategies currently being used to design antiangiogenesis agents are aimed at blocking angiogenic factors (or enhancing negative regulators) or acting on endothelial cells to block cell surface receptors or prevent them from breaking down the surrounding matrix.

Besides cetuximab and other EGFR targeting mAbs, there are other receptors and non-receptor tyrosine kinase inhibitors, which might play an important role in the future treatment of HNSCC. Many investigatons have been carried out to solve the problem of multi-drug resistance in HNSCC progenitor cells. Cetuximab, as an epidermal growth factor receptor-specific monoclonal antibody, plus radiation were shown to improve survival rate as compared to radiation treatment alone (Bonner, et al., 2006). However, one retrospective study suggests the duration of progression free survival and overall survival is shorter in patient receiving cetuximab plus radiation than those with cisplatin plus radiation (Pignon, et al., 2009).

It is prostulated that VEGF targeted therapy has the potential to fulfill both anti-angiogenic and anti-tumorigenic functions (Tong, et al., 2008). As reported, CD44 certainly posseses a valid target for anti-cancer therapy. CD44 targeting members of several relevant pathways might be used to induce apoptosis or inhibit tumour angiogenesis and metastatic spread. Immunotherapy for HNSCC is a relatively new but promising therapeutic strategy. In HNSCC, immunotherapy has been implemented successfully in patients, especially in patients with end-stage metastasising disease, who had undergone a variety of other therapeutic modalities. Despite this fact, both clinical and translational trials with cytokines, monoclonal antibodies, and various kinds of other strategies have yielded promising results with little evidence of host toxicity. Future efforts will be foucusing on finding ways to circumvent immune tolerance and overcome malignancy-related immune dysfunction to produce regimens with better efficacy.

6. References

Alavi, S., Namazie, A., Sercarz, J. A., Wang, M. B. & Blackwell, K. E. (1999). Distant lymphatic metastasis from head and neck cancer. Annals of Otology Rhinology and Laryngology. Vol 108. No (9). pp: 860-863.ISSN 0003-4894

Alvarez Marcos, C. A., Llorente Pendas, J. L., Franco Gutierrez, V., Hermsen, M., Cuesta Albalad, M. P., Fernandez Espina, H. & Suarez Nieto, C. (2006). Distant metastases in head and neck cancer. Acta Otorrinolaringol Esp. Vol 57. No (8). pp: 369-372.ISSN 0001-6519

Amer, M. H., Al-Sarraf, M. & Vaitkevicius, V. K. (1979). Factors that affect response to chemotherapy and survival of patients with advanced head and neck cancer. Cancer. Vol 43. No (6). pp: 2202-2206.ISSN 0008-543X

Arcangeli, G., Giovinazzo, G., Saracino, B., D'Angelo, L., Giannarelli, D. & Micheli, A. (1998). Radiation therapy in the management of symptomatic bone metastases: the effect of total dose and histology on pain relief and response duration. International Journal of Radiation Oncology Biology Physics. Vol 42. No (5). pp: 1119-1126.ISSN 0360-3016

Basu, D., Siegel, B. A., McDonald, D. J. & Nussenbaum, B. (2007). Detection of occult bone metastases from head and neck squamous cell carcinoma: impact of positron emission tomography computed tomography with fluorodeoxyglucose F 18. Archives of Otolaryngology-Head & Neck Surgery.. Vol 133. No (8). pp: 801-805. ISSN 0886-4470

Bonner, J. A., Harari, P. M., Giralt, J., Azarnia, N., Shin, D. M., Cohen, R. B., Jones, C. U., Sur, R., Raben, D., Jassem, J., Ove, R., Kies, M. S., Baselga, J., Youssoufian, H., Amellal, N., Rowinsky, E. K. & Ang, K. K. (2006). Radiotherapy plus cetuximab for squamous-cell carcinoma of the head and neck. The New England Journal of Medicine. Vol 354. No (6). pp: 567-578.ISSN 1533-4406 (Electronic)

Buckley, J. G. (2000). The future of head and neck surgery. Journal of Laryngology and Otology. Vol 114. No (5). pp: 327-330.ISSN 0022-2151

Byers, R. M., Wolf, P. F. & Ballantyne, A. J. (1988). Rationale for elective modified neck dissection. Head & Neck Surgery. Vol 10. No (3). pp: 160-167.ISSN 0148-6403

Candela, F. C., Kothari, K. & Shah, J. P. (1990). Patterns of cervical node metastases from squamous carcinoma of the oropharynx and hypopharynx. New York Head and Neck Society. Vol 12. No (3). pp: 197-203.ISSN 1043-3074

Candela, F. C., Shah, J., Jaques, D. P. & Shah, J. P. (1990). Patterns of cervical node metastases from squamous carcinoma of the larynx.Archives of otolaryngology-head & neck surgery.. Vol 116. No (4). pp: 432-435.ISSN 0886-4470

Capote, A., Escorial, V., Munoz-Guerra, M. F., Rodriguez-Campo, F. J., Gamallo, C. & Naval, L. (2007). Elective neck dissection in early-stage oral squamous cell carcinoma--does it influence recurrence and survival? New York Head and Neck Society. Vol 29. No (1). pp: 3-11.ISSN 1043-3074

Chen, Z., Smith, C. W., Kiel, D. & Van Waes, C. (1997). Metastatic variants derived following in vivo tumor progression of an in vitro transformed squamous cell carcinoma line acquire a differential growth advantage requiring tumor-host interaction. Clinical & Experimental Metastasis. Vol 15. No (5). pp: 527-537. ISSN 0262-0898

Civantos, F. J., Gomez, C., Duque, C., Pedroso, F., Goodwin, W. J., Weed, D. T., Arnold, D. & Moffat, F. (2003). Sentinel node biopsy in oral cavity cancer: correlation with PET scan and immunohistochemistry. New York Head and Neck Society. Vol 25. No (1). pp: 1-9. ISSN 1043-3074

Civantos, F. J., Moffat, F. L. & Goodwin, W. J. (2006). Lymphatic mapping and sentinel lymphadenectomy for 106 head and neck lesions: contrasts between oral cavity and cutaneous malignancy. Laryngoscope. Vol 112. No (3 Pt 2 Suppl 109). pp: 1-15. ISSN 0023-852X

Coatesworth, A. P. & MacLennan, K. (2002). Squamous cell carcinoma of the upper aerodigestive tract: the prevalence of microscopic extracapsular spread and soft tissue deposits in the clinically N0 neck. New York Head and Neck Society. Vol 24. No (3). pp: 258-261. ISSN 1043-3074

Davidson, B. J., Kulkarny, V., Delacure, M. D. & Shah, J. P. (1993). Posterior triangle metastases of squamous cell carcinoma of the upper aerodigestive tract. American Journal of Surgery. Vol 166. No (4). pp: 395-398. ISSN 0002-9610

de Mulder, P. H. (1999). The chemotherapy of head and neck cancer. Anticancer Drugs. Vol 10 Suppl 1. No pp: S33-37. ISSN 0959-4973

Dennington, M. L., Carter, D. R. & Meyers, A. D. (1980). Distant metastases in head and neck epidermoid carcinoma. Laryngoscope. Vol 90. No (2). pp: 196-201. ISSN 0023-852X

Di, B., Li, X. M., Shang, Y. D., Song, Q., Li, J., Shen, Y. P. & Cheng, J. M. (2009). Clinicopathologic aspects of locoregional recurrence of hypopharyngeal cancer and their implication on the survival of patients. Zhonghua Er Bi Yan Hou Tou Jing Wai Ke Za Zhi. Vol 44. No (9). pp: 716-721. ISSN 1673-0860

Dunne, A. A., Jungclas, H. & Werner, J. A. (2001). Intraoperative sentinel node biopsy in patients with squamous cell carcinomas of the head and neck--experiences using a well-type NaI detector for gamma ray spectroscopy. The Polish Otolaryngology. Vol 55. No (2). pp: 127-134. ISSN 0030-6657

Ellis, U. (2008). Harrison's principles of internal medicine. Choice: Current Reviews for Academic Libraries. Vol 46. No (1). pp: 138-138. ISSN 00094978

Fidler, I. J. & Hart, I. R. (1982). Biological diversity in metastatic neoplasms: origins and implications. Science. Vol 217. No (4564). pp: 998-1003. ISSN 0036-8075

Fisch, U. P. (1964). Cervical Lymphography in Cases of Laryngo-Pharyngeal Carcinoma. Journal of Laryngology and Otology. Vol 78. No pp: 715-726. ISSN 0022-2151

Folkman, J. (1990). What is the evidence that tumors are angiogenesis dependent? Journal of the National Cancer Institute. Vol 82. No (1). pp: 4-6. ISSN 0027-8874

Folkman, J. (1992). The role of angiogenesis in tumor growth. Seminars in Cancer Biology. Vol 3. No (2). pp: 65-71. ISSN 1044-579X

Folkman, J. (1996). Fighting cancer by attacking its blood supply. Scientific American. Vol 275. No (3). pp: 150-154. ISSN 0036-8733

Gebbia, V., Agostara, B., Callari, A., Zerillo, G., Restivo, G., Speciale, R., Cupido, G., Ingria, F., Spatafora, G., Fazio, L. & et al. (1993). Head and neck carcinoma with distant metastases: a retrospective analysis of 44 cases treated with cisplatin-based chemotherapeutic regimens. Anticancer Research. Vol 13. No (4). pp: 1129-1131. ISSN 0250-7005

Godden, D. R., Ribeiro, N. F., Hassanein, K. & Langton, S. G. (2002). Recurrent neck disease in oral cancer. Journal of Oral and Maxillofacial Surgery. Vol 60. No (7). pp: 748-753; discussion 753-745. ISSN 0278-2391

Gowen, G. F. & Desuto-Nagy, G. (1963). The incidence and sites of distant metastases in head and neck carcinoma. Surgery, Gynecology & Obstetrics. Vol 116. No pp: 603-607. ISSN 0039-6087

Gray, L., Woolgar, J. & Brown, J. (2000). A functional map of cervical metastases from oral squamous cell carcinoma. Acta Oto-laryngologica. Vol 120. No (7). pp: 885-890. ISSN 0001-6489

Hannen, E. J. & Riediger, D. (2004). The quantification of angiogenesis in relation to metastasis in oral cancer: a review. International Journal of Oral and Maxillofacial Surgery. Vol 33. No (1). pp: 2-7. ISSN 0901-5027

Hiratsuka, H., Miyakawa, A., Nakamori, K., Kido, Y., Sunakawa, H. & Kohama, G. (1997). Multivariate analysis of occult lymph node metastasis as a prognostic indicator for patients with squamous cell carcinoma of the oral cavity. Cancer. Vol 80. No (3). pp: 351-356. ISSN 0008-543X

Hoegler, D. (1997). Radiotherapy for palliation of symptoms in incurable cancer. Current Problems in Cancer. Vol 21. No (3). pp: 129-183. ISSN 0147-0272

Homer, J. J., Greenman, J. & Stafford, N. D. (2002). Circulating angiogenic cytokines as tumour markers and prognostic factors in head and neck squamous cell carcinoma. Clinical Otolaryngology and Allied Sciences. Vol 27. No (1). pp: 32-37. ISSN 0307-7772

Hosal, A. S., Carrau, R. L., Johnson, J. T. & Myers, E. N. (2000). Selective neck dissection in the management of the clinically node-negative neck. Laryngoscope. Vol 110. No (12). pp: 2037-2040.ISSN 0023-852X

Hsu, Y. B., Chu, P. Y., Liu, J. C., Lan, M. C., Chang, S. Y., Tsai, T. L., Huang, J. L., Wang, Y. F. & Tai, S. K. (2008). Role of chest computed tomography in head and neck cancer. Archives of Otolaryngology-Head & Neck Surgery. Vol 134. No (10). pp: 1050-1054. ISSN 1538-361X (Electronic)

Jeong, H. S., Baek, C. H., Son, Y. I., Ki Chung, M., Kyung Lee, D., Young Choi, J., Kim, B. T. & Kim, H. J. (2007). Use of integrated 18F-FDG PET/CT to improve the accuracy of initial cervical nodal evaluation in patients with head and neck squamous cell carcinoma. New York Head and Neck Society. Vol 29. No (3). pp: 203-210. ISSN 1043-3074

John, D. G., Anaes, F. C., Williams, S. R., Ahuja, A., Evans, R., To, K. F., King, W. W. & van Hasselt, C. A. (1993). Palpation compared with ultrasound in the assessment of malignant cervical lymph nodes. Journal of Laryngology and Otology. Vol 107. No (9). pp: 821-823.ISSN 0022-2151

Johnstone, S. & Logan, R. M. (2007). Expression of vascular endothelial growth factor (VEGF) in normal oral mucosa, oral dysplasia and oral squamous cell carcinoma. International Journal of Oral and Maxillofacial Surgery. Vol 36. No (3). pp: 263-266. ISSN 0901-5027

Kishimoto, K., Sasaki, A., Yoshihama, Y., Mese, H., Tsukamoto, G. & Matsumura, T. (2003). Expression of vascular endothelial growth factor-C predicts regional lymph node metastasis in early oral squamous cell carcinoma. Oral Oncology. Vol 39. No (4). pp: 391-396. ISSN 1368-8375

Kowalski, L. P. (2001). Noncervical lymph node metastasis from head and neck cancer. ORL; Journal for Oto-rhino-laryngology and Its Related Specialties. Vol 63. No (4). pp: 252-255. ISSN 0301-1569

Kruse, A. L. & Gratz, K. W. (2009). Cervical metastases of squamous cell carcinoma of the maxilla: a retrospective study of 9 years. New York Head and Neck Society Oncol. Vol 1. No pp: 28.ISSN 1758-3284 (Electronic)

Kurokawa, H., Yamashita, Y., Takeda, S., Zhang, M., Fukuyama, H. & Takahashi, T. (2002). Risk factors for late cervical lymph node metastases in patients with stage I or II carcinoma of the tongue. New York Head and Neck Society. Vol 24. No (8). pp: 731-736. ISSN 1043-3074

Leon, X., Quer, M., Orus, C., del Prado Venegas, M. & Lopez, M. (2000). Distant metastases in head and neck cancer patients who achieved loco-regional control. New York Head and Neck Society. Vol 22. No (7). pp: 680-686. ISSN 1043-3074

Leong, S. P., Cady, B., Jablons, D. M., Garcia-Aguilar, J., Reintgen, D., Jakub, J., Pendas, S., Duhaime, L., Cassell, R., Gardner, M., Giuliano, R., Archie, V., Calvin, D., Mensha, L., Shivers, S., Cox, C., Werner, J. A., Kitagawa, Y. & Kitajima, M. (2006). Clinical patterns of metastasis. Cancer Metastasis Rev. Vol 25. No (2). pp: 221-232. ISSN 0167-7659

Li, X., Di, B., Shang, Y., Zhou, Y., Cheng, J. & He, Z. (2009). Clinicopathologic risk factors for distant metastases from head and neck squamous cell carcinomas. European Journal of Surgical Oncology. Vol 35. No (12). pp: 1348-1353. ISSN 1532-2157 (Electronic)

Li, X. M., Wei, W. I., Guo, X. F., Yuen, P. W. & Lam, L. K. (1996). Cervical lymph node metastatic patterns of squamous carcinomas in the upper aerodigestive tract. Journal of Laryngology and Otology. Vol 110. No (10). pp: 937-941. ISSN 0022-2151

Lim, S. C., Zhang, S., Ishii, G., Endoh, Y., Kodama, K., Miyamoto, S., Hayashi, R., Ebihara, S., Cho, J. S. & Ochiai, A. (2004). Predictive markers for late cervical metastasis in stage I and II invasive squamous cell carcinoma of the oral tongue. Clinical Cancer Research. Vol 10. No (1 Pt 1). pp: 166-172. ISSN 1078-0432

Lim, Y. C., Koo, B. S., Lee, J. S., Lim, J. Y. & Choi, E. C. (2006). Distributions of cervical lymph node metastases in oropharyngeal carcinoma: therapeutic implications for the N0 neck. Laryngoscope. Vol 116. No (7). pp: 1148-1152. ISSN 0023-852X

Lim, Y. C., Lee, J. S., Koo, B. S., Kim, S. H., Kim, Y. H. & Choi, E. C. (2006). Treatment of contralateral N0 neck in early squamous cell carcinoma of the oral tongue: elective neck dissection versus observation. Laryngoscope. Vol 116. No (3). pp: 461-465. ISSN 0023-852X

Lindberg, R. (1972). Distribution of cervical lymph node metastases from squamous cell carcinoma of the upper respiratory and digestive tracts. Cancer. Vol 29. No (6). pp: 1446-1449. ISSN 0008-543X

Markus, G. (1988). The relevance of plasminogen activators to neoplastic growth. A review of recent literature. Enzyme. Vol 40. No (2-3). pp: 158-172. ISSN 0013-9432

Menda, Y. & Graham, M. M. (2005). Update on 18F-fluorodeoxyglucose/positron emission tomography and positron emission tomography/computed tomography imaging of squamous head and neck cancers. Seminars in Nuclear Medicine. Vol 35. No (4). pp: 214-219.ISSN 0001-2998

Merino, O. R., Lindberg, R. D. & Fletcher, G. H. (1977). An analysis of distant metastases from squamous cell carcinoma of the upper respiratory and digestive tracts. Cancer. Vol 40. No (1). pp: 145-151. ISSN 0008-543X

Miyajima, Y., Nakano, R. & Morimatsu, M. (1995). Analysis of expression of matrix metalloproteinases-2 and -9 in hypopharyngeal squamous cell carcinoma by in situ hybridization. Annals of Otology Rhinology and Laryngology. Vol 104. No (9 Pt 1). pp: 678-684. ISSN 0003-4894

Munoz-Guerra, M. F., Marazuela, E. G., Martin-Villar, E., Quintanilla, M. & Gamallo, C. (2004). Prognostic significance of intratumoral lymphangiogenesis in squamous cell carcinoma of the oral cavity. Cancer. Vol 100. No (3). pp: 553-560. ISSN 0008-543X

Murakami, R., Uozumi, H., Hirai, T., Nishimura, R., Shiraishi, S., Ota, K., Murakami, D., Tomiguchi, S., Oya, N., Katsuragawa, S. & Yamashita, Y. (2007). Impact of FDG-PET/CT imaging on nodal staging for head-and-neck squamous cell carcinoma. International Journal of Radiation Oncology Biology Physics. Vol 68. No (2). pp: 377-382. ISSN 0360-3016

Myers, E. N. & Fagan, J. F. (1999). Management of the neck in cancer of the larynx. Annals of Otology Rhinology and Laryngology. Vol 108. No (9). pp: 828-832. ISSN 0003-4894

Nagata, M., Fujita, H., Ida, H., Hoshina, H., Inoue, T., Seki, Y., Ohnishi, M., Ohyama, T., Shingaki, S., Kaji, M., Saku, T. & Takagi, R. (2003). Identification of potential biomarkers of lymph node metastasis in oral squamous cell carcinoma by cDNA microarray analysis. International Journal of Cancer. Vol 106. No (5). pp: 683-689. ISSN 0020-7136

Nelson, W. R. & Sisk, M. (1994). Axillary metastases from carcinoma of the larynx: a 25-year survival. New York Head and Neck Society. Vol 16. No (1). pp: 83-87.ISSN 1043-3074

Ng, S. H., Yen, T. C., Liao, C. T., Chang, J. T., Chan, S. C., Ko, S. F., Wang, H. M. & Wong, H. F. (2005). 18F-FDG PET and CT/MRI in oral cavity squamous cell carcinoma: a prospective study of 124 patients with histologic correlation. Journal of Nuclear Medicine. Vol 46. No (7). pp: 1136-1143. ISSN 0161-5505

Nikitakis, N. G., Rivera, H., Lopes, M. A., Siavash, H., Reynolds, M. A., Ord, R. A. & Sauk, J. J. (2003). Immunohistochemical expression of angiogenesis-related markers in oral squamous cell carcinomas with multiple metastatic lymph nodes. American Journal of Clinical Pathology. Vol 119. No (4). pp: 574-586. ISSN 0002-9173

O'Brien, C. J., Traynor, S. J., McNeil, E., McMahon, J. D. & Chaplin, J. M. (2000). The use of clinical criteria alone in the management of the clinically negative neck among patients with squamous cell carcinoma of the oral cavity and oropharynx. Archives of Otolaryngology-Head & Neck Surgery.. Vol 126. No (3). pp: 360-365. ISSN 0886-4470

O'Reilly, M. S., Boehm, T., Shing, Y., Fukai, N., Vasios, G., Lane, W. S., Flynn, E., Birkhead, J. R., Olsen, B. R. & Folkman, J. (1997). Endostatin: an endogenous inhibitor of angiogenesis and tumor growth. Cell. Vol 88. No (2). pp: 277-285. ISSN 0092-8674

Orian-Rousseau, V. CD44, a therapeutic target for metastasising tumours. European Journal of Cancer . Vol 46. No (7). pp: 1271-1277. ISSN 1879-0852 (Electronic)

Parkin, D. M., Bray, F., Ferlay, J. & Pisani, P. (2005). Global cancer statistics, 2002. Journal of Cancer Research and Clinical Oncology. Vol 55. No (2). pp: 74-108. ISSN 0007-9235

Patel, B. P., Shah, S. V., Shukla, S. N., Shah, P. M. & Patel, P. S. (2007). Clinical significance of MMP-2 and MMP-9 in patients with oral cancer. New York Head and Neck Society. Vol 29. No (6). pp: 564-572. ISSN 1043-3074

Pentenero, M., Gandolfo, S. & Carrozzo, M. (2005). Importance of tumor thickness and depth of invasion in nodal involvement and prognosis of oral squamous cell carcinoma: a review of the literature. New York Head and Neck Society. Vol 27. No (12). pp: 1080-1091. ISSN 1043-3074

Peters, L. J., Goepfert, H., Ang, K. K., Byers, R. M., Maor, M. H., Guillamondegui, O., Morrison, W. H., Weber, R. S., Garden, A. S., Frankenthaler, R. A. & et al. (1993). Evaluation of the dose for postoperative radiation therapy of head and neck cancer: first report of a prospective randomized trial. International Journal of Radiation Oncology Biology Physics. Vol 26. No (1). pp: 3-11. ISSN 0360-3016

Pignon, J. P., le Maitre, A., Maillard, E. & Bourhis, J. (2009). Meta-analysis of chemotherapy in head and neck cancer (MACH-NC): an update on 93 randomised trials and 17,346 patients. Radiotherapy and Oncology . Vol 92. No (1). pp: 4-14. ISSN 1879-0887 (Electronic)

Prim, M. P., De Diego, J. I., Hardisson, D., Madero, R., Nistal, M. & Gavilan, J. (1999). Extracapsular spread and desmoplastic pattern in neck lymph nodes: two prognostic factors of laryngeal cancer. Annals of Otology Rhinology and Laryngology. Vol 108. No (7 Pt 1). pp: 672-676.ISSN 0003-4894

Riedel, F., Gotte, K., Schwalb, J., Bergler, W. & Hormann, K. (2000). Expression of 92-kDa type IV collagenase correlates with angiogenic markers and poor survival in head and neck squamous cell carcinoma. International Journal of Oncology. Vol 17. No (6). pp: 1099-1105. ISSN 1019-6439

Robbins, K. T., Clayman, G., Levine, P. A., Medina, J., Sessions, R., Shaha, A., Som, P. & Wolf, G. T. (2002). Neck dissection classification update: revisions proposed by the American Head and Neck Society and the American Academy of Otolaryngology-Head and Neck Surgery.Archives of Otolaryngology-Head & Neck surgery.. Vol 128. No (7). pp: 751-758. ISSN 0886-4470

Ruokolainen, H., Paakko, P. & Turpeenniemi-Hujanen, T. (2004). Expression of matrix metalloproteinase-9 in head and neck squamous cell carcinoma: a potential marker for prognosis. Clinical Cancer Research. Vol 10. No (9). pp: 3110-3116. ISSN 1078-0432

Shah, J. P. & Andersen, P. E. (1994). The impact of patterns of nodal metastasis on modifications of neck dissection. Annals of Surgical Oncology. Vol 1. No (6). pp: 521-532. ISSN 1068-9265

Shah, J. P., Candela, F. C. & Poddar, A. K. (1990). The patterns of cervical lymph node metastases from squamous carcinoma of the oral cavity. Cancer. Vol 66. No (1). pp: 109-113. ISSN 0008-543X

Shah, J. P. & Gil, Z. (2009). Current concepts in management of oral cancer--surgery. Oral Oncology. Vol 45. No (4-5). pp: 394-401.ISSN 1368-8375

Shingaki, S., Takada, M., Sasai, K., Bibi, R., Kobayashi, T., Nomura, T. & Saito, C. (2003). Impact of lymph node metastasis on the pattern of failure and survival in oral carcinomas. American Journal of Surgery . Vol 185. No (3). pp: 278-284. ISSN 0002-9610

Shintani, S., Li, C., Ishikawa, T., Mihara, M., Nakashiro, K. & Hamakawa, H. (2004). Expression of vascular endothelial growth factor A, B, C, and D in oral squamous cell carcinoma. Oral Oncology. Vol 40. No (1). pp: 13-20. ISSN 1368-8375

Sigg, M. B., Steinert, H., Gratz, K., Hugenin, P., Stoeckli, S. & Eyrich, G. K. (2003). Staging of head and neck tumors: [18F]fluorodeoxyglucose positron emission tomography compared with physical examination and conventional imaging modalities.Journal of Oral and Maxillofacial Surgery. Vol 61. No (9). pp: 1022-1029. ISSN 0278-2391

Sim, F. H., Frassica, F. J. & Frassica, D. A. (1992). Metastatic bone disease: current concepts of clinicopathophysiology and modern surgical treatment. Annals of the Academy of Medicine, Singapore. Vol 21. No (2). pp: 274-279. ISSN 0304-4602

Simental, A. A., Jr., Johnson, J. T. & Myers, E. N. (2006). Cervical metastasis from squamous cell carcinoma of the maxillary alveolus and hard palate. Laryngoscope. Vol 116. No (9). pp: 1682-1684. ISSN 0023-852X

Smith, B. D., Smith, G. L., Carter, D., Sasaki, C. T. & Haffty, B. G. (2000). Prognostic significance of vascular endothelial growth factor protein levels in oral and oropharyngeal squamous cell carcinoma. Journal of Clinical Oncology. Vol 18. No (10). pp: 2046-2052. ISSN 0732-183X

Snow, J. B., Jr., Gelber, R. D., Kramer, S., Davis, L. W., Marcial, V. A. & Lowry, L. D. (1980). Randomized preoperative and postoperative radiation therapy for patients with carcinoma of the head and neck: preliminary report. Laryngoscope. Vol 90. No (6 Pt 1). pp: 930-945. ISSN 0023-852X

Sparano, A., Weinstein, G., Chalian, A., Yodul, M. & Weber, R. (2004). Multivariate predictors of occult neck metastasis in early oral tongue cancer. Otolaryngol Head & Neck Surgery. Vol 131. No (4). pp: 472-476. ISSN 0194-5998

Spector, G. J. (2001). Distant metastases from laryngeal and hypopharyngeal cancer. ORL; journal for oto-rhino-laryngology and its related specialties. Vol 63. No (4). pp: 224-228. ISSN 0301-1569

Steenland, E., Leer, J. W., van Houwelingen, H., Post, W. J., van den Hout, W. B., Kievit, J., de Haes, H., Martijn, H., Oei, B., Vonk, E., van der Steen-Banasik, E., Wiggenraad, R. G., Hoogenhout, J., Warlam-Rodenhuis, C., van Tienhoven, G., Wanders, R., Pomp, J., van Reijn, M., van Mierlo, I. & Rutten, E. (1999). The effect of a single fraction compared to multiple fractions on painful bone metastases: a global analysis of the Dutch Bone Metastasis Study. Radiotherapy and Oncology . Vol 52. No (2). pp: 101-109. ISSN 0167-8140

Stoeckli, S. J., Steinert, H., Pfaltz, M. & Schmid, S. (2002). Is there a role for positron emission tomography with 18F-fluorodeoxyglucose in the initial staging of nodal negative oral and oropharyngeal squamous cell carcinoma. New York Head and Neck Society. Vol 24. No (4). pp: 345-349. ISSN 1043-3074

Stuckensen, T., Kovacs, A. F., Adams, S. & Baum, R. P. (2000). Staging of the neck in patients with oral cavity squamous cell carcinomas: a prospective comparison of PET, ultrasound, CT and MRI. Journal of Cranio-maxillo-facial Surgery . Vol 28. No (6). pp: 319-324. ISSN 1010-5182

Su, Y. X., Zheng, J. W., Zheng, G. S., Liao, G. Q. & Zhang, Z. Y. (2008). Neoadjuvant chemotherapy of cisplatin and fluorouracil regimen in head and neck squamous cell carcinoma: a meta-analysis. Chinese Medical Journal . Vol 121. No (19). pp: 1939-1944. ISSN 0366-6999

Sugawara, T. & Kaneta, K. (1983). [Radiation therapy of pulmonary metastases]. Gan no rinsho. Japan Journal of Cancer Clinics. Vol 29. No (6). pp: 567-571. ISSN 0021-4949

Takes, R. P., Righi, P., Meeuwis, C. A., Manni, J. J., Knegt, P., Marres, H. A., Spoelstra, H. A., de Boer, M. F., van der Mey, A. G., Bruaset, I., Ball, V., Weisberger, E., Radpour, S., Kruyt, R. H., Joosten, F. B., Lameris, J. S., van Oostayen, J. A., Kopecky, K., Caldemeyer, K., Henzen-Logmans, S. C., Wiersma-van Tilburg, J. M., Bosman, F. T., van Krieken, J. H., Hermans, J. & Baatenburg de Jong, R. J. (1998). The value of ultrasound with ultrasound-guided fine-needle aspiration biopsy compared to computed tomography in the detection of regional metastases in the clinically negative neck. International Journal of Radiation Oncology Biology Physics. Vol 40. No (5). pp: 1027-1032. ISSN 0360-3016

Tauzin, M., Rabalais, A., Hagan, J. L., Wood, C. G., Ferris, R. L. & Walvekar, R. R. (2010). PET-CT staging of the neck in cancers of the oropharynx: patterns of regional and retropharyngeal nodal metastasis. World Journal of Surgical Oncology. Vol 8. No pp: 70. ISSN 1477-7819 (Electronic)

Teichgraeber, J. F. & Clairmont, A. A. (1984). The incidence of occult metastases for cancer of the oral tongue and floor of the mouth: treatment rationale. Head & Neck Surgery. Vol 7. No (1). pp: 15-21. ISSN 0148-6403

Tong, M., Lloyd, B., Pei, P. & Mallery, S. R. (2008). Human head and neck squamous cell carcinoma cells are both targets and effectors for the angiogenic cytokine, VEGF. Journal of Cellular Biochemistry. Vol 105. No (5). pp: 1202-1210. ISSN 1097-4644 (Electronic)

Troell, R. J. & Terris, D. J. (1995). Detection of metastases from head and neck cancers. Laryngoscope. Vol 105. No (3 Pt 1). pp: 247-250.ISSN 0023-852X

Uppelschoten, J. M., Wanders, S. L. & de Jong, J. M. (1995). Single-dose radiotherapy (6 Gy): palliation in painful bone metastases. Radiotherapy and Oncology . Vol 36. No (3). pp: 198-202. ISSN 0167-8140

van den Brekel, M. W., Stel, H. V., Castelijns, J. A., Nauta, J. J., van der Waal, I., Valk, J., Meyer, C. J. & Snow, G. B. (1990). Cervical lymph node metastasis: assessment of radiologic criteria. Radiology. Vol 177. No (2). pp: 379-384.ISSN 0033-8419

Vikram, B., Strong, E. W., Shah, J. P. & Spiro, R. (1984). Failure at distant sites following multimodality treatment for advanced head and neck cancer. Head & Neck Surgery. Vol 6. No (3). pp: 730-733.ISSN 0148-6403

Wallwork, B. D., Anderson, S. R. & Coman, W. B. (2007). Squamous cell carcinoma of the floor of the mouth: tumour thickness and the rate of cervical metastasis. Anz Journal of Surgery. Vol 77. No (9). pp: 761-764. ISSN 1445-1433

Warburton, G., Nikitakis, N. G., Roberson, P., Marinos, N. J., Wu, T., Sauk, J. J., Jr., Ord, R. A. & Wahl, S. M. (2007). Histopathological and lymphangiogenic parameters in relation to lymph node metastasis in early stage oral squamous cell carcinoma.Journal of Oral and Maxillofacial Surgery. Vol 65. No (3). pp: 475-484. ISSN 0278-2391

Wedman, J., Balm, A. J., Hart, A. A., Loftus, B. M., Hilgers, F. J., Gregor, R. T., van Zandwijk, N. & Zoetmulder, F. A. (1996). Value of resection of pulmonary metastases in head and neck cancer patients. New York Head and Neck Society. Vol 18. No (4). pp: 311-316.ISSN 1043-3074

Werner, J. A., Sapundzhiev, N. R., Teymoortash, A., Dunne, A. A., Behr, T. & Folz, B. J. (2004). Endoscopic sentinel lymphadenectomy as a new diagnostic approach in the N0 neck. European Archives of Oto-rhino-laryngology. Vol 261. No (9). pp: 463-468. ISSN 0937-4477

Wild, D., Eyrich, G. K., Ciernik, I. F., Stoeckli, S. J., Schuknecht, B. & Goerres, G. W. (2006). In-line (18)F-fluorodeoxyglucose positron emission tomography with computed tomography (PET/CT) in patients with carcinoma of the sinus/nasal area and orbit. Journal of Cranio-maxillo-facial Surgery . Vol 34. No (1). pp: 9-16. ISSN 1010-5182

2

Advanced Squamous Cell Carcinoma of the Skin

Vinicius Vazquez, Sergio Serrano and Renato Capuzzo
Barretos Cancer Hospital
Brazil

1. Introduction

The squamous cell carcinoma of the skin (SCCS) is one of the most common cancers around the world.(Ries, Melbert et al. 2007; 2008) It affects mostly the sun exposed areas of people with fair skin. The majority of cases are easily treatable by simple excision or radiotherapy with a good chance of achieving cure. Despite this, the aging population process associated to chronic ultraviolet radiation (U.V.) exposition is raising the SCCS incidence and consequently the number of patients with advanced tumors.(Staples, Elwood et al. 2006) This is a devastating presentation of the disease, where the lack of information occurs and even the professionals in the field are a few. Local disease progression, local and regional recurrence, lymph node or distant metastases are the focus of this review chapter. The characteristics of the tumors arising in the trunk and extremities are different from those in the head and neck, and they are described and discussed separately.

2. Advanced squamous cell carcinoma of the skin of the trunk and extremities

2.1 Definition

We consider as patients with advanced squamous cell carcinoma of the skin of the trunk and extremities, those with T3/T4 (tumor invading deep structures/axial esqueleton) or N1/2/3 (regional lymph node metastasis) tumors according the 7th UICC TNM classification(Sobin and Compton). Tumors arising from genital or anus are not considered.

2.2 Epidemiology, clinical presentation, diagnostic methods and defining a risk population

There are some clinical conditions associated to locally advanced disease. The patients are typically old, with risk conditions to skin carcinomas (chronic U.V. exposition and fair skin) and may have other local disease as burn scars, chronic skin ulcer and systemic pathologies related to immune system suppression (organ transplant receptors, hematopoietic disorders)(Cherpelis, Marcusen et al. 2002; Trakatelli, Ulrich et al. 2007). Low economic and educational status or difficult access to the health system may also play a role to the presentation of advanced cases, but not confirmed in studies.

The usual presentation is a patient with a long story of a "chronic ulcer" with many previous local treatments. Some present with pathological bone fractures or lymph node metastasis. (de Lima Vazquez, Sachetto et al. 2008)

TX Primary tumor cannot be assessed
T0 No evidence of primary tumor
Tis Carcinoma in situ
T1 Tumor ≤ 2 cm in greatest dimension with 2 high-risk features*
T2 Tumor > 2 cm in greatest dimension with or without one additional high-risk feature,* or any size with ≥ 2 high-risk features*
T3 Tumor with invasion of maxilla, mandible, orbit, or temporal bone
T4 Tumor with invasion of skeleton (axial or appendicular) or perineural invasion of skull base

*High-risk features include depth (> 2-mm thickness; Clark level ≥ IV); perineural invasion; location (primary site ear; primary site nonglabrous lip); and differentiation (poorly differentiated or undifferentiated).

Table 1. Definition of cutaneous squamous cell carcinoma tumor (T) staging system in 7th edition of American Joint Committee on Cancer

NX. Regional lymph nodes cannot be assessed
N0. No regional lymph node metastasis
N1. Metastasis in a single ipsilateral lymph node, 3 cm or less in greatest dimension
N2. Metastasis in a single ipsilateral lymph node, more than 3 cm but not more than 6 cm in greatest dimension; or in multiple ipsilateral lymph nodes, none more than 6 cm in greatest dimension; or in bilateral or contralateral lymph nodes, none more than 6 cm in greatest dimension
N2a. Metastasis in a single ipsilateral lymph node, more than 3 cm but not more than 6 cm in greatest dimension
N2b. Metastasis in multiple ipsilateral lymph nodes, none more than 6 cm in greatest dimension
N2c. Metastasis in bilateral or contralateral lymph nodes, none more than 6 cm in greatest dimension
N3. Metastasis in a lymph node more than 6 cm in greatest dimension

Table 2. Definition of cutaneous squamous cell carcinoma Nodes (N) staging system in 7th edition of American Joint Committee on Cancer

2.3 Factors related to prognosis

2.3.1 Clinical

The clinical factors classically related to prognosis are the tumor size and regional lymph node status (TNM stage). Many studies have confirmed both tumor size our local infiltration and presence and number of lymph node metastasis as the main prognosticator for advanced disease. The incidence of lymph node metastasis varys according the population studied from 4.5 to 17%(North, Spellman et al. 1997; Cherpelis, Marcusen et al. 2002; Mullen, Feng et al. 2006). Other factors have being pointed but the association is uncertain as anatomic location and previous chronic disease locally on the skin (i.e. Marjolin ulcer). (Collins, Nickoonahand et al. 2004)

2.3.2 Pathological

A detailed histopathological descriptive classification considering all subtypes of squamous cell carcinoma of the skin was proposed by Cassarino (Cassarino, Derienzo et al. 2006), categorized tumors as low, intermediated and high risk, but it was not confirmed by well designed studies. The tumor length in millimeters (Breslow measurement) is associated with prognosis in some studies, but not confirmed(Breuninger, Black et al. 1990). The tumor grade, proposed by Broders and simplified to grade I, II and III (I well differentiated and III undifferentiated) is other controversial factor related to the prognosis, as well as the mitotic index and the Intratumoral lymphocytic infiltrate (ILI). In our retrospective study, the tumor grade was related to prognosis and the ILI was related to the lymph node metastasis.(de Lima Vazquez , Scapulatempo et al. 2011)

2.3.3 Molecular

With the advent of the molecular diagnosis, some authors looked at the relation of molecular changes and disease progression. Knowledge of the role of molecular markers in tumor progression and metastasis is limited. The tyrosine kinases Human Epidermal Receptor (HER) family (EGFR - Epidermal Growth Factor Receptor, HER-2, HER-3 and HER-4) are transmembrane glycoproteins related to cell proliferation, differentiation and apoptosis. Altered expression of the HER family is associated with several epithelial tumors such as breast carcinoma and esophageal squamous cell carcinoma. Small studies have also shown altered HER expression in localized squamous cell carcinoma when compared to normal skin. HER 2 expression in advanced CSCC of the trunk and extremities is not well studied and may be related to prognosis allowing the use of target therapies that block the HER pathway(Krahn, Leiter et al. 2001). E-cadherin is a transmembrane glycoprotein and it is a mediator of calcium-dependent cell-cell adhesion in normal cells. Reduced cell-cell adhesiveness is considered important in both early and late carcinogenis. High E-cadherin expression in cell cytoplasm and low expression in the cell membrane is associated with tumor aggressiveness in different cancers.(Koseki, Aoki et al. 1999) Podoplanin is a membrane protein found on lymphatic vessel endothelium. Its function is poorly understood although it may govern endothelial motility and its absence in animal studies is associated with lymphedema and malformation of lymphatic vessels.(Schacht, Ramirez et al. 2003)

In our study with 55 patients with advanced cutaneous squamous cell carcinoma (CSCC) of the trunk and extremities, Primary tumor positivity was 25.5% for EGFR, 87.3% for HER-3 and 48.1% for HER-4. Metastases were positive for EGFR in 41.7%, for HER-3 in 83.3% and HER-4 in 43.5%. HER-2 was negative in all samples. Membrane E-cadherin and cytoplasmic E-cadherin were positive in 47.3% and 30.2% of primary tumors and 45.5%and 27.3% of metastases respectively. Podoplanin was positive in 41.8% of primary tumors and 41.7% of metastases. The hiperexpression of Podoplanin in the primary tumor was related to lower survival rates. The HER family and the E-cadherin were not related to prognosis. The HER-4 hiperexpression in the lymph node metastasis was associated to lower survival and showed that the HER family may play a role in the disease progression.(de Lima Vazquez , Scapulatempo et al. 2011)

2.4 The treatment modalities

2.4.1 Surgery

Surgery is the classic treatment for skin cancers and for advanced tumors it is still the most effective treatment. Unfortunately, in advanced cases amputations and extensive resections and dissections (i.e. extensive lymph node dissection with skin resection) are usual and have a high morbidity and sometimes mortality rate. Complex reconstructions with surgical flaps (figure 1) and other advanced techniques may be applied but local and clinical suboptimal conditions contraindicate them frequently. Local control is the goal, and the main objectives are to obtain clear margins and in case of lymph node metastasis, to clear completely the lymphatic chain (i.e. axilla or groin). Due the tumor characteristics of local and regional dissemination, aggressive approaches are indicated if clinical conditions are satisfactory. Recurrence rate vary in the literature achieving 50% {de Lima Vazquez, 2008}.

2.4.2 Radiation therapy

When surgery is not an option for advanced tumours, i.e - patient refusal, clinical adverse conditions - radiation may be applied, but with limited results. The main role of the radiation therapy is when incomplete resection occurs, and in the adjuvant setting, when tumour margins are not sufficient or after resection of bulky lymph node metastasis. Indications are personalised since there is no standard care with this method.

3. Head and neck tumors

3.1 Introduction

Squamous cell carcinoma accounts for 20% of non-melanoma cancers of the head and neck (Alam and Ratner 2001). In most cases, these tumors are cured with surgical treatment and / or radiotherapy, but a small portion of these patients had unfavorable outcomes with high rates of metastases and regional recurrence after treatment, which is associated with 20% of deaths from skin cancer (Alam and Ratner 2001). This more aggressive presentation is found in patients referred for high risk, which the literature has discussed the factors involved in this group (Veness 2007). In head and neck surgery, it is particularly associated with the presence of regional metastasis and invasiveness of the primary tumor. The latest edition of the UICC AJCC, published in 2010 (Edge and Compton 2010), showed major changes in the staging of nonmelanoma skin cancers, remarking lymph node staging aligned with the other sites of head and neck and including new factors for classification of the primary tumor.

This part of the chapter will present some specific features of the therapy of skin cancers of the head and neck that often overlap with those found in other regions of the body, but in advanced tumors may limit surgical treatment and carry a poor prognosis for these tumors.

3.2 Advanced tumors: Characteristics of primary tumor

The following factors define a high risk of metastasis and recurrence in skin cancers (Edge and Compton 2010):

Size of the primary tumor greater than 2 cm
Breslow tumor thickness greater than 2 mm, Clark level IV or greater

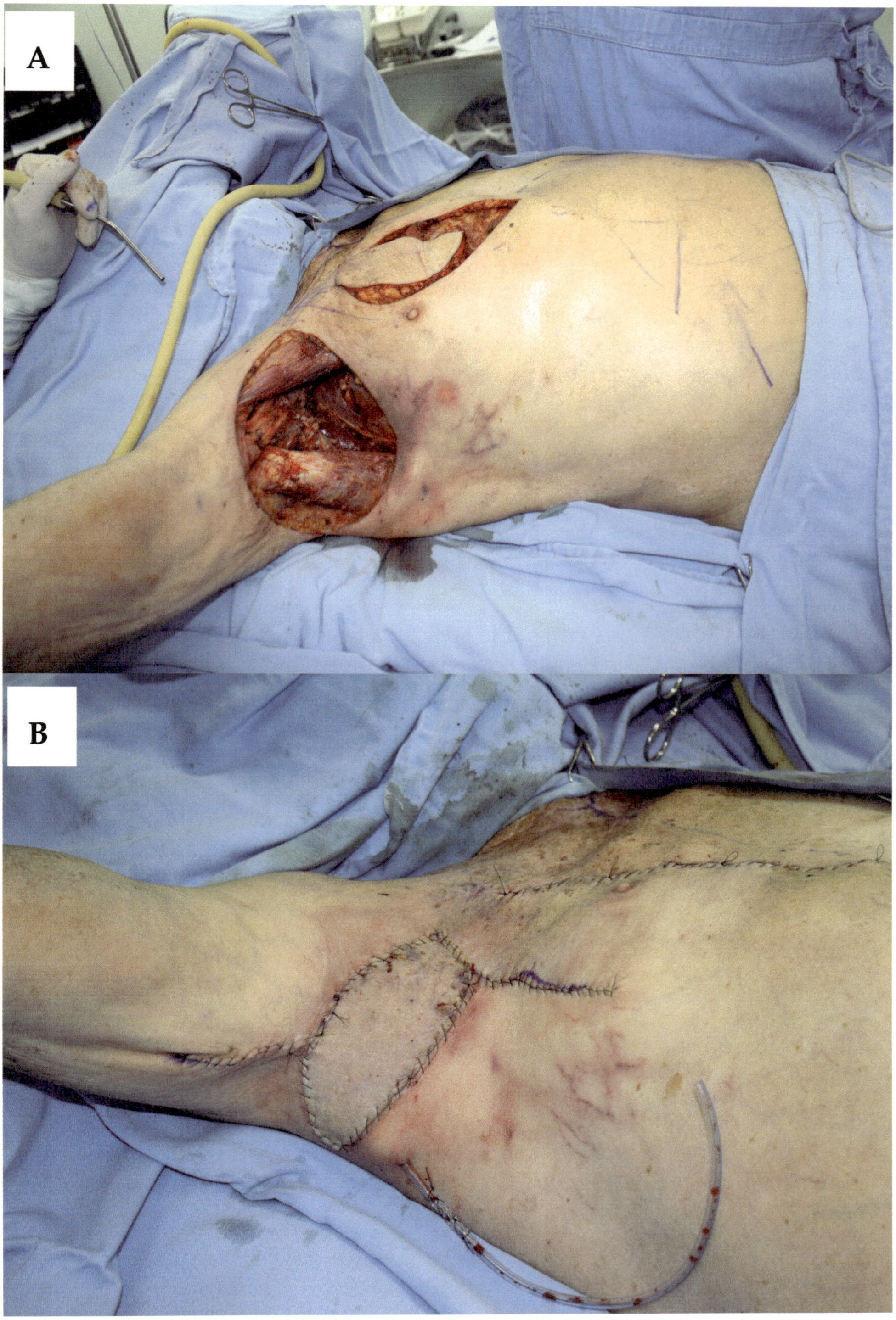

Fig. 1. A - Axilar lymphadenectomy with skin resection and miocutaneous flap prepared for the reconstruction. Fig. 1. B - Final aspect of the reconstruction

Perineural invasion (PNI)
Poor differentiation
Anatomic sites that which carry high risk for recurrence or metastasis
Immunocompromised state of the patient

These changes are based on data-derived, evidence-based medicine and some changed in the last edition of the AJCC and will be detailed below.

Tumor size: this parameter does not present a linear correlation of increased risk of metastasis and recurrence, according to tumor growth, however a limit of 2 cm is shown in several articles as a risk factor for locoregional recurrence. In the sixth edition of the AJCC edition, the limit of 5 cm separated the tumors in T2 and T3, however this limit did not have enough evidence to be sustained and was abolished in the seventh edition, being replaced by parameters more related to the invasiveness than the diameter of tumor (Farasat, Yu et al. 2011).

Tumor depth and PNI: Even the tumor thickness and depth of invasion are important risk factors to SCCHN metastasis and local recurrence (Farasat, Yu et al. 2011). So, in the last edition of AJCC, Breslow depth and Clark level were incorporated. These changes directly affected head and neck tumors that invade the facial bones or skull base, being classified as advanced tumors, with higher risk of metastases and local recurrence (Edge and Compton 2010).

Another factor was added is the perineural invasion of nerves at the base of the skull, which often restricts a craniofacial resection with clear margins and is associated with a worse prognosis. Although based on retrospective studies, PNI showed a higher association with tumors in the face, lower degree of differentiation, tumors larger than 2 cm and recurrent tumors (Leibovitch, Huilgol et al. 2005). There is evidence of an increased incidence of cervical lymphadenopathy and distant metastasis, along with significantly reduced survival in patients with tumors that showed PNI(Farasat, Yu et al. 2011).

A careful radiological preoperative assessment may reveal tumor invasion of branches of the trigeminal or facial nerve. The use of CT and MRI in invasive tumors of the skull base shows high accuracy in detecting perineural invasions, when correlated with intraoperative and pathological findings (Gandhi, Panizza et al. 2010).

Immunosuppression: Although not a specific factor that affects tumor staging, AJCC, in his last edition, highlights this as a risk factor for increased aggressiveness of skin tumors. Organ transplant recipients are 65 times greater risk of developing squamous cell carcinoma of the skin than the general population and have much more aggressive evolution.

Location of primary tumor: some anatomical sites are more associated with worse outcomes in head and neck. This can be seen in sites that drain to the parotid gland like external ear, temple, forehead and anterior scalp. The lower lip also has an increased risk of nodal metastasis.(Veness 2007)

Some series showed a poor outcome of cutaneous squamous cell carcinoma of external ear (Brantsch, Meisner et al. 2008; Turner, Morgan et al. 2009). Faustina et al found 24,3% of regional metastasis in 111 patients with squamous cell carcinoma of the eyelid and periocular region, advising close observation of parotid after the treatment of this site(Faustina, Diba et al. 2004)

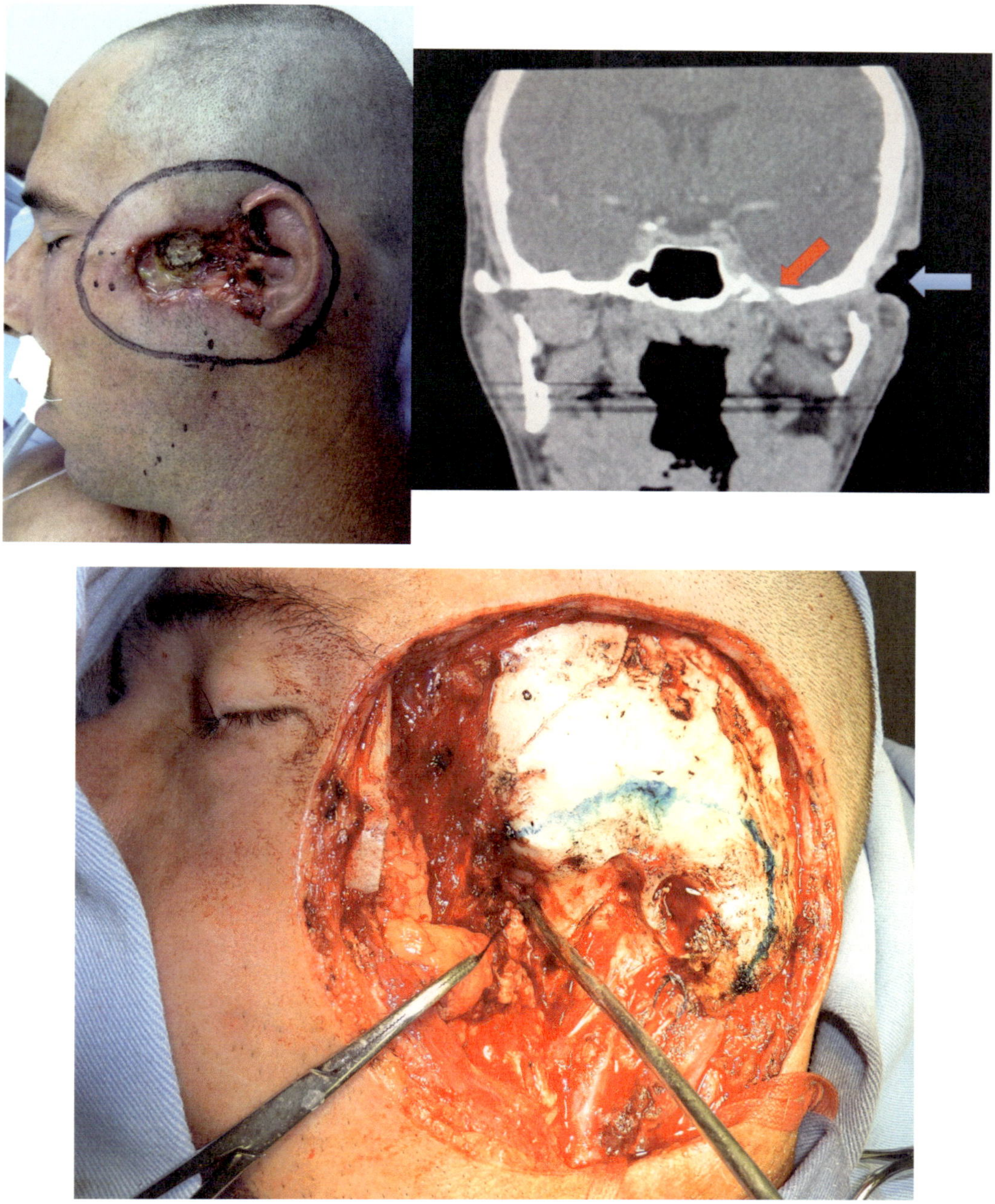

Fig. 2. A (On the left): Clinical aspect of the patient with invasive skin tumor and bone exposure of the zigomatic arc with installed facial nerve paralysis. Fig. 2. B (right): The red arrow reveals perineural invasion of V3 and the blue arrow shows the skin tumor of temporal region. Fig. 2. C: Surgical aspect after removal of skin tumor, with sacrifice of the facial nerve, zigomatic arc, ascending mandible and parotid gland. The blue line delimits the temporal bone resection by the neurosurgical team and the instruments pointing V3 at skull base, with perineural invasion

Histopathological differentiation grade: tumors less differentiated are associated with a more aggressive outcome. This item also has changed in the last edition of the AJCC, becoming one of the high risk factors, opposed to being a separate classification as in the sixth edition. (Farasat, Yu et al. 2011)

Lymph node metastases

SCCHN that develop nodal metastasis in the parotid gland or the neck is an aggressive disease and show poor outcomes. Some studies these prognosis revealing 5-years overall survival rates from 22 to 36% (Khurana, Mentis et al. 1995; Kraus, Carew et al. 1998).

Untill the sixth edition of AJCC, the nodal staging of squamous carcinoma of skin only separate the presence of nodal metastasis or no. This classification was pointed by several authors as insufficient, what have already indicated the need of a new proposal for lymph nodes staging, including a P stage for parotid metastasis and stratification of nodal disease (O'Brien, McNeil et al. 2002; Ch'ng, Maitra et al. 2006). The seventh edition of AJCC incorporated some changes in nodal classification aligning with the staging of lymph nodes from others sites of head and neck but the P staging has not been implemented, because of the benefit of having subgroups of P and N stage is uncertain, but further research may demonstrate the need of this staging system (Palme, MacKay et al. 2007; Forest, Clark et al. 2010; O'Hara, Ferlito et al. 2010)

In a survey of tertiary treatment centers, about 5% of squamous cell carcinomas present skin present metastasis, usually to regional lymph nodes of the parotid and cervical level II. (2, 5). Sites such as cheek, ear, forehead, temple and lateral scalp are the most implicated in the onset of regional disease, which usually occurs on an average of 13 months of primary treatment, but may occur until 2 to 3 years later (Hong, Kriesel et al. 2005). The rate of regional metastases in head and neck can be between 10 and 20% when clinical and pathological characteristics of high-risk primary tumor are present.

When parotid metastasis with clinical negative neck are present, the risk of occult metastases in the cervical lymph nodes reaches 35-50%, which justifies elective neck dissection in the presence of parotid involvement(O'Hara, Ferlito et al. 2010). The data by Vauterin revealed when positive pathological neck is observed, level II is involved in 79% of cases and external jugular chain lymph nodes are particularly at risk, what should have not be forgot to be included in the neck dissection. (Vauterin, Veness et al. 2006).

Levels IV and V are only involved in massive lymph node disease to the neck, except in situations where the primary is located in the posterior scalp, in which the involvement of this code chain can be isolated. Metastases to the level I is present alone when the primary occurs in the anterior region of the face (O'Hara, Ferlito et al. 2010).

The radiological search of metastases to the parotid and neck should be performed only in patients at high risk, which can use CT, MRI and USG-guided FNA (O'Hara, Ferlito et al. 2010).

The use of sentinel lymph node in squamous cell carcinoma in head and neck is not yet defined and is not routinely used in cancer not melanoma, due to the low risk of nodal metastasis, but has potential for improved survival in patients at high risk (O'Hara, Ferlito et al. 2010). The sentinel lymph node study in the parotid region should be done with caution because it adds a possible morbidity due to the risk of facial nerve injury.

3.3 Treatment

3.3.1 Treatment of primary tumor

The treatment of advanced SCCHN tumors usually involves surgical resection and adjuvant radiotherapy. The goal of surgical treatment is tumor resection with clear margins. Tumors that fail to be cleared surgically often recur despite radiation. In contrast, high-risk SCCHN with clear surgical margins has documented excellent outcomes when compared to those with unreported margin status (local recurrence 5% vs. 8%, nodal metastasis 5% vs. 14%, distant metastases 1% vs. 7%, and disease-specific death 1% vs. 7%).

Skin squamous cell carcinoma with invasion of skull base are treated with craniofacial resections and have worse survival when compared to basal cell carcinomas. (Backous, DeMonte et al. 2005). Backous used as contraindication criteria for this type of resection encasement of the carotid artery or optic chiasm, cavernous sinus invasion or distant metastasis. Factors found to reduce survival are perineural invasion, intracranial extension with invasion of brain parenchyma and impossibility of adjuvant radiotherapy because of previous radiation.

Immunosuppressed patients should receive more aggressive surgical treatment and adjuvant radiotherapy should be strongly considered.

A multisciplinary aproach is recommended for the treatment of SCCHN, with combination of head and neck surgeon and plastic surgery, so that the reconstrution should not carry a limiting resection.

3.3.2 Treatment of regional metastasis

The published evidence suggests that the optimum treatment for metastatic SCCHN should be surgical resection with adjuvant radiotherapy. (O'Hara, Ferlito et al. 2010)

The most common site of metastases in the head and neck is the parotid gland. Usually when performing parotidectomy is associated the dissection of cervical levels I-III in negative neck and a radical neck dissection in positive necks (14, 18). This treatment option can save adjuvant irradiation in the pathologically negative neck restricting the field of radiation only to the parotid field, but another option is the radiation of the clinically negative neck.

In patients undergoing parotidectomy, Ebrahimi recommends selective neck dissection including level I to III for facial primaries, level II and III for anterior scalp and external ear primaries, and levels II to V for posterior scalp and neck primaries(Ebrahimi, Moncrieff et al. 2010). Isolated metastases of level V and primary region of the scalp or posterior subocipital region, a posterior lateral neck dissection (II to V) is recommended. (O'Hara, Ferlito et al. 2010)

Cervical neck node disease without parotid involvement can be seen in 18 to 41% of patients.(Andruchow, Veness et al. 2006; Vauterin, Veness et al. 2006) In this situation, the recommendation is the treatment of the neck with classic or modified radical dissection associated with elective parotidectomy in primaries of anterior regions of scalp and lateral face (Barzilai, Greenberg et al. 2005; Jennings and Schmults 2010).

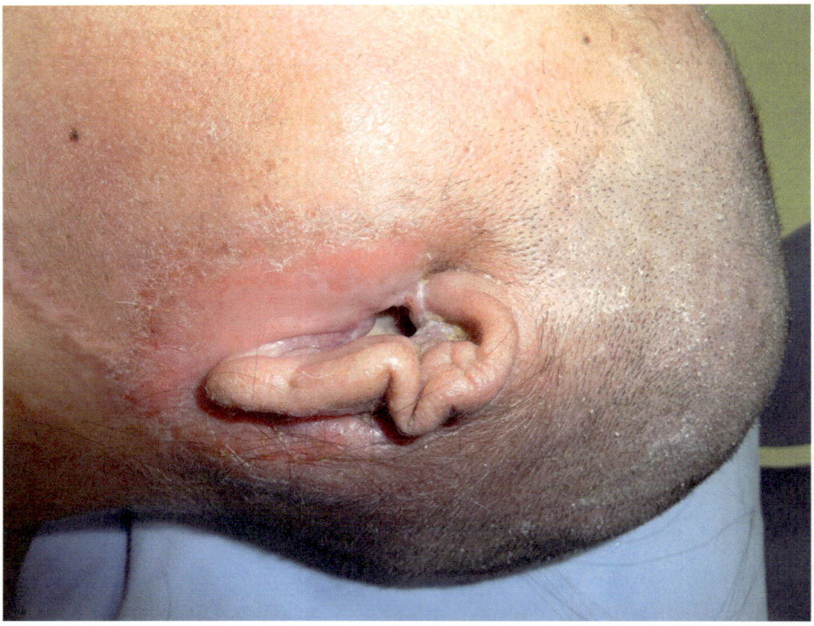

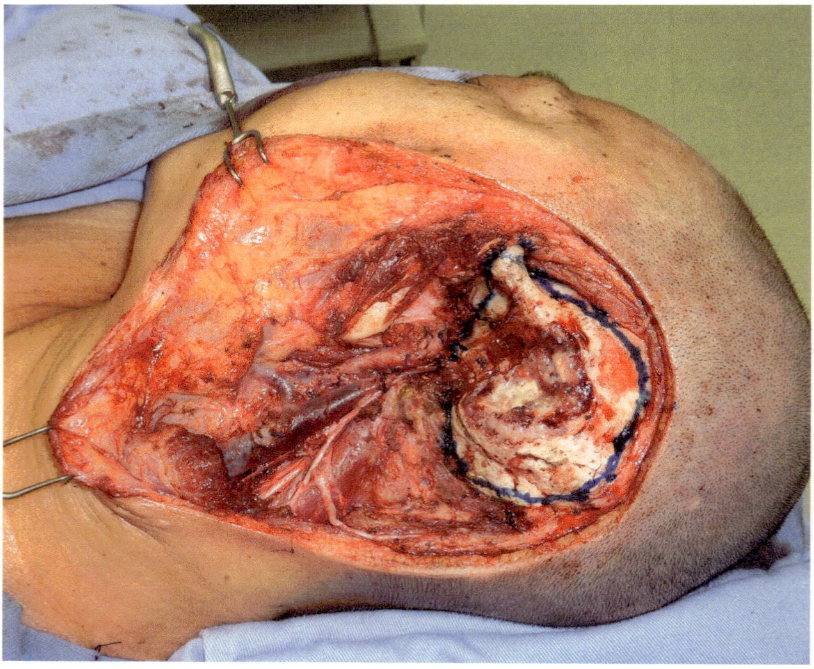

Fig. 3. A: Example of multidisciplinary aproach: recurrent squamous cell carcinoma after local excision and radiation therapy. Facial nerve paralysis and intratemporal perineural nerve spread. Fig. 3. B: Surgical field of total parotidectomy and sacrifice of the facial nerve and ascending portion of mandible and neck dissection of levels I-III with sacrifice of sternocleidomastoid muscle. The blue line delimits the temporal bone resection by the neurosurgical team, with frozen sections of the nerve stump.

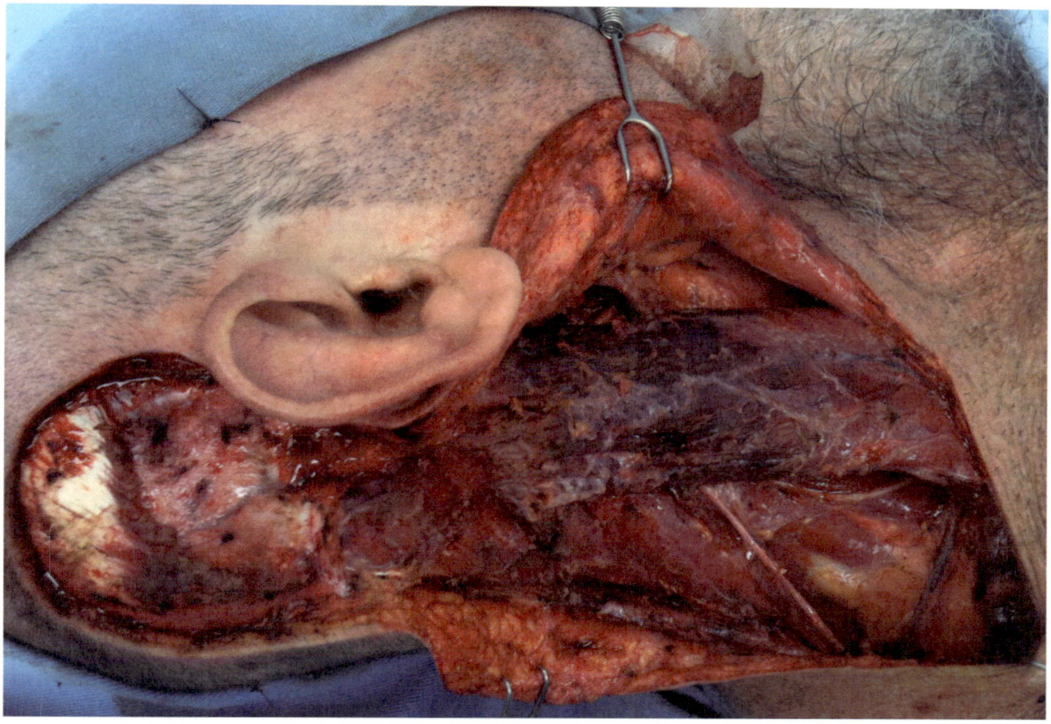

Fig. 4. Surgical treatment aspect of a posterior scalp skin tumor with posterior lateral neck dissection (cervical levels II-V), sparing the spinal acessory nerve

Although some anatomical regions have an increased risk of developing regional metastases, it is difficult to recommend elective neck dissection as a routine base, because of the low rate of nodal spread and high prevalence of these skin cancers. Others risk factors should be added to consider elective regional treatment like immunnocompromised host, poorly diferentiated grade (Veness 2007). Elective parotidectomy for patients without clinical or radiological evidence of metastasis of the neck or parotid is not recommended by most authors (Osborne, Shaw et al. 2008).

Intraparotid metastasis to lymph nodes may be attached to the facial nerve, which is at risk of sacrifice in some situations. All facial nerve not functioning in the preoperative evaluation or completely surrounded by tumor should be sacrificed but it should rarely be done when it has normal function before surgery. According to Iyer, surgical approaches to the parotid metastatic cancers shall, as far as possible, spare the facial nerve with normal function, even if that causes resection with microscopic involved margins and the need for adjuvant radiotherapy. Such strategie do not generate differences in the rates of recurrence and overall survival compared with patients undergoing resection with microscopically free margins. However, this study shows no statistical difference between groups, but shows a tendency to a worse local control and survival, which could have significance with a larger number of cases. In fact, free surgical margins greater than 5 mm are rarely obtained due to the proximity of parotidectomy metastasis with the facial nerve (Iyer, Clark et al. 2009).

Parotidectomy may be associated with resection of skin tumors of the parotid region and the series of Lai reveals perineural invasion of the facial nerve in 6 of the 23. Lai recommends

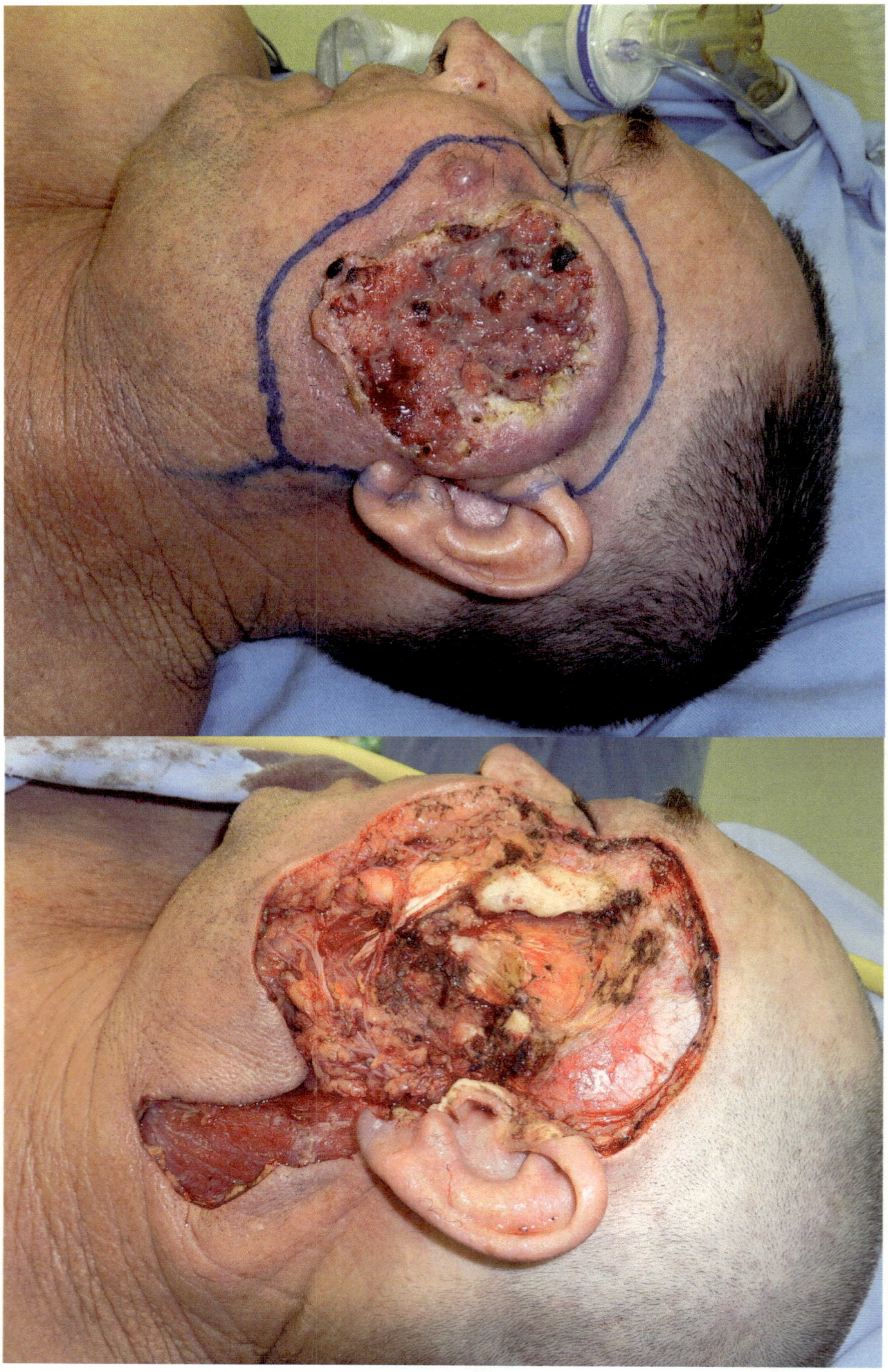

Fig. 5. A: Squamous cell carcinoma of skin of parotid region, with in transit metastasis. Fig. 5. B: Surgical field after ressection including superficial parotidectomy and the zigomatic arc with sacrifice of the superior branch of facial nerve that was involved by the tumor.

parotidectomy depending on the depth of the primary lesion, especially in the preauricular region. Similarly, facial nerve dissection is necessary in superficial parotidectomy for nodal involvement or deep invasion from preauricular primary lesions. As the facial nerve is identified, areas of gross tumor involvement may necessitate partial or total facial nerve resection. When there is sacrifice of the facial nerve, some authors recommend frozen sections of the facial nerve stumps, to ensure free margins before a microsurgical nerve reconstruction (Lai, Weinstein et al. 2002).

3.3.3 Radiotherapy

Primary radiation for SCCHN can be an alternative treatment when the surgucal defect causes challenging reconstructions and should be used in lesions with little invasiveness. Local tumor control in small lesions rivals that of surgical resection, even in recurrent disease. However, as T stage increases, local control decreases when compared to surgical excision.(Mendenhall, Amdur et al. 2009)

The treatment of neck or parotid metastasis, surgery and adjuvant radiotherapy should be done rather than radiation alone(Palme, O'Brien et al. 2003). Multiple studies have noted decreased disease-specific survival in patients treated with RT alone (delCharco, Mendenhall et al. 1998; Veness, Palme et al. 2003)

The use of adjuvant radiation should be strongly considered in incomplete excision or positive margins, perineural invasion, multiple nodal involvement and recurrent tumors. (Veness 2007)

4. Systemic therapy (for all tumors)

4.1 Adjuvant therapy for high risk SCCS

The risk of locoregional recurrence and regional or distant metastasis is the most important factor in determining the treatment for cutaneous SCC. In a large review of studies of SCC of the skin, lip and ear, between 1940 and 1992 it was observed that recurrence rates double from 7.4% to 15.2% for tumors greater than 2 cm in diameter, and that tumors less than 4 mm in depth are at low risk for metastasis compared with tumors deeper than 4 mm (6.7% and 45.7%, respectively). (Rowe, Carroll et al. 1992) Also, 30% of locally recurrent SCCS develop metastases. Long-term prognosis for metastatic disease is extremely poor. Ten-year survival rates are less than 20% for patients with regional lymph node involvement and less than 10% for patients with distant metastases. (Cherpelis, Marcusen et al. 2002).

Histopathologic features associated with an increased risk of local failure or metastasis include large lesion size, perineural invasion, and involvement beyond the subcutaneous tissue. (Clayman, Lee et al. 2005)]

Chemotherapy in the management of high-risk SCCS remains relatively unexplored. (Jennings and Schmults 2010) The role of retinoids, which are known to decrease new cancer formation, but do not alter the course of an existing tumor, as prophylactic agents in patients with diffuse actinic damage or recurrent CSCCs is well established, especially in organ transplant recipients (OTRs). (Harwood, Leedham-Green et al. 2005) Unfortunately, randomized trials of retinoids, either used alone for the adjuvant-treatment of established mucosal SCC of the head and neck (Toma, Bonelli et al. 2004) or in combination with interferon (Brewster, Lee et al. 2007) for established SCCS, have shown no benefit.

Many of the available agents with activity demonstrated in advanced SCCS, including EGRF inhibitors and oral capecitabine, are well tolerated with relatively low risks, and are potential candidates for adjuvant therapy in highest-risk cases. Further work remains to identify patient subsets likely to benefit from adjuvant chemotherapy and to define optimal regimens. Collaborative clinical trials are needed to establish standardized prognostic or treatment models to assist clinicians in most effectively identifying and managing patients at risk for poor outcomes. (LeBoeuf and Schmults 2011)

4.2 Systemic therapy for advanced SCCS

The use of systemic therapy is limited to patients with distant metastases or locally advanced disease that cannot be adequately managed with surgery or radiotherapy. Because of the rarity of metastatic squamous cell cancers of the skin, the approach to systemic treatment is based primarily upon isolated case reports, with only a few small case series.

Treatment of metastatic SCC may include systemic chemotherapy or treatment with biologic response modifiers. The efficacy of these methods has not been established.

Wollina and colleagues (Wollina, Hansel et al. 2005) reported 4 patients with advanced SCC of the skin who were treated with oral capecitabine and IFN subcutaneously, resulting in complete remission in 2 patients and partial response in the other 2. IFN may act synergistically to capecitabine by causing a forced accumulation of 5-FU in tumor cells as a result of stimulation of dThdPase. In another report the use of oral capecitabine alone for the treatment of 14 patients with advanced cutaneous SCC resulted in 2 partial remissions and 3 minimal remissions. (Cartei, Cartei et al. 2000)

Cisplatin-based combinations appear to be the most active regimens in the published experience. Most regimens that have been studied for the treatment of advanced SCCS were adapted from those used for squamous cell cancers arising in other sites. Sadek et al. reported on the treatment of 14 patients with advanced squamous cell carcinoma of the skin or lip with a combination of bolus cisplatin, plus a five-day infusion of bleomycin and 5-fluorouracil. (Sadek, Azli et al. 1990) Four complete and seven partial responses were observed and in seven patients, tumor regression permitted subsequent definitive local treatment with either surgery or radiation therapy.

Using a combination of cisplatin daily times four plus a four day continuous infusion of bleomycin to treat five patients with locally advanced disease of the head and neck (three squamous cell and two basal cell), Denic observed one complete response and 3 partial responses. (Denic 1999) One patient had disease progression.

Multiple targeted therapies are being developed for many malignancies, including those with squamous cell histologies. These may ultimately have utility in patients with advanced or metastatic non melanoma skin cancers. The primary targets of molecular inhibition in squamous cell carcinoma include the epidermal growth factor receptor (EGFR), the vascular endothelial growth factor (VEGF) and its receptor, and tyrosine kinase (TK). (O'Bryan and Ratner 2011) Molecular studies have demonstrated that these molecules are overexpressed in a subset of SCCS and may be associated with more aggressive clinical behavior. (Detmar, Velasco et al. 2000; Maubec, Duvillard et al. 2005; Ch'ng, Low et al. 2008)

Intracellular signal transduction mediated by the epidermal growth factor receptor (EGFR) has been one of the most studied pathways in carcinogenesis. The phosphorylation of EGFR activates multiple biological processes, including apoptosis, differentiation, cellular proliferation, motility, invasion, adhesion, DNA repair, and survival. EGFR is a transmembrane tyrosine kinase receptor involved in the proliferation and survival of many cancer cells and is one of the first molecular target against which monoclonal antibodies have been developed for cancer therapy. EGFR plays an important role in tumorigenesis of non melanoma skin cancer, especially metastatic squamous cell carcinoma, via mechanisms similar to those of other visceral tumors. (Khan, Alam et al. 2011)

Several case reports suggest that Cetuximab, a monoclonal antibody that targets the epidermal growth factor receptor (EGFR), has antitumor activity in patients with advanced squamous cell carcinoma of the skin. (Bauman, Eaton et al. 2007; Suen, Bressler et al. 2007; Arnold, Bruckner-Tuderman et al. 2009)

Maubec and colleagues reported the results of a phase II study that included 36 patients with advanced squamous cell carcinoma of the skin treated with cetuximab in the first line setting. (Maubec, Duvillard et al. 2010) In this study, cetuximab was administered on a weekly schedule (400 mg/m2 on week 1 and then 250 mg/m2 weekly). Eight partial and two complete responses were observed, and 21 had stable disease for an overall disease control rate of 69 percent. Furthermore, three patients were able to undergo complete resection of their tumor following systemic treatment with cetuximab. Similarly to what is reported in other malignancies, patients developing acneiform rash apparently had a better outcome.

The combination of cetuximab with chemotherapy is a promising approach. Association with platinum-based chemotherapy and 5-FU in patients with recurrent or metastatic SCC of the head and neck (SCCHN) has shown benefit in a large prospective randomized trial. (Vermorken, Mesia et al. 2008) In this study, 442 eligible patients with untreated recurrent or metastatic SCCHN were randomized to receive 5-FU with cisplatin or carboplatin, with or without cetuximab. The ORR was 36% versus 20% with and without cetuximab ($P = 0.001$). Survival increased from 7.4 to 10.1 months with the addition of cetuximab ($P = 0.04$), and progression-free survival increased from 3.3 to 5.6 months ($P \leq 0.0001$).

Other targeted EGFR inhibitors are also currently under investigation in clinical trials mainly for the treatment of SCCHN, including Panitumumab (Vectibix, Amgen, Thousand Oaks, CA) which is a fully human monoclonal antibody to EGFR. (Lacouture and Melosky 2007; AMGEN 2011; AMGEN 2011)

Additionally, many targeted molecular therapies to VEGF and VEGF TKs have proven efficacy in other malignancies. Research into their use for SCCHN is growing and these agents may also be useful for the treatment of SCCS. (Wang and Agulnik 2008) Bevacicumab (Avastin, Genentech, South San Francisco, CA) is a fully human monoclonal antibody against VEGF, and is being tested for recurrent and metastatic SCCHN in a phase 3 trial comparing chemotherapy alone versus chemotherapy plus bevacizumab. (Wang and Agulnik 2008) There is hope that the combination of EGFR and VEGF pathway inhibitors will provide an increased clinical benefit in such patients. This alternative is being studied in an ongoing phase 2 trial, cituximab, radiotherapy, and pemetrexed with or without bevacizumab is being tested in patients with locally advanced SCCHN. (Gold, Lee et al. 2009)

As mentioned earlier, the vast majority of studies focus on the use of molecular inhibitors in SCCHN. More research is needed, for the development of new treatment modalities and to establish their role in treating patients with advanced or aggressive CSCC.

5. References

(2008). "Cancer incidence in five continents." *IARC Sci Publ* IX(160): 1-837.

Alam, M. and D. Ratner (2001). "Cutaneous squamous-cell carcinoma." *N Engl J Med* 344(13): 975-83.

AMGEN. (2011, April 7, 2011). "PARTNER: Panitumumab Added to Regimen for Treatment of Head aNd Neck Cancer Evaluation of Response." Retrieved July 14, 2011, from http://clinicaltrials.gov/ct2/show/record/NCT00454779.

AMGEN. (2011, January 20, 2011). "PRISM (Panitumumab Regimen In Second-line Monotherapy of Head and Neck Cancer)." Retrieved July 14, 2011, from http://clinicaltrials.gov/ct2/show/record/NCT00446446.

Andruchow, J. L., M. J. Veness, et al. (2006). "Implications for clinical staging of metastatic cutaneous squamous carcinoma of the head and neck based on a multicenter study of treatment outcomes." *Cancer* 106(5): 1078-83.

Arnold, A. W., L. Bruckner-Tuderman, et al. (2009). "Cetuximab therapy of metastasizing cutaneous squamous cell carcinoma in a patient with severe recessive dystrophic epidermolysis bullosa." *Dermatology* 219(1): 80-3.

Backous, D. D., F. DeMonte, et al. (2005). "Craniofacial resection for nonmelanoma skin cancer of the head and neck." *Laryngoscope* 115(6): 931-7.

Barzilai, G., E. Greenberg, et al. (2005). "Pattern of regional metastases from cutaneous squamous cell carcinoma of the head and neck." *Otolaryngol Head Neck Surg* 132(6): 852-6.

Bauman, J. E., K. D. Eaton, et al. (2007). "Treatment of recurrent squamous cell carcinoma of the skin with cetuximab." *Arch Dermatol* 143(7): 889-92.

Brantsch, K. D., C. Meisner, et al. (2008). "Analysis of risk factors determining prognosis of cutaneous squamous-cell carcinoma: a prospective study." *Lancet Oncol* 9(8): 713-20.

Breuninger, H., B. Black, et al. (1990). "Microstaging of squamous cell carcinomas." *Am J Clin Pathol* 94(5): 624-7.

Brewster, A. M., J. J. Lee, et al. (2007). "Randomized trial of adjuvant 13-cis-retinoic acid and interferon alfa for patients with aggressive skin squamous cell carcinoma." *J Clin Oncol* 25(15): 1974-8.

Cartei, G., F. Cartei, et al. (2000). "Oral 5-fluorouracil in squamous cell carcinoma of the skin in the aged." *Am J Clin Oncol* 23(2): 181-4.

Cassarino, D. S., D. P. Derienzo, et al. (2006). "Cutaneous squamous cell carcinoma: a comprehensive clinicopathologic classification. Part one." *J Cutan Pathol* 33(3): 191-206.

Ch'ng, S., I. Low, et al. (2008). "Epidermal growth factor receptor: a novel biomarker for aggressive head and neck cutaneous squamous cell carcinoma." *Hum Pathol* 39(3): 344-9.

Ch'ng, S., A. Maitra, et al. (2006). "Parotid metastasis--an independent prognostic factor for head and neck cutaneous squamous cell carcinoma." *J Plast Reconstr Aesthet Surg* 59(12): 1288-93.

Cherpelis, B. S., C. Marcusen, et al. (2002). "Prognostic factors for metastasis in squamous cell carcinoma of the skin." *Dermatol Surg* 28(3): 268-73.

Clayman, G. L., J. J. Lee, et al. (2005). "Mortality risk from squamous cell skin cancer." *J Clin Oncol* 23(4): 759-65.

Collins, G. L., N. Nickoonahand, et al. (2004). "Changing demographics and pathology of nonmelanoma skin cancer in the last 30 years." *Semin Cutan Med Surg* 23(1): 80-3.

de Lima Vazquez, V., T. Sachetto, et al. (2008). "Prognostic factors for lymph node metastasis from advanced squamous cell carcinoma of the skin of the trunk and extremities." *World J Surg Oncol* 6: 73.

de Lima Vazquez , V., C. Scapulatempo, et al. (2011). "Prognostic and Risk Factors in Patients with Locally Advanced Cutaneous Squamous Cell Carcinoma of the Trunk and Extremities " *Journal of Skin Cancer* 2011: 9

delCharco, J. O., W. M. Mendenhall, et al. (1998). "Carcinoma of the skin metastatic to the parotid area lymph nodes." *Head Neck* 20(5): 369-73.

Denic, S. (1999). "Preoperative treatment of advanced skin carcinoma with cisplatin and bleomycin." *Am J Clin Oncol* 22(1): 32-4.

Detmar, M., P. Velasco, et al. (2000). "Expression of vascular endothelial growth factor induces an invasive phenotype in human squamous cell carcinomas." *Am J Pathol* 156(1): 159-67.

Ebrahimi, A., M. D. Moncrieff, et al. (2010). "Predicting the pattern of regional metastases from cutaneous squamous cell carcinoma of the head and neck based on location of the primary." *Head Neck* 32(10): 1288-94.

Edge, S. B. and C. C. Compton (2010). "The American Joint Committee on Cancer: the 7th edition of the AJCC cancer staging manual and the future of TNM." *Ann Surg Oncol* 17(6): 1471-4.

Farasat, S., S. S. Yu, et al. (2011). "A new American Joint Committee on Cancer staging system for cutaneous squamous cell carcinoma: Creation and rationale for inclusion of tumor (T) characteristics." *J Am Acad Dermatol* 64(6): 1051-9.

Faustina, M., R. Diba, et al. (2004). "Patterns of regional and distant metastasis in patients with eyelid and periocular squamous cell carcinoma." *Ophthalmology* 111(10): 1930-2.

Forest, V. I., J. J. Clark, et al. (2010). "N1S3: a revised staging system for head and neck cutaneous squamous cell carcinoma with lymph node metastases: results of 2 Australian Cancer Centers." *Cancer* 116(5): 1298-304.

Gandhi, M. R., B. Panizza, et al. (2010). "Detecting and defining the anatomic extent of large nerve perineural spread of malignancy: comparing "targeted" MRI with the histologic findings following surgery." *Head Neck* 33(4): 469-75.

Gold, K. A., H. Y. Lee, et al. (2009). "Targeted therapies in squamous cell carcinoma of the head and neck." *Cancer* 115(5): 922-35.

Harwood, C. A., M. Leedham-Green, et al. (2005). "Low-dose retinoids in the prevention of cutaneous squamous cell carcinomas in organ transplant recipients: a 16-year retrospective study." *Arch Dermatol* 141(4): 456-64.

Hong, T. S., K. J. Kriesel, et al. (2005). "Parotid area lymph node metastases from cutaneous squamous cell carcinoma: implications for diagnosis, treatment, and prognosis." *Head Neck* 27(10): 851-6.

Iyer, N. G., J. R. Clark, et al. (2009). "Outcomes following parotidectomy for metastatic squamous cell carcinoma with microscopic residual disease: implications for facial nerve preservation." *Head Neck* 31(1): 21-7.

Jennings, L. and C. D. Schmults (2010). "Management of high-risk cutaneous squamous cell carcinoma." *J Clin Aesthet Dermatol* 3(4): 39-48.

Khan, M. H., M. Alam, et al. (2011). "Epidermal Growth Factor Receptor Inhibitors in the Treatment of Nonmelanoma Skin Cancers." *Dermatol Surg*.

Khurana, V. G., D. H. Mentis, et al. (1995). "Parotid and neck metastases from cutaneous squamous cell carcinoma of the head and neck." *Am J Surg* 170(5): 446-50.

Koseki, S., T. Aoki, et al. (1999). "An immunohistochemical study of E-cadherin expression in human squamous cell carcinoma of the skin: relationship between decreased expression of E-cadherin in the primary lesion and regional lymph node metastasis." *J Dermatol* 26(7): 416-22.

Krahn, G., U. Leiter, et al. (2001). "Coexpression patterns of EGFR, HER2, HER3 and HER4 in non-melanoma skin cancer." *Eur J Cancer* 37(2): 251-9.

Kraus, D. H., J. F. Carew, et al. (1998). "Regional lymph node metastasis from cutaneous squamous cell carcinoma." *Arch Otolaryngol Head Neck Surg* 124(5): 582-7.

Lacouture, M. E. and B. L. Melosky (2007). "Cutaneous reactions to anticancer agents targeting the epidermal growth factor receptor: a dermatology-oncology perspective." *Skin Therapy Lett* 12(6): 1-5.

Lai, S. Y., G. S. Weinstein, et al. (2002). "Parotidectomy in the treatment of aggressive cutaneous malignancies." *Arch Otolaryngol Head Neck Surg* 128(5): 521-6.

LeBoeuf, N. R. and C. D. Schmults (2011). "Update on the management of high-risk squamous cell carcinoma." *Semin Cutan Med Surg* 30(1): 26-34.

Leibovitch, I., S. C. Huilgol, et al. (2005). "Cutaneous squamous cell carcinoma treated with Mohs micrographic surgery in Australia II. Perineural invasion." *J Am Acad Dermatol* 53(2): 261-6.

Maubec, E., P. Duvillard, et al. (2010). Cetuximab as first-line monotherapy in patients with skin unresectable squamous cell carcinoma: Final results of a phase II multicenter study (abstract #8510). *ASCO*. Chicago. 28: 613s.

Maubec, E., P. Duvillard, et al. (2005). "Immunohistochemical analysis of EGFR and HER-2 in patients with metastatic squamous cell carcinoma of the skin." *Anticancer Res* 25(2B): 1205-10.

Mendenhall, W. M., R. J. Amdur, et al. (2009). "Radiotherapy for cutaneous squamous and basal cell carcinomas of the head and neck." *Laryngoscope* 119(10): 1994-9.

Mullen, J. T., L. Feng, et al. (2006). "Invasive squamous cell carcinoma of the skin: defining a high-risk group." *Ann Surg Oncol* 13(7): 902-9.

North, J. H., Jr., J. E. Spellman, et al. (1997). "Advanced cutaneous squamous cell carcinoma of the trunk and extremity: analysis of prognostic factors." *J Surg Oncol* 64(3): 212-7.

O'Brien, C. J., E. B. McNeil, et al. (2002). "Significance of clinical stage, extent of surgery, and pathologic findings in metastatic cutaneous squamous carcinoma of the parotid gland." *Head Neck* 24(5): 417-22.

O'Bryan, K. W. and D. Ratner (2011). "The role of targeted molecular inhibitors in the management of advanced nonmelanoma skin cancer." *Semin Cutan Med Surg* 30(1): 57-61.

O'Hara, J., A. Ferlito, et al. (2010). "Cutaneous squamous cell carcinoma of the head and neck metastasizing to the parotid gland-A review of current recommendations." *Head Neck.*

Osborne, R. F., T. Shaw, et al. (2008). "Elective parotidectomy in the management of advanced auricular malignancies." *Laryngoscope* 118(12): 2139-45.

Palme, C. E., S. G. MacKay, et al. (2007). "The need for a better prognostic staging system in patients with metastatic cutaneous squamous cell carcinoma of the head and neck." *Curr Opin Otolaryngol Head Neck Surg* 15(2): 103-6.

Palme, C. E., C. J. O'Brien, et al. (2003). "Extent of parotid disease influences outcome in patients with metastatic cutaneous squamous cell carcinoma." *Arch Otolaryngol Head Neck Surg* 129(7): 750-3.

Ries, L. A. G., D. Melbert, et al. (2007). "SEER Cancer Statistics Review, 1975-2005." Retrieved November, 2007, 2007, from http://seer.cancer.gov/csr/1975_2005/.

Rowe, D. E., R. J. Carroll, et al. (1992). "Prognostic factors for local recurrence, metastasis, and survival rates in squamous cell carcinoma of the skin, ear, and lip. Implications for treatment modality selection." *J Am Acad Dermatol* 26(6): 976-90.

Sadek, H., N. Azli, et al. (1990). "Treatment of advanced squamous cell carcinoma of the skin with cisplatin, 5-fluorouracil, and bleomycin." *Cancer* 66(8): 1692-6.

Schacht, V., M. I. Ramirez, et al. (2003). "T1alpha/podoplanin deficiency disrupts normal lymphatic vasculature formation and causes lymphedema." *EMBO J* 22(14): 3546-56.

Sobin, L. H. and C. C. Compton "TNM seventh edition: what's new, what's changed: communication from the International Union Against Cancer and the American Joint Committee on Cancer." *Cancer* 116(22): 5336-9.

Staples, M. P., M. Elwood, et al. (2006). "Non-melanoma skin cancer in Australia: the 2002 national survey and trends since 1985." *Med J Aust* 184(1): 6-10.

Suen, J. K., L. Bressler, et al. (2007). "Cutaneous squamous cell carcinoma responding serially to single-agent cetuximab." *Anticancer Drugs* 18(7): 827-9.

Toma, S., L. Bonelli, et al. (2004). "13-cis retinoic acid in head and neck cancer chemoprevention: results of a randomized trial from the Italian Head and Neck Chemoprevention Study Group." *Oncol Rep* 11(6): 1297-305.

Trakatelli, M., C. Ulrich, et al. (2007). "Epidemiology of nonmelanoma skin cancer (NMSC) in Europe: accurate and comparable data are needed for effective public health monitoring and interventions." *Br J Dermatol* 156 Suppl 3: 1-7.

Turner, S. J., G. J. Morgan, et al. (2009). "Metastatic cutaneous squamous cell carcinoma of the external ear: a high-risk cutaneous subsite." *J Laryngol Otol* 124(1): 26-31.

Vauterin, T. J., M. J. Veness, et al. (2006). "Patterns of lymph node spread of cutaneous squamous cell carcinoma of the head and neck." *Head Neck* 28(9): 785-91.

Veness, M. J. (2007). "High-risk cutaneous squamous cell carcinoma of the head and neck." *J Biomed Biotechnol* 2007(3): 80572.

Veness, M. J., C. E. Palme, et al. (2003). "Cutaneous head and neck squamous cell carcinoma metastatic to cervical lymph nodes (nonparotid): a better outcome with surgery and adjuvant radiotherapy." *Laryngoscope* 113(10): 1827-33.

Vermorken, J. B., R. Mesia, et al. (2008). "Platinum-based chemotherapy plus cetuximab in head and neck cancer." *N Engl J Med* 359(11): 1116-27.

Wang, L. X. and M. Agulnik (2008). "Promising newer molecular-targeted therapies in head and neck cancer." *Drugs* 68(12): 1609-19.

Wollina, U., G. Hansel, et al. (2005). "Oral capecitabine plus subcutaneous interferon alpha in advanced squamous cell carcinoma of the skin." *J Cancer Res Clin Oncol* 131(5): 300-4.

3

Sarcomatoid Squamous Cell Carcinoma

Charmaine C. Anderson, Brian H. Le and Bernice Robinson-Bennett
The Reading Hospital and Medical Center
USA

1. Introduction

Although much has been characterized about squamous cell carcinoma of the lower female reproductive tract, there is limited knowledge and experience with cases demonstrating squamous cell carcinoma with sarcomatoid features. Sarcomatoid squamous cell carcinoma (SSCC) is mainly found in the upper aerodigestive tract with the larynx being the most common site in the head and neck region. (Otay et al., 2011) The esophagus and skin are other well known affected sites. In these sites, risk factors include, smoking, alcohol consumption, and previous irradiation of the head and neck region. (Otay et al., 2011) Risk factors for skin involvement include prolonged sun exposure and the effects of toxins and irradiation.

True sarcomas of the lower female genital tract arising in the vulva, vagina, and cervix, are extremely rare. They comprise only 1-2% of vulvar cancers, 2% of vaginal cancers (Temkin et.al,2007), 2-3% of cervical cancers, and 3% of endometrial cancers. They tend to be heterogeneous, rapidly progressive, with a high rate of recurrence and distant metastasis to organs such as liver and lungs. For the vulva and vagina, the main sites of occurrence are the labium majus and upper vagina, respectively. Leiomyosarcomas are the most common type of sarcoma in the female genital tract where several factors have been demonstrated to play a role in recurrence including tumor diameter, cytologic atypia, mitotic index, and infiltrating margins. Although there are no specific treatment guidelines, the mainstay of therapy has been surgical excision followed by chemotherapy. Neoadjuvant chemotherapy has been used in patients who have bulky tumors in which surgical debulking had not been optimal. Currently, some believe that neoadjuvant chemotherapy can also be used as primary therapy followed by surgical debulking regardless of tumor. It is thought that this treatment strategy can optimize surgical excision, giving rise to less morbidity, and a longer disease-free interval. (Temkin et.al,2007) The role of radiation therapy has been controversial as some believe that sarcomas themselves are induced by a history of radiation therapy or exposure. Nevertheless, there have been reports of radiation lengthening the time interval to local recurrence.

Sarcomatoid squamous cell carcinoma of the female genital tract has been reported in very small numbers. Human Papilloma Virus (HPV) has been known to be a major causal factor for the development of SCC. High risk subtypes of Human Papilloma Virus, 16 and 18, have been demonstrated in not only the squamous cell component of SSCC but also in the sarcomatoid component. Making immunohistochemical assays of this cancer a hallmark to diagnosis to differentiate pure squamous cell carcinoma from a pure sarcoma.

Like pure sarcomas, Sarcomatoid Squamous Cell Carcinoma has a very poor prognosis, short disease-free intervals, and is diagnosed at later stages of disease. Even with optimal treatment and follow up, SSCC recur rapidly and metastasize to regions such as the peritoneum, kidney, and subcutaneous tissue. Most cases of SSCC of the female genitalia have been reported to arise from the cervix and vulva. There are currently 16 cases of cervical and vulvar SSCC reported in the English literature to date. (Tae-Wook Kong et. al., 2010 and Dong-Seok Choi et. al., 2006), with our current case of vulvar SSCC making up the 17th case.

SSCC of the Cervix Literature Review

Author	No. of Cases	Age	FIGO	Tumor Diameter(cm)	Primary treatment	Outcome after primary treatment	Survival (months)
Steeper et al (1983)	1	67	III	10	ERT	PD	2, DOD
Pang (1998)	2	65 61	N/A N/A	6 5	RAH+CRT RAH+CRT	PD RD	2, DOD 14, DOD
Rodriques et al (2000)	1	39	IB2	6	ERT+RAH	RD	12, DOD
Brown et al (2003)	9	29 32 34 39 47 57 59 59 76	IB2 IB2 IB1 IB IIA IVA IVB IVB IIA	4 8 1,6 N/A 3 N/A N/A N/A 5	RAH+ERT ERT RAH+CRT ERT ERT ERT+exenteration TAH+CTx ERT ERT	RD CR CR RD CR RD RD RD CR	N/A 42, NED 5, NED N/A 40, NED N/A N/A N/A 22, NED
Lin et al (2006)	1	31	N/A	6	RAH	CR	20, NED
Mohan et al (2008)	1	75	IIB	5,6	ERT	CR	10, NED
Kumar et al (2008)	1	54	IIIB	4	CRT	CR	6, NED
Tae-Wook King et al (2011)	1	26	IB1	2	LRH	CR	18, NED

Table 1. **SSCC of the Cervix Reported Cases in the Literature (Tae-Wook King et al, 2010)** N/A= not available, ER= external pelvic radiation therapy, RAH= radical abdominal hysterectomy, CRT= chemoradiation therapy, TAH= total abdominal hysterectomy, LRH= laparoscopic radical hysterectomy, PD= progressive disease, RD= recurrent disease, CR= complete remission, DOD= dead of disease, NED= no evidence of disease

Authors	No	Age	FIGO stage	Histologic report	IF-LN	P-LN	Primary treatment	Adjuvant therapy	DFI	Survival
Way (1960)	6	-	-	Epithelioma of very unusual type	NA	NA	Surgical treatment	-	NA	No longer than 4.5 years
Gosling et al (1961)	2	-	-	Spindled SCC	NA	NA	Surgical treatment	-	NA	NA
Copas et al (1982)	1	54	III	Poorly differentiated spindle cell carcinoma	+	-	RV with bilateral groin and pelvic LND	CTx with RTx	1 month	2-3 months
Steeper et al (1983)	1	89	-	Pseudosarcomatous SCC	NA	NA	RTx	Simple vulvectomy	9 months	2.5 months
LiVolsi et al (1987)	2	-	-	Carcinoma with sarcomatoid features	NA	NA	NA	NA	NA	NA
Santeusanio et al (1991)	1	77	IV	Poorly differentiated carcinoma with sarcoma-like features	+	NA	RV with bilateral femoral inguinal LND	-	15 days	1 month
Parham et al (1991)	1	54	I	Mixed soft tissue sarcoma with atypical squamous cells	NA	NA	Local excision	-	3 years	More than 6 years
Cooper et al (2002)	1	73	III	Sarcomatoid SCC	+	NA	RV with bilateral inguinal LND	RTx	5 months	NA
Dong-Seok et al (2006)	1	43	II	Poorly differentiated SCC with extensive sarcomatoid features	-	NA	Radical local excision and bilateral groin LND	NA	NED	More than 2 years
Case Number Two Below	1	78	I	Poorly differentiated SSCC	-	-	Bilateral simple hemivulvectomy	NA	NED	Alive at present date

IF-LN= inguino-femoral lymph node metastasis, P-LN= pelvic lymph node metastasis, DFI= disease free interval, NA= not available, SCC= squamous cell carcinoma, NED= no evidence of disease, RV= radical vulvectomy, LND= lymph node dissection, CTx= chemotherapy, RTx= radiation therapy

Table 2. SSCC of the Vulva Reported Cases in the Literature (D.-S. Choi et al, 2006)

Four cases of vaginal SSCC have been reported, with our current case constituting the fifth.

Authors	Age	Site	FIGO Stage	Initial Diagnosis	Treatment	Follow up
Steeper et al (1983)	54	Fornices bilaterally	II	Malignant fibrous histiocytoma	8500 rads with F/U Adriamycin/vincristine DTIC	Died 11 months after diagnosis
	81	Lower 1/3 anterior, extending to labium minus	Positive right inguinal nodes	Carcinosarcoma	55mg of intravaginal radium, 9990 rad to vaginal surface, and 5075 rad to right pelvic lymph nodes	Free of recurrence 4 years after diagnosis
Motoyama et al (1989)	74	Middle 1/3 left lateral	II	Sarcomatous spindle cell tumor	7000 rad external radiation with F/U vinicristine, actinomycin D, cyclophosphamide	Died 1 year after diagnosis with local recurrence and lung metastasis
Raptis et al (1993)	25	Upper 1/3 left lateral wall	II	Sarcoma	4600 CGw external radiation, and high dose brachytherapy 3x 800 cGw	No evidence of disease 6 months after diagnosis
Case number 1 below	67		III	Leiomyosarcoma	Radiation, Chemo	Metastatic disease at 2 years

Table 3. SSCC of the Vagina Reported Cases in the Literature (Raptis et al, 1993)

The low volume of cases poses a dilemma in that institutional encounters of such cases are sporadic and as such, there are no established guidelines for diagnosis or treatment. These cancers have traditionally been treated and staged similar to squamous cell carcinomas of their respective sites using the FIGO staging system. There has been reported success in long term survival rates of patients who present earlier in the disease and whose tumors could be fully resected. These presentations are rare, as patients tend to present with long standing bulky tumors and with metastasis.

2. Case report

Two cases of sarcomatoid squamous cell carcinoma, one of the vagina and one of the vulva, will be utilized as illustrative examples of this rare entity.

Case number one: 67 year old, Gravida 7 Para 6 woman status post total abdominal hysterectomy 13 years prior for reportedly benign fibroids, presented with profuse vaginal bleeding. Examination revealed a vaginal lesion which was biopsied, revealing a high-grade, malignant sarcomatoid neoplasm with no concurrent precursor lesion, such as an in-situ component. Pathologic assessment suggested that this was a sarcoma, specifically, a leiomyosarcoma, as evidence of smooth muscle differentiation was demonstrated by immunohistochemisty. However, with subsequent demonstration of pelvic sidewall and pelvic lymph node involvement, features not typically associated with sarcomas, immunohistochemistry for p16 and in situ hybridization for high risk human Papilloma virus (HPV) subtypes was performed; this demonstrated that the tumor was, indeed, an HPV-driven malignancy compatible with sarcomatoid squamous cell carcinoma. Following a course of chemotherapy and radiation therapy, the patient presented two years later with deep vein thrombosis and obstructive uropathy, with subsequent biopsy demonstrating recurrent metastatic squamous cell carcinoma involving the ureter.

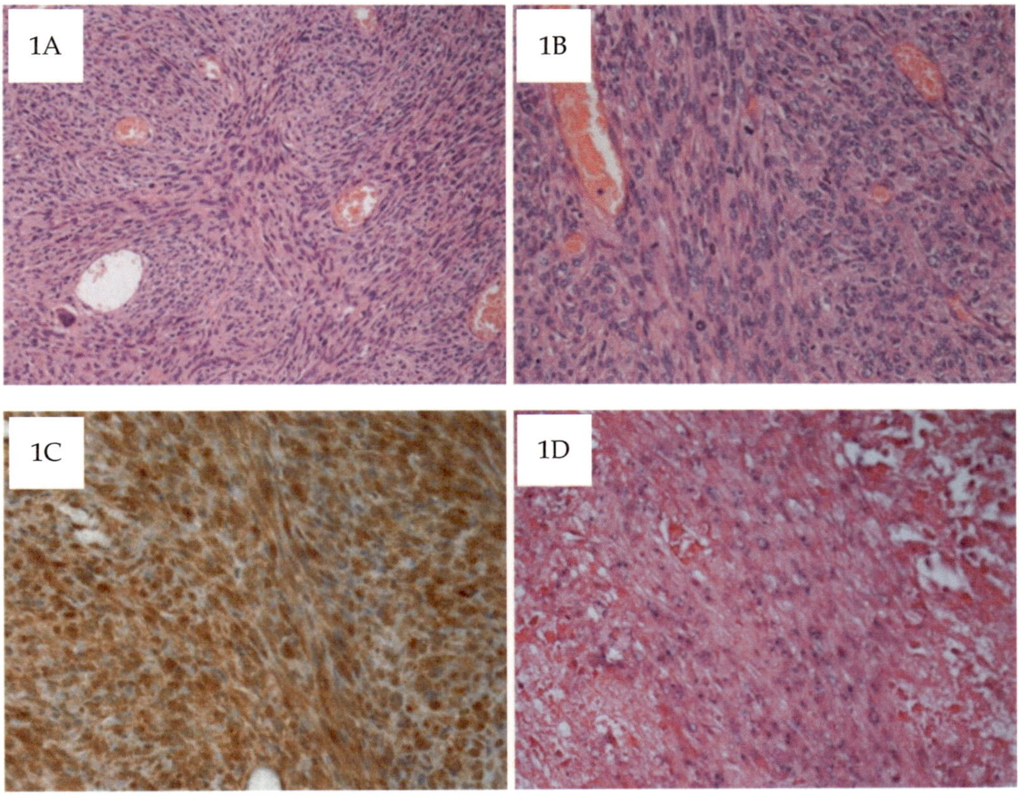

Fig. 1. Sarcomatoid squamous cell carcinoma of the vagina. (A) The lesion is characterized exclusively by spindled cells, architecturally arranged in fascicles. No in situ or conventional squamous cell morphology is apparent [200x original magnification]. (B) High-power magnification shows spindled cells with abundant mitotic figures [400x original magnification]. (C) Neoplastic cells show diffuse nuclear reactivity for p16, indicative of a HPV-driven tumor [400x original magnification]. (D) Chromogenic in situ hybridization for high-risk HPV subtypes demonstrates diffuse nuclear chromogenic labeling (in blue dot pattern) [400x original magnification].

Case number two: 78 year old Para 1 woman with long-standing vulvar irritation presented with a 4cm vulvar lesion. She underwent biopsies that demonstrated a high-grade vulvar intraepithelial lesion (VIN III, carcinoma in situ), and subsequent wide local excision showed involved margins. Four years later, she re-presented with a 4cm, enlarging vulva mass; excision of this mass revealed an invasive, poorly differentiated Sarcomatoid Squamous Cell Carcinoma (SSCC), again with positive margins. She subsequently underwent a bilateral simple hemivulvectomy with pathology demonstrating involvement of the urethral margin, with other margins uninvolved. A metastatic evaluation was negative. Other comorbidities rendered the patient to be a poor candidate for additional surgical intervention.

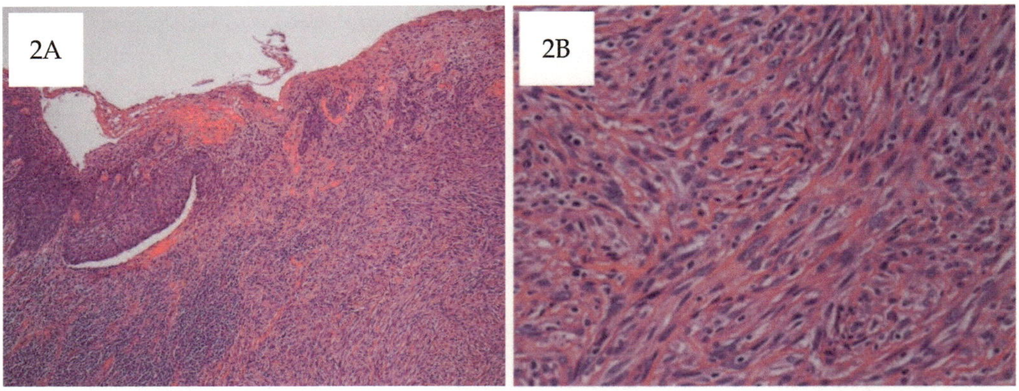

Fig. 2. (A) Sarcomatoid squamous cell carcinoma of the vulva. The lesion has an interface with an in situ component (left side of image), and transitions to a tumor of predominant spindled cell morphology (right side of image) [100x original magnification]. (B) High-power magnification shows spindle cell morphology in a fascicular architectural pattern, imparting a mesenchymal-like, sarcomatoid morphology [400x original magnification].

3. Incidence

The incidences of SSCC has not been well established but is deemed to be very low from the isolated published case reports, constituting, at most only 1-2% of all gynecologic malignancies overall. There have been more reported cases of vulvar and cervical SSCC than cases from the vagina. This trend is also seen in squamous cell carcinomas of the female genital tract, with cervix and vulvar being more common than vagina. In general, SSCC are observed in more frequency with advancing age, and there is a correlation between vaginal cancers in women who have undergone a hysterectomy for malignant disease. It would be interesting to see if this is also true in SSCC. A possibility for the low incidence of SSCC is that the sarcomatoid component is under recognized, or under reported as part of the pathology report.

4. Risk factors

Risk factors for SSCC of the female genital tract are assumed to be the same as risk factors for Squamous cell carcinoma. This is even more so if the belief that SSCC transforms from SCC. Risk factors include HPV infection, high risk sexual behavior, cigarette smoking, specific vitamin deficiencies, and immunosupression.

Human Papillomavirus (HPV) is a well known causal factor for the development of squamous cell carcinoma of the vulva, vagina, cervix, anus, and oropharynx.It is the most frequently diagnosed sexually transmitted disease in the United States. HPV subtypes 16 and 18 in particular have a high known oncogenic potential and are thus called "high risk"subtypes, accounting for approximately 80% of cases of invasive cervical cancer. (Bereck and Hacker, 2010). HPV has been reported to affect roughly 20 million people in the U.S. and is the most frequently diagnosed STD. This number is expected to decrease as more young 2A 2B Sarcomatoid Squamous Cell Carcinoma 7 women and men are being offered the Gardasil and Cervarix injections. These injections are FDA improved and are aimed at immunizing against some of the "high risk" human papillomavirus types that predispose to cancer and the "low risk" subtypes of human papillomavirus that cause genital warts. Despite relatively wide availability, less than 30% of patients receive the recommended three doses. (NCI Cancer Bulletin, 2011) Even though the rates of HPV infection decrease sharply after 30 years of age, older women are less likely to clear an infection with a high risk subtype of HPV. The older the patient at presentation the more likely the patient will have a more advanced stage (Berek and Hacker 201

High risk sexual behavior is a risk factor due to the increase in exposure to sexually transmitted infections (STI). The more sexual partners one has the higher the chance that they will become infected with an STI. This is partly due to the fact that some STI's cause disruption of the epithelial cell layer that can facilitate the transport of infectious material. When the cervix is exposed to infection it undergoes reparative metaplastic changes that can also increase susceptibility of and STI. (Bereck and Hacker, 2010)

Cigarette smokers are known to be at increased risk of cancer of the lungs and other body organs including the cervix and vulva. Cigarette smoke is an independent risk factor for cervical cancer. (Nishino, K. et al, 2008) The pathogenesis is due to the elevated levels of genotoxic breakdown products that are in the cigarettes, including nicotine, cotinine, hydrocarbons, and tars, that have mutagenic properties that are present in cervical mucus and cells. (Berek and Hacker, 2010) Coker et al (2009) found that smokers were 21% more likely to succumb to cervical cancer compared to those who did not smoke at all, suggesting that it expedites the disease process due to the inhibited epithelial immune response.

Although there has been a lack of sound evidence that vitamins and minerals has a clinically significant affect on the progression and prevention of cancer (World Cancer Research Fund, 2007), there have been several studies that have shown a benefit of certain nutrients and vitamins. Research continues to find a correlation between essential vitamin and nutrient intake and the progression/prevention of breast, cervical, prostate, and colon cancer. Vitamins A, C, D, and E have been depicted to have protective properties. Vitamin A has some role in regulating differentiation, growth, and apoptosis of normal as well as malignant cells. (Cui et al, 2008) The role of Vitamin C has been in the foraging of free radicals. Vitamin E works in conjunction with vitamins A and C to regulate cell differentiation and proliferation, to scavenge free radicals and oxidants, and may reduce the persistence of HPV as well as inhibit cervical carcinogenesis by augmenting immunological function and modulating the inflammatory response to infection. (Kim et al, 2010) Toner and Milner (2010) found that even though Vitamin D has been shown to be beneficial in cancer prevention the problem lies in finding a standard and most beneficial dosage and also showed that there were risk with overexposure.

There are several disease states that can result in immunosupression. These include HIV, transplant patients, cancer patients undergoing chemotherapy, congenital immunodeficiency disorders, and immunosuppressive drugs, among others. The main physiological function of the immune cells is to monitor tissue homeostasis, to protect against invading pathogens, and to eliminate transformed or damaged cells. (Bremmes et al, 2011) When the physiologic function of immune cells are interrupted in any way, the body has an impeded response to the recognition and response to cancer cells. This delayed response and recognition aides in the more rapid progression of cancer. Studies on immunotherapy in cancer patients have been ongoing and there have been great advances, giving validity that the immune response is an important mediator in preventing and fighting off cancer.

5. Pathogenesis

There have been many hypotheses about the pathogenesis of SSCC, including the basis of its aggressiveness. The theory that is longstanding and the most accepted is that there is a transformation from the squamous cell carcinoma component into a spindle cell cancer. This is mainly due to parallel immunohistochemical, molecular, and ultrastructural characteristics. In 1960, Hay-Roe et al found that the epithelial portion of SSCC of the esophagus had an apparent tendency to become spindled in tissue culture. This was also reported by Sherwin et al (1963) which also stated there is a probable loss of unity of the epithelial cells in the basal layer and this was the major feature causing the spindle cell transformation. Raptis et. al (1993) showed a relative decrease in desmosomes and tonofilaments within the spindled component therefore lacking the structural foundation of ordinary squamous cell carcinoma and might be more susceptible to the compressing effect of surrounding stroma. The fact that the spindle cells have desmosomes and tonofilaments confirms the squamous cell origin. Lastly, there has been speculation that the spindle cell component and the squamous cell component arise concurrently from distinct stem cell lines and thus SSCC has been termed a "collision" tumor and not a single tumor with conversion to a spindled cell type. (Otay et al. 2011)

6. Presentation

The disease process of Sarcomatoid Squamous Cell Carcinoma is very aggressive, patients typically present with extensive local disease or with metastasis on imaging and during surgery. The clinical signs and symptoms do not correlate to the severity of disease. Early nonspecific symptoms can include fatigue, anemia, pelvic pain, pelvic pressure, constipation, bloating, weight loss, and loss of appetite.

The most common presenting symptom of cervical SSCC was abnormal vaginal bleeding. There have also been cases of patients complaining of a foul smelling discharge (Brown et al 2003), postcoital spotting (Kong et al, 2010). In all of the cases of cervical SSCC there was a visible cervical lesion ranging from 1.6cm to 10cm. Vaginal lesions can present in a similar fashion with vaginal bleeding and a yellowish-white vaginal discharge. On physical exam a mass was usually palpable. Vulvar lesions usually present with the patient reporting a lesion that bleeds, is expanding, and/or is worrisome. In a small percentage of patients, there were no signs or symptoms of a genital mass. SSCC lesions of the cervix, vagina, and vulva, were all described similarly in the text as being ulceroproliferative, friable, of polypoid configuration, and necrotic in areas.

7. Diagnosis

The hallmark of diagnosing this disease is biopsy of the lesion. It is important to get an adequate specimen to increase the probability of accurately diagnosing the cancer. There is no consensus as to the diameter and depth of specimen that gives the highest yield for proper pathological evaluation.

An excisional biopsy is one in which the entire mass is removed with a margin of normal tissue. This is done in the OR for the most part under sedation or if the lesion is small enough in the office with local anesthesia. Since the lesion is friable, supplies for bleeding should be readily available. Excisional biopsy is preferred for smaller lesions in which margins are available and do not interfere with surrounding structures. An incisional biopsy, in which the surgeon removes a portion of the mass, may be done in the office or in the operating room. This is utilitized in the event the mass is too large to obtain normal margin of surrounding tissue.

7.1 Histology

In general, the histopathological diagnosis of SSCC rests upon demonstration of a malignancy with regions of classic squamous cell carcinoma morphology, merging with those exhibiting a prominent spindle cell component. In cases where such a transition occurs, and/or where a squamous cell carcinoma in situ interface is evident, the diagnosis can be confidently rendered on morphologic grounds alone.

However, in situations where the spindled cell component predominates, without areas of classic squamous morphology or an interface with an in situ carcinoma component, the diagnosis is particularly challenging, as key differential diagnostic considerations would include a sarcoma. Such was the case with the current vaginal lesion, which was a tumor demonstrating exclusive spindled cell morphology; as immunohistochemistry for muscle markers (smooth muscle actin) was positive, the lesion was initially thought to reflect a leiomyosarcoma. In review of the cases, some report round to polygonal cells, scanty eosinophilic cytoplasm, irregular nuclei, prominent nucleoli, numerous mitosis, and areas of necrosis with interlacing bundles of spindle cells on microscopic exam.

7.2 Immunohistochemical methodologies including HPV detection

There are many tools in modern immunohistochemistry that may aid in facilitating the diagnosis of SSCC, but may also pose significant nuances. In our case of SSCC of the vagina, tumor cells which are exclusively spindled in morphology, were positive for markers associated with both, mesenchymal and epithelial differentiation, including cytokeratin, vimentin, desmin and smooth muscle actin. Indeed, while one report indicates that neoplastic cells of SSCC do not show reactivity for smooth muscle actin (C-P, Lin et al. 2006), another reports that this marker may be positive in tumor cells. (Brown et al., 2003). In our particular case of SSCC from the vagina, the tumor initially thought to reflect a leiomyosarcoma, was ultimately demonstrated to harbor high-risk HPV subtypes by in situ hybridization, as well as expression of p16, a tumor suppressor protein implicated in the HPV tumorigenesis pathway. These latter findings, despite the morphologic appearance of the tumor and the ambiguous immunophenotype, permitted a definitive final diagnosis of SSCC.

8. Staging

Due to the rarity of this cancer, the FIGO staging system that is used for squamous cell carcinoma is also used to stage SSCC of the vulva, vagina, and cervix.

Stage I	Tumor confined to the vulva
• **IA**	Lesions ≤2 cm in size, confined to the vulva or perineum and with stromal invasion ≤1.0 mm*, no nodal metastasis
• **IB**	Lesions >2 cm in size or with stromal invasion >1.0 mm*, confined to the vulva or perineum, with negative nodes
Stage II	Tumor of any size with extension to adjacent perineal structures (1/3 lower urethra, 1/3 lower vagina, anus)
Stage III	Tumor of any size with or without extension to adjacent perineal structures (1/3 lower urethra, 1/3 lower vagina, anus) with positive inguino-femoral lymph nodes
• **IIIA**	i. With 1 lymph node metastasis (≥5 mm), or ii. 1-2 lymph node metastasis(es) (<5 mm)
• **IIIB**	i. With 2 or more lymph node metastases (≥5 mm), or ii. 3 or more lymph node metastases (<5 mm)
• **IIIC**	With positive nodes with extracapsular spread
Stage IV	Tumor invades other regional (2/3 upper urethra, 2/3 upper vagina), or distant structures
• **IVA**	Tumor invades any of the following: i. upper urethral and/or vaginal mucosa, bladder mucosa, rectal mucosa, or fixed to pelvic bone, or ii. fixed or ulcerated inguino-femoral lymph nodes
• **IVB**	Any distant metastasis including pelvic lymph nodes

*The depth of invasion is defined as the measurement of the tumor from the epithelial-stromal junction of the adjacent most superficial dermal papilla to the deepest point of invasion. (**FIGO Committee on Gynecologic Oncology.** 2009)

Table 4. Carcinoma of the Vulva FIGO Staging. (2008)

Stage I	The carcinoma is limited to the vaginal wall
Stage II	The carcinoma has involved the subvaginal tissue but has not extended to the pelvic wall
Stage III	The carcinoma has extended to the pelvic wall
Stage IV	The carcinoma has extended beyond the true pelvis or has involved the mucosa of the bladder or rectum; bullous edema as such does not permit a case to be allotted to stage IV
• **IVA**	Tumor invades bladder and/or rectal mucosa and/or direct extension beyond the true pelvis
• **IVB**	Spread to distant organs

(**FIGO Annual Report.** 2006)

Table 5. Carcinoma of the Vagina FIGO Nomenclature

Cervical cancer is still staged clinically, which is not always very accurate in portraying the extent of the disease. Clinical staging can include palpation, inspection, colposcopy, endocervical curettage, hysteroscopy, cystoscopy, proctoscopy, intravenous urography, and e-ray examination of the lungs and skeletal system. (Berek and Hacker, 2010) CT and MRI are also utilized often as this can give a better idea of extent of disease, margins, lymphadenopathy, and other organ involvement. Positron emission tomography (PET) is mainly utilized for nodal status.

Stage I	The carcinoma is strictly confined to the cervix (extension to the corpus would be disregarded)
• **IA**	Invasive carcinoma which can be diagnosed only by microscopy, with deepest invasion ≤5 mm and largest extension ≤7 mm
IA1	Measured stromal invasion of ≤3.0 mm in depth and extension of ≤7.0 mm
IA2	Measured stromal invasion of >3.0 mm and not >5.0 mm with an extension of not >7 mm
• **IB**	Clinically visible lesions limited to the cervix uteri or pre-clinical cancers greater than stage IA*
IB1	Clinically visible lesion ≤4.0 cm in greatest dimension
IB2	Clinically visible lesion >4.0 cm in greatest dimension
Stage II	Cervical carcinoma invades beyond the uterus, but not to the pelvic wall or to the lower third of the vagina
• **IIA**	Without parametrial invasion
IIA1	Clinically visible lesion ≤4.0 cm in greatest dimension
IIA2	Clinically visible lesion >4.0 cm in greatest dimension
• **IIB**	With obvious parametrial invasion
Stage III	The tumor extends to the pelvic wall and/or involves lower third of the vagina and/or causes hydronephrosis or non-functioning kidney**
• **IIIA**	Tumor involves lower third of vagina, with no extension to the pelvic sidewall
• **IIIB**	Extension to the pelvic wall and/or hydronephrosis or non-functioning kidney
Stage IV	The carcinoma has extended beyond the true pelvis or has involved (biopsy proven) the mucosa of the bladder or rectum. A bullous edema, as such, does not permit a case to be allotted to Stage IV
• **IVA**	Spread of the growth to adjacent organs
• **IVB**	Spread to distant organs

**All macroscopically visible lesions-even with superficial invasion-are allotted to stage IB carcinomas. Invasion is limited to a measured stromal invasion with a maximal depth of 5.00 mm and a horizontal extension of not >7.00 mm. Depth of invasion should not be >5.00 mm taken from the base of the epithelium of the original tissue-squamous or glandular. The depth of invasion should always be reported in mm, even in those cases with "early (minimal) stromal invasion" (~1 mm). the involvement of vascular/lymphatic spaces should not change the stage allotment)*
***On rectal examination, there is no cancer-free space between the tumor and the pelvic wall. All cases with hydronephrosis or non-functioning kidney are included, unless they are known to be due to another cause.*

(**FIGO Committee on Gynecologic Oncology.** 2009)

Table 6. Carcinoma of the Cervix Uteri (2008)

9. Therapy

The rarity of these malignancies makes recommendations for standard treatments a formidable endeavor. In general, the stage of the cancer will dictate therapy.

In early stage disease of the vulva, vagina and cervix the role for surgery is more clearly defined. These lesions are usually treated with radical surgery followed by radiation therapy and/or chemotherapy in certain cases. Size, margin status, and local tumor biology might dictate the need for radiotherapy. Brown et al (2003) treated all Stage I and Stage II women with radiation therapy alone and this was successfully able to eradicate the tumor. This proves radiation to be an effective treatment option, even though some believe it to be a source of the transition of this cancer from SCC to the intermingling of the spindle shaped cells. In 2010, Kong et al reported a case of IB1 SSCC of the cervix in a young patient, being treated by laparoscopic radical hysterectomy, bilateral pelvic lymph node biopsy, peritoneal washing cytology and transposition of both ovaries without adjuvant therapy. Despite the initial treatment for low stage cancers, recurrent cancer did not respond to second line therapy (Brown et al, 2003) which leads some to take a more aggressive approach with surgery and adjuvant therapy, especially since time from recurrence to death is less than a year as reported in the literature.

In more advanced stages, patients present with such extensive disease that surgery is usually done on a palliative basis if indicated. These tumors are usually treated with concurrent chemotherapy and radiation, extrapolating from the pure squamous counterparts. In contradiction to these lesions where there exist more robust standard treatment recommendations the response to similar treatment is largely unknown and the risk for recurrence is very significant with a very short disease free interval.

10. Prognosis

Prognosis of SSCC is very poor. It is a very aggressive cancer, is usually diagnosed at a later stage, and most recur within one year despite aggressive combined therapy. As with the majority of solid tumors, the survival of patients that were detected at early stages is very reassuring. Patients who are diagnosed at Stage I have a higher survival rate at 5 years, approaching 90%. In contrast, those who present at Stage IV, according to the studies, have a survival rate of less than 5% at five years, according to the review of the case reports. Prognostic factors have not been uniformed in any of the studies. Lane believed the extent of the grossly carcinomatous element was the best predictor of survival. Friedel et al found that not only was the degree of differentiation of the carcinomatous component an important prognostic factor but also the extent of invasiveness. Some suggest size and location are the sole factors impacting prognosis. (Randall et al.) Brown et al found that the younger patients tended to present at an earlier stage. Of these women who presented at stage 1, all were free of disease with the longest interval reported at 42 months. They also found that all patients less than 40 presented at Stage I and not a more advanced stage III or IV. One explanation for the fact that younger patients present at a lesser stage is that they are more prone to go to the doctors for acute visits and are more likely to voice there concerns over abnormal changes in their bodies. This is different to the belief that women >40 are more apt to cope with the symptoms and only present when the condition is debilitating or they are urged by family.

11. Conclusion

SSCC is a very rare cancer that has an aggressive and rapidly fatal course. Due to its rarity, there is no distinct staging or guidelines to direct therapy and care. As more cases become available and follow up is documented on patients with early FIGO stages, treatments, and surveillance decisions there will be a better chance of developing a set of guidelines based on the evidence. Since this cancer is most accepted as being a variant of SCC, the FIGO staging and treatment guidelines for squamous cell carcinoma are also used for SSCC.

Human papillomavirus has been implicated in SCC and is also found in the spindle cell component of SSCC. Even with the use of the widely available HPV vaccine and better screening modalities, it is difficult to discern which squamous cell cancers will transition to SSCC so no risk prevention can be done. One would assume that with the reduction in squamous cell carcinoma cases of the female genital tract that there will be a parallel reduction of SSCC.

Diagnosis has traditionally been difficult due to the large ratio of sarcomatous to squamous cell component. Immunohistochemistry and ancillary testing, such as in situ hybridization for high-risk HPV subtypes are very important for the precise diagnosis which can guide treatment and counseling of the patient. One should perform immunohistochemistry for squamous epithelial markers as well as in situ hybridization for HPV when encountering a sarcomatoid neoplasm to rule out SSCC.

As with any cancer, the lower the FIGO stage at diagnosis the better the prognosis. Unfortunately even when adequately treated according to unset standards, recurrence is very prevalent with disease free interval to death being very rapid. Once recurrence occurs there is very little recourse as the cancer does not respond to second line therapy and has usually extended out of the pelvis to distant organs. There have been few cases of a FIGO stage greater than II in which there has been long term survival but not enough to effectively alter the inevitable outcome.

12. Acknowledgements

The authors of this chapter have no financial acknowledgments.

13. References

Bereck, J.; Hacker, N. (2010) *Gynecologic Oncology* (5th), Lippincott, Williams, and Wilkins, ISBN 978-0-7817-9512-8, Philadelphia, Pennsylvania.

Bremnes, R.; Al-Shibli, K.; Donnem, T.; Sirera, R.; Al-Saad, S.; Anderson, S.; Stenvold, H.; Camps, C.; Busund, L. (2011) The Role of Tumor-Infiltrating Immune Cells And Chronic Inflammation at the Tumor Site on Cancer Development, Progression, and Prognosis: Emphasis on Non-small Cell Lung Cancer. *Journal of Thoracic Oncology.* Vol. 6, No. 4, (April 2011), pp. 824-33, ISSN 1556-0864

Brown, J.; Broaddus, R.; Koeller, M.; Burke,T.; Gershenson, D.; Bodurka, D. (2003). Sacrcomatoid Carcinoma of the Cervix. *Gynecologic Oncology,* Vol. 90, No. 1,(July 2003), pp. 23-28, ISSN 0090-8258

Choi, D.-S.; Lee, J.-W.; Lee, S.-J.; Choi, C.-H., Kim, T.-J.; Lee, J.-H.; Bae, D.-S.; Ahn, G.; Kim, B.-G. (2006). Squamous Cell Carcinoma with Sarcomatoid Features of the Vulva: A case Report and Review of the Literature. *Gynecologic Oncology,* Vol. 103, No. 1, (October 2006), pp. 363-67, ISSN 0090-8258

Coker, AL; DeSimone, CP; Eggleston, KS; Hopenhayn, C; Nee, J; Tucker, T. (2009) Smoking And survival among Kentucky women diagnosed with invasive cervical Cancer: 1995-2005. *Gynecologic Oncology,* Vol. 112, No. 2, (February 2009), pp. 365-69, ISSN 1095-6859.

Cui, Y.; Shikany, JM.; Liu, S.; Shagufta, Y.; Rohan, TE. (2008) Selected antioxidants and risk Of hormone receptor-defined invasive breast cancers among post menopausal Women in the Women's Health Initiative Observational Study. *American Journal of Clinical Nutrition.* Vol. 87, No. 4, (April 2008), pp. 1009-18, ISSN 0002-9165

Hay-Roe, V.; Hill, R.; Civin, W. (1960) An Unclassified Tumor of the Esophagus: Case Review. *Journal of Thoracic and Cardiovascular Surgery.* Vol. 40, (July 1960), pp. 107-13, ISSN 0022-5223

Iwata, H. (2008). Spindle Cell Squamous Cell Carcinoma Showing Epithelial Mesenchymal Transition. *Journal of the European Academy of Dermatology and Venerology.* Vol 23, No. 2, (February 2009), pp. 214-15, ISSN 1468-3083

Kim, J.; Kim, M.; Lee, J.; Kim, J-H.; Son, S.; Song, E-S.; Lee, K.; Lee, J.P.; Lee, J.M.; Yun, Y. Intakes of Vitamin A, C, E, and Beta-Carotene are Associated with Risk Of Cervical Cancer: A Case-Control Study in Korea. *Nutrition and Cancer.* Vol. 62, No. 2, (April 2009), pp. 181-89, ISSN 0163-5581.

Kong, T.-W.; Kim, J.-H.; Chang, S.-J.; Chang, K.-H.; Ryu, H.-S.; Joo, H.-J. (2010). Sarcomatoid Squamous Cell Carcinoma of the Uterine Cervix Successfully Treated by Laparoscopic radical Hysterectomy. *Journal of Reproductive Medicine,* Vol. 55, No. 8-9, (Sep-Oct 2010), 99. 445-48, ISSN 0024-7758

Kumar, M.; Bahl, A.; Sharma, D.; Agarwal, S.; Halanaik, D.; Kumar, R.; Raht, G. (2008) Sarcomatoid Squamous cell Carcinoma of Uterine Cervix: Pathology, imaging, and treatment. *Journal of Cancer Research and Therapeutics,* Vol. 4, No. 1, (Jan-Mar 2008), pp. 39-41, ISSN 0973-1482

Lin, C.-P.; Ho, C.-L.; Shen, M.-R.; Huang, L.-H.; Chou, C.-Y. (2006) Evidence of Human Papillomavirus Infection, Enhanced Phosphorylation of Retinoblastoma Protein, and Decreased Apoptosis in Sarcomatoid Squamous Cell Carcinoma Of Uterine Cervix. *International Journal of Gynecologic Cancer,* Vol. 16, No. 1, (Jan-Feb 2006), pp. 336-40, ISSN 1525-1438

Nishino, Koji.; Sekine, M.; Kodama, S.; Sudo, N.; Aoki, Y.; Seki, N.; Tanaka, K. (2008) Cigarette smoking and *glutathione S-transferase* M1 polymophism associated With risk for uterine cervical cancer. *Japan Society of Obstetrics and Gynecology.* Vol. 34, No. 6, (December 2008), pp. 994-1001, ISSN 1447-0756

Otay, M. (2011). Spindle Cell Carcinoma of the Tongue: A Rare Tumor in an Unusual Location. *Pathology Research International.* Vol. 2011, (01/2011), pp., ISSN 572381

Phillips, C. (2011) Use and Acceptance of HPV Vaccine Still a Work in Progress. *NCI Cancer Bulletin,* Vol. 8, No. 9, (March 2011), pp. 6, National Cancer Institute. Retrieved From http://www.cancer.gov/ncicancerbulletin/050311/page6

Raptis, S.; Haber, G.; Ferenczy, A. (1993). Vaginal Squamous Cell Carcinoma with Sarcomatoid Spindle Cell Features. *Gynecologic Oncology,* Vol. 49, No. 1, (April 1993), pp. 100-06, ISSN 0090-8288

Santeusanio, G.; Schiaroli, S.; Anemona, L.; Sesti, F.; Valli, E.; Piccione, E.; Spagnoli, L. (1991) Carcinoma of the Vulva with Sarcomatoid Features: A Case Report with Immunohistochemical Study. *Gynecologic Oncology,* Vol. 40. No. 2, (February 1991), pp. 160-63, ISSN 0090-8258

Sherwin, R.; Strong, M.; Vaughn, C. (1963). Polypoid and Junctional Squamous Cell Carcinoma of the Tongue and Larynx with Spindle Cell Carcinoma ("pseudocarcinoma"). *Cancer,* Vol. 16, (January 1963), pp. 51-60. ISSN 0008-543X

Steeper, T.; Piscioli, F.; Rosai, J. (1983). Squamous Cell Carcinoma with Sarcoma-Like Stroma of the Female Genital Tract: Clinicopathologic Study of Four Cases. *Cancer.* Vol. 52, No. 5, (September 1983), pp. 890-98, ISSN 0008-543X

Temkin, SM; Hellmann, M; Lee, Y; Abulafia, O. (2007) Primary Spindle Cell Sarcoma of the Vagina Treated with Neoadjuvant Radiation and Pelvic Exenteration. *Journal Of Lower Genital Tract Disease.* Vol. 11, No. 2, pp. 105-07, ISSN 1089-2591

Toner, C.; Milner, J. (2010). The Vitamin D and Cancer Conundrum: aiming at a moving Target. *Journal of the American Dietetic Association.* Vol. 110, No. 10, (October 2010), pp. 1492-500, ISSN 0002-8223

4

Basaloid Squamous Cell Carcinoma

Jasim Radhi
Department of Pathology and
Molecular Medicine McMaster University
Hamilton, Ontario
Canada

1. Introduction

Squamous cell carcinoma is the second most common cancer of the skin. This tumor arises predominantly in sun exposed actinically damaged areas. Implicated as predisposing factors, in addition to sunlight, these are industrial carcinogens, chronic ulcers, and ionizing radiation [1]. They are common cancer in immunocompromised and renal transplant patients [2]. Squamous cell carcinomas are known to be the most prevalent malignant tumor of the head and neck region [3]. They are also reported in many organs including cervix, lung, bladder, uterus, ovary, esophagus and teratomas [4;5;6,7].

Squamous cell carcinoma is characterized by squamous cells with large nuclei and abundant eosinophilic cytoplasm. The cells exhibit prominent intracellular bridges and variable keratin formation, depending on the degree of differentiation. Poorly differentiated tumors lack keratinization and usually form solid sheets of cells with marked pleomorphism to the extent that require special studies to establish the nature of the tumor.

2. Histologic variants of squamous cell carcinoma

Several histologic variant of squamous cell carcinoma are identified. These variants are based on certain morphological features accordingly, which may or may not have prognostic implications. The following are the most reported variant in the literature and include basaloid, warty verrucous, papillary, spindle cell, adenosquamous, clear cell, acantholytic and lymphoepithelioma-like type.

Spindle cell carcinoma is rather rare and is composed of atypical spindle cells with whorled arrangement (Fig 1), which mostly come from immunosuppressed renal transplant patients. The tumor needs to be differentiated from desmoplastic melanoma, atypical fibroxanthoma or metastatic carcinoma with spindle cell features. Immunohistochemistry is of value in differentiating these entities [8].

Clear squamous cell carcinoma is another variant first described as squamous cell carcinoma with extensive hydropic changes. The cells appear glassy looking, due to accumulation of fluid, and can be easily mistaken for sebaceous cell carcinoma. The differential also includes other clear cell tumors such as clear cell acanthoma, clear cell hidradenoma, metastatic renal cell carcinoma, balloon cell nevus and melanoma [9].

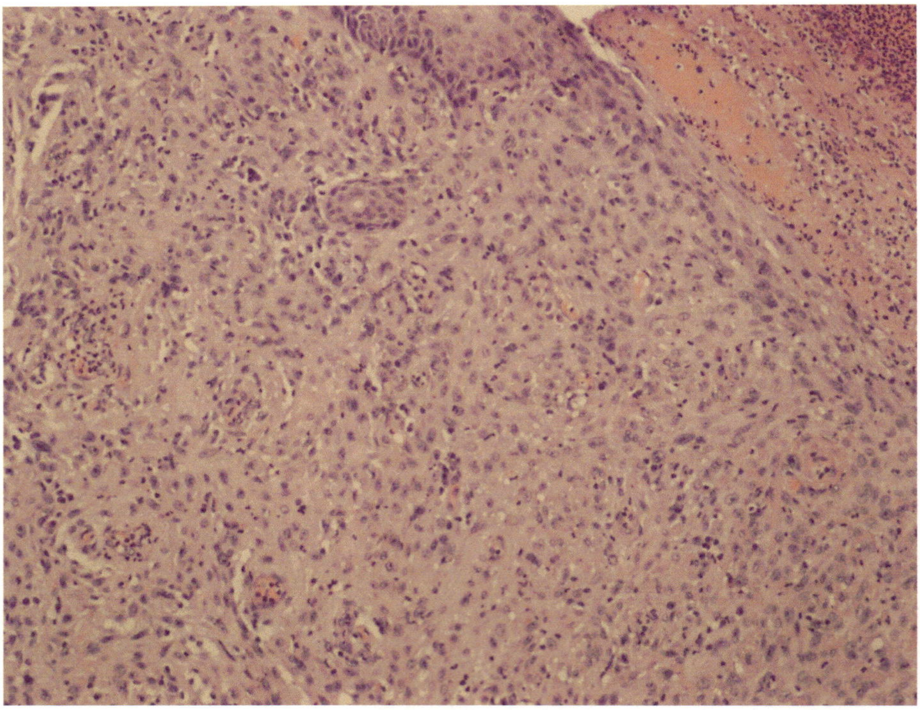

Fig. 1. Spindle cell variant of squamous cell carcinoma

Verrucous squamous cell carcinoma presents with rather non dysplastic epithelium with hyperkeratosis and elongation of the rete pegs. This is in contrast to the **papillary variant** of squamous cell carcinoma, which is characterized by malignant looking epithelium with papillary or exophytic architecture [10]. **Adenosquamous** cell carcinoma is very rare subtype, which is composed of admixed adenocarcinoma with squamous cell carcinoma. Mucin stain usually highlights the adenocarcinoma component.

Basaloid basal cell carcinoma is a rare variant of squamous cell carcinoma with more cases, which have been published since its first description in 1986 by Wain et al (11). These tumors affect both sexes but with predominance of male patients. They are frequently seen in the aerodigestive tract with most of the cases to be found in the tongue, floor of the mouth, the pyriform sinus, tonsil, and larynx [12]. These tumors have also been described in a variety of sites including nasopharynx, trachea, skin, cervix, bladder, thymus, anus, conjunctiva, and lung [13,14,15,16]. Clinically, patients have similar presentation to conventional squamous cell carcinoma depending on the site of the lesion.

Etiology and pathogenesis of basaloid cell carcinoma is similar to conventional squamous carcinoma. Most patients have a long history of smoking and alcohol drinking. In some cases there was a history of previous radiation to the head and neck region [17]. Both represent independent risk factors for the development of squamous cell carcinoma. Smokeless tobacco and other exogenous carcinogens such as occupational, environmental and nutritional factors may also play role in the pathogenesis of this cancer. EBV was detected in few cases using in situ hybridization technique from nasopharyngeal sites.

Recent studies detected a higher frequency of HPV and HSV in basaloid tumors than in conventional squamous cell carcinomas of the head and neck [18]. Basaloid squamous cell carcinoma in non smoker young patients revealed infection with HPV, high risk genotype 16. The expression is so significant, to the extent that it led some authors to consider the expression may be important for the diagnosis of this type of squamous cell carcinoma. The prognosis of HPV induced carcinoma appeared to have better outcome than the HPV negative cases [19]. It is not practical to perform in situ hybridization and sequencing techniques on every single case of basaloid squamous carcinoma as this is technically demanding and can be performed mostly in special centers [20]. The cell of origin of these tumors has been suggested to be a multipotential cell, which is able to differentiate into multiple cell type. However, the most acceptable origin for these cells is that they are from the surface epithelium since there is dysplastic or carcinoma in situ changes with direct continuity within the invasive component.

The tumor is considered by many authors as high grade with more aggressive behavior [11.16]. These lesions are capable of distant metastases, deep invasion, local recurrence and lymph node involvement. The most common sites for distant metastasis are the lung and liver. Multifocal disease includes other sites in the head and neck, which were also documented [17] However, some controversy is still present regarding the prognosis and conflicting results, which have appeared in recent literature. Some published papers claimed they have similar prognosis to traditional squamous cell carcinoma [21]. The majority of these cases are found at an advanced stage, which could explain the poor clinical outcome and prognosis. No general guidelines are present regarding the management of this disease; however, most published reports recommend a combination of surgery and postoperative radiotherapy, in order to prevent local recurrence and distant metastases [12,14].

3. Pathology of basal squamous cell carcinoma

Macroscopic appearances of these tumors show flat or slightly raised or polypoid exophytic lesions with or without a central ulceration in most cases reported in the literature [3] Microscopic examination of these lesions show characteristic invasive growth appearance, shared by most lesions. Generally they are composed of ribbons and or cords of basaloid cells with peripheral palisading and closely resemble traditional basal cell carcinoma figure 2. This lesion comes from rare urinary bladder flat lesion from a 66-year-old man seen on cystoscopy. In addition, the cellular arrangements of these lesions can closely mimic adenoid cystic carcinoma, due to the glandular or cribriform pattern, and have a tendency to have intracellular deposition of eosinophilic hyaline material figure 3. One of the major features of this tumor is that the cells exhibit high nucleocytoplasmic ratio and often have dense hyperchromatic nuclei and comedonecrosis may be seen in these tumor, figure 4, which was seen in a patient who presented with nasal sinus mass. This appearance represents common features of these lesions. Mitotic figures may be high and may include atypical forms. Careful search will reveal focal squamous differentiation with intercellular bridges or keratin formation, which is important for the accurate pathological assessment of these tumors. Another important feature of these lesions is dysplasia of the surface epithelium in cutanous neoplasm. Sometimes the tumor show true neural type rosette formation and other tumors may exhibit spindle shaped pleomorphic cells with elongated nuclei. Vascular or lymphatic invasion may also be present. In recent publication of cutanous basaloid squamous cell carcinoma, this tumor may also have rather large pleomorphic cells with big nuclei widely scattered throughout the lesion. These pleomorphic cells present no significant biological behavior. The immunoprofile of these tumors show consistent positive staining to high molecular weight cytokeratin antibody 34βE12, KL1, and MNF116, and focal staining for vimentin, EMA, CAM5.2, CK7, CEA, S100 and GFAP, and negative immunostaining for CK20, chromogranin, synaptophysin, BCL2, and Ber-EP4. Actin staining was positive in the basaloid cells and some cases were positive for CD99. More recent studies confirm strong and diffuse staining for P63 immunomarker in this tumor figure 5. Lastly, electron microscopic examination of samples may show tonofilaments and desmosome and do not demonstrate any characteristic findings, as the malignant cells show mainly undifferentiated cellular features, and the organelles are rather poorly developed(22).

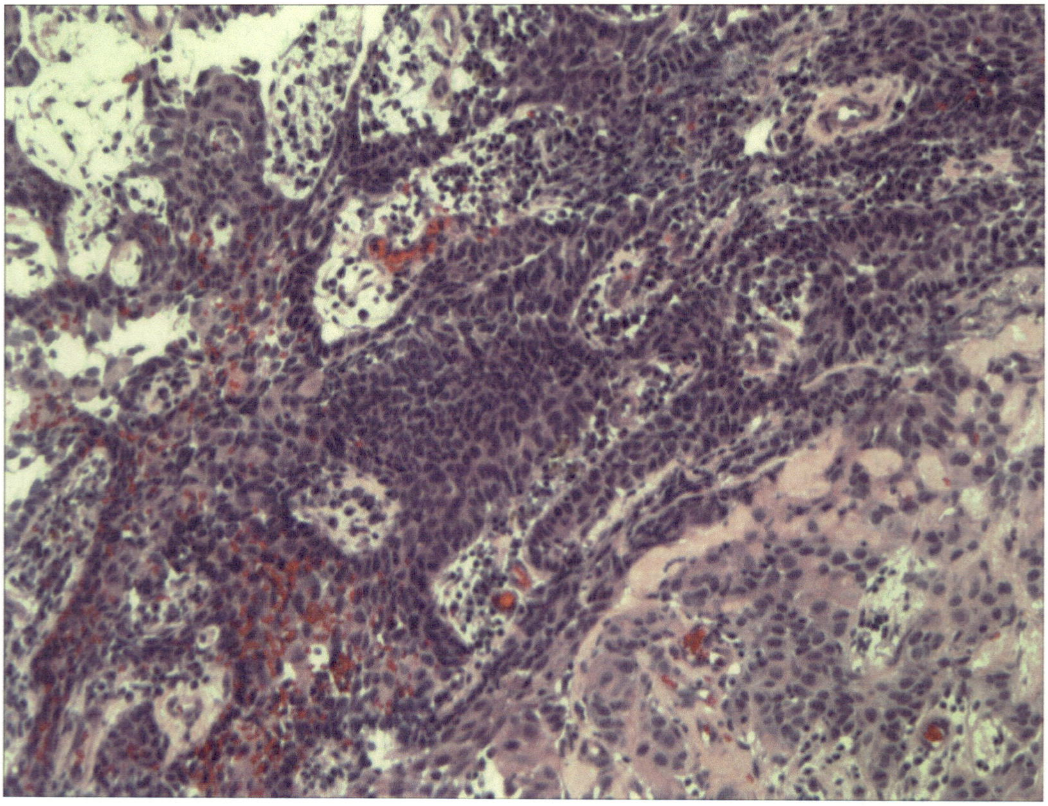

Fig. 2. Basaloid squamous cell carcinoma with peripheral palisading

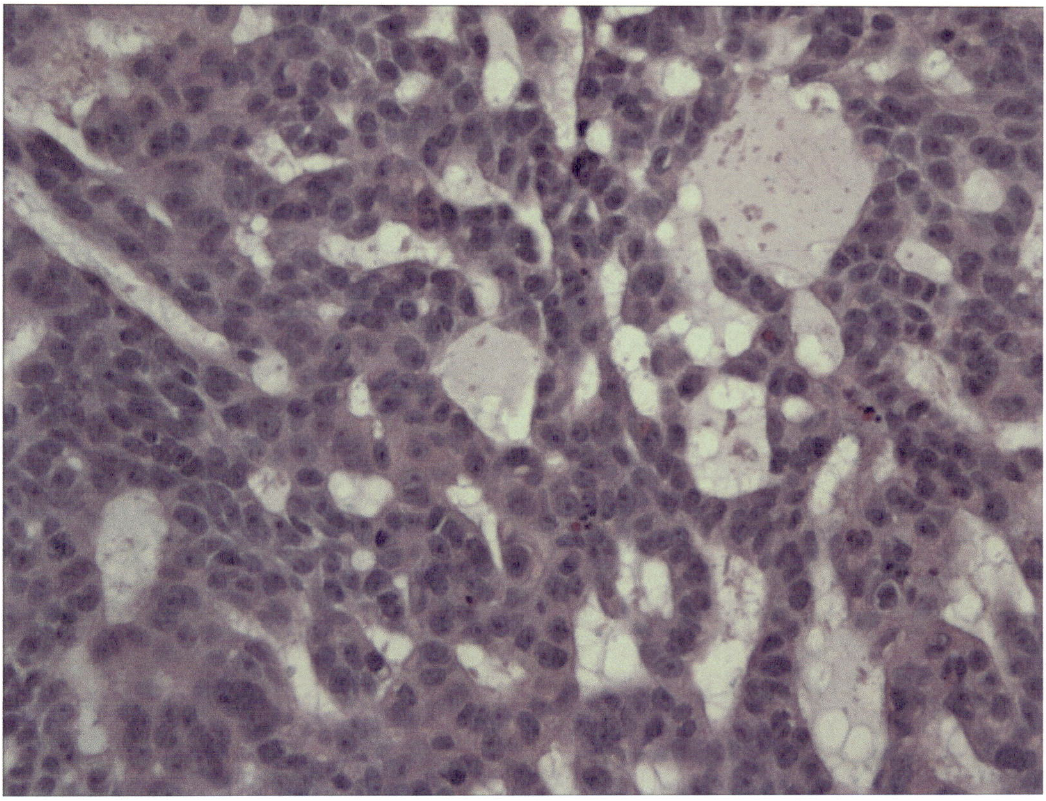

Fig. 3. Basaloid squamous carcinoma with glandular pattern

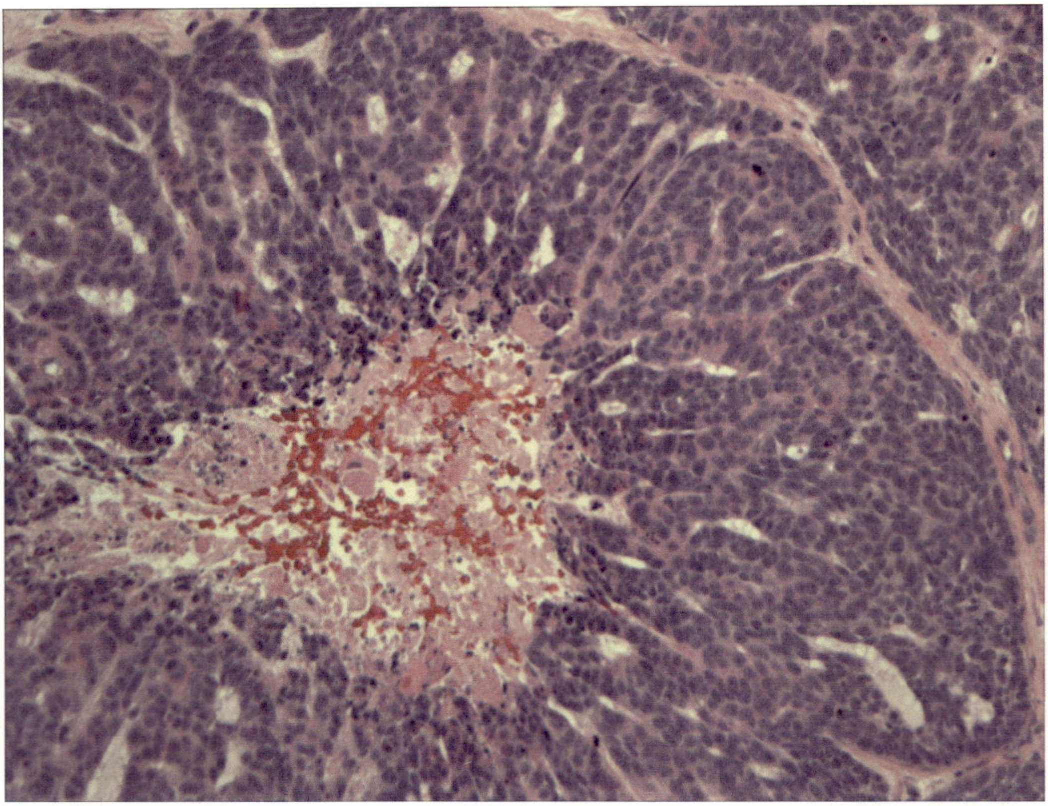

Fig. 4. The lesion shows prominent central necrosis

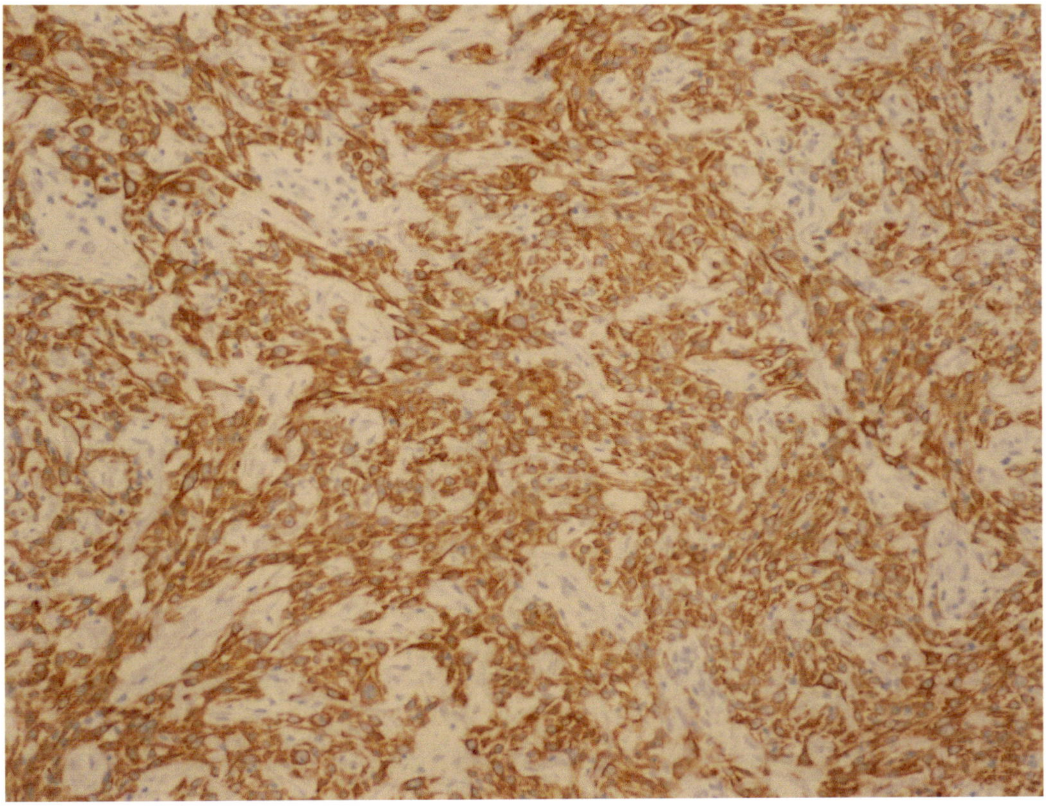

Fig. 5. Immunostaining with 34βE12

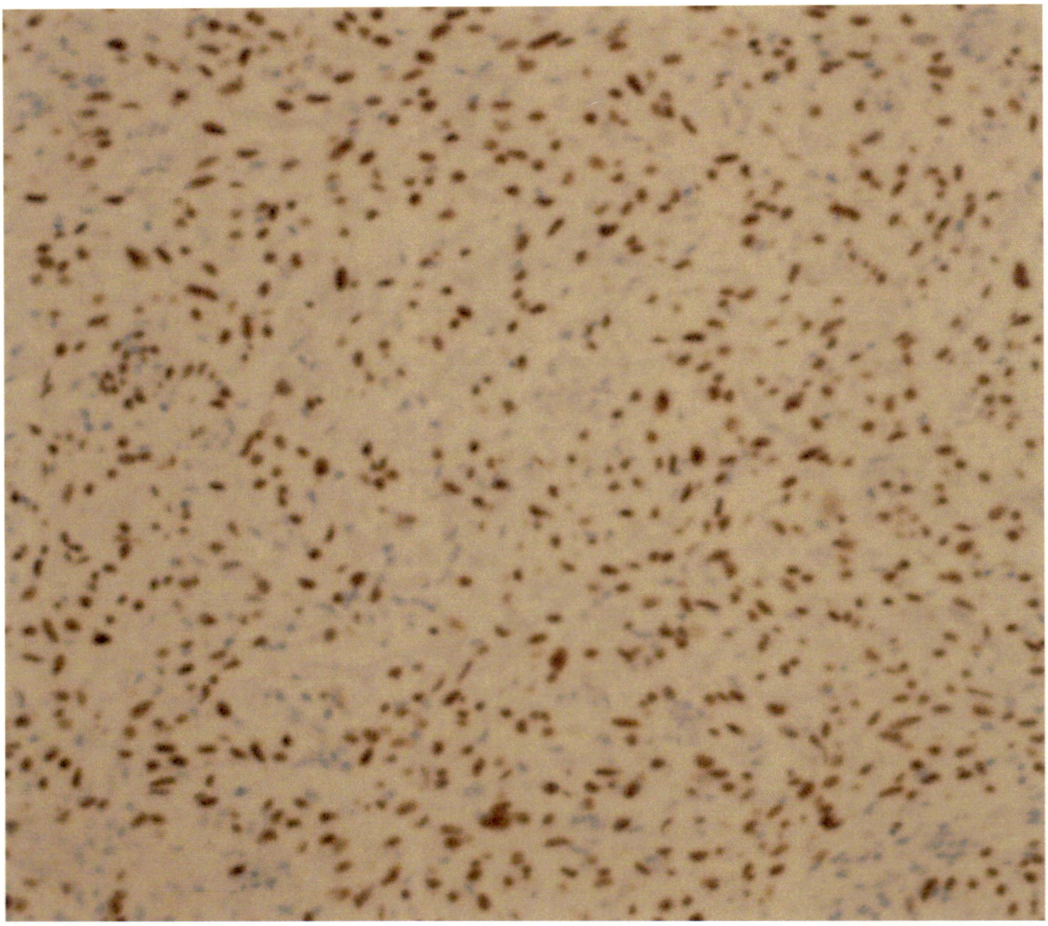

Fig. 6. Showing diffuse p63 positive malignant cell

The differential diagnosis of these tumors includes adenoid cystic carcinoma, small cell neuroendocrine carcinoma and other carcinomas depending on the anatomical sites.

Adenoid cystic carcinoma is characterized by basaloid-looking cells with predominant myoepithelial cells forming cribriform, solid or tubular structure. The tumor is slowly growing, less aggressive and with infrequent lymph node metastasis. Perineural invasion is a common feature of this lesion [23]. Immunohistochemistry show positive staining of the myoepthelial cells for S100, actin and calponin. The epithelial ductal cells of the tumor stain for cytokeratin, CEA and EMA. The stromal hyaline material can be highlighted with collagen IV and laminin. Small cell carcinoma is a more aggressive lesion with a different treatment approach. The tumor cells are positive for chromogranin, synaptophysin and dot-like staining for cytokeratin. These tumors are negative for 34βE12 marker, which is normally present in basaloid squamous cell carcinoma [17]. Skin basal cell carcinoma share histologic features with basaloid squamous cell carcinoma and need to be differentiate; however it lacks surface epithelial dysplasia, pleomorphism and the comedonecrosis seen in basaloid squamous cell carcinoma [17]. Adenosquamous carcinoma, which comprised of squalors and glandular differentiation, can have surface epithelial dysplasia. These lesions contain mucin and lack basaloid cells and peripheral palisading [24].

In conclusion, this variant of squamous cell carcinoma is reported in many sites and organs and present unique pathological and clinical features. This neoplasm is currently under more investigation to determine the nature and clinical behavior. The pathology of this entity is characterized by closely packed basaloid-looking cells with scanty cytoplasm. The cells are arranged in ribbons or with trabecular pattern. Occasional foci of squamous-looking cells are identified. The immunoprofile of these tumors are helpful to distinguish them from basal cell carcinoma, adenoid cystic carcinoma and small cell neuroendocrine carcinoma. The tumor cells are positive for epithelial marker 34B E12, EMA and P63.

Management of basaloid squamous cell carcinoma which is considered by many authors as more aggressive tumor requires radical excision followed by locoregional radiation and chemotherapy. For advance cases combination of radiotherapy and chemotherapy is a logical approach to control the disease. The overall disease free survival rate statically is slightly lower than in the conventional type of squamous cell carcinoma. Meanwhile some studies concluded that the prognosis is comparable to conventional type but the number of cases is to small to draw a definite conclusion. Metastatic disease is recorded in many patients with basaloid squamous cell carcinoma and it is advisable to perform metastatic work up. In conclusion the disease appears in most reported cases in the literature as more aggressive and capable of distant metastasis. [17, 25].

4. References

[1] Hurt, M.A, Santa Cruz, D.J Tumors of the skin in Daignostic histopathology of tumors 2nd Edition, Vol 2, Churchill Livingstone 2000.

[2] Glover MT, Deeks JJ, Raftery MJ, Cunningham J, Leigh IM. Immunosuppression and risk of non-melanoma skin cancer in renal transplant recipients. Lancet 1997;349:398.

[3] Ereño C, Gaafar A, Garmendia M, Etxezarraga C, Bilbao FJ, López JI Basaloid squamous cell carcinoma of the head and neck: a clinicopathological and follow-up study of 40 cases and review of the literature. Head neck pathol, 2008 Jun; 2(2):83-91. Epub 2008 Mar 21

[4] Silverberg SG, Ioffe OB. Pathology of cervical cancer. Cancer J. 2003 Sep-Oct;9(5):335-47

[5] Shinton NK. The histological classification of lower respiratory tract tumors. Br J Cancer. 1963, 17:213-21

[6] Radhi JM, Awad SM.Bilateral squamous cell carcinoma of the ovary;case report Br J Obstet Gynaecol. 1990 Sep;97(9):855-6.

[7] Powell JL, Stinson JA, Connor GP, Shiro BS, Mattison M. Squamous cell carcinoma arising in a dermoid cyst of the ovary Gynecol Oncol. 2003 Jun;89(3):526-

[8] Kanner WA, Brill LB 2nd, Patterson JW, Wick MR. CD10, p63 and CD99 expression in the differential diagnosis of atypical fibroxanthoma, spindle cell squamous cell carcinoma and desmoplastic melanoma J Cutan Pathol. 2010 Jul;37(7):744-50

[9] Requena L, Sánchez M, Requena I, Alegre V, Sánchez Yus E. Clear cell squamous cell carcinoma. A histologic, immunohistologic, and ultrastructural study J Dermatol Surg Oncol. 1991 Aug; 17(8):656-60.

[10] Chaux A, Soares F, Rodríguez I, Barreto J, Lezcano C, Torres J, Velazquez EF, Cubilla AL. Papillary squamous cell carcinoma, not otherwise specified (NOS) of the penis:

clinicopathologic features, differential diagnosis, and outcome of 35 cases Am J Surg Pathol. 2010 Feb;34(2):223-30.

[11] Wain, S. L., R. Kier, R. T. Vollmer, and E. H. Bossen. 1986. Basaloid-squamous carcinoma of the tongue, hypopharynx, and larynx: report of 10 cases. Hum Pathol 17:1158-66.

[12] Choussy, O., M. Bertrand, A. Francois, E. Blot, H. Hamidou, and D. Dehesdin. Basaloid squamous cell carcinoma of the head and neck: report of 18 cases. J Laryngol Otol:1-6.

[13] Kwon, Y. S., Y. M. Kim, G. W. Choi, Y. T. Kim, and J. H. Nam. 2009. Pure basaloid squamous cell carcinoma of the uterine cervix: a case report. J Korean Med Sci 24:542-5.

[14] Nagakawa, H., K. Hiroshima, Y. Takiguchi, M. Yatomi, Y. Takahashi, M. Mikami, Y. Nakatani, and T. Kuriyama. 2006. Basaloid squamous-cell carcinoma of the lung in a young woman. Int J Clin Oncol 11:66-8.

[15] Neves, T. R., M. J. Soares, P. G. Monteiro, M. S. Lima, and H. G. Monteiro. Basaloid squamous cell carcinoma in the urinary bladder with small-cell carcinoma. J Clin Oncol 29:e440-2.

[16] Vasudev, P., O. Boutross-Tadross, and J. Radhi. 2009. Basaloid squamous cell carcinoma: two case reports. Cases J 2:9351.

[17] Wieneke JA, Thompson L, Weng BM Basaloid squamous cell carcinoma of sinonasal tract, cancer 1999;85.841-854

[18] Kleist B, Bankau A, Lorenz G, Jäger B, Poetsch M. Laryngoscope 2004 Different risk factors in basaloid and common squamous head and neck cancer.114(6):1063-8.

[19] Thariat, J., C. Badoual, C. Faure, C. Butori, P. Y. Marcy, and C. A. Righini. Basaloid squamous cell carcinoma of the head and neck: role of HPV and implication in treatment and prognosis. J Clin Pathol 63:857-66.

[20] Friedrich RE, Sperber C, Jäkel T, Röser K, Löning T Basaloid lesions of oral squamous epithelial cells and their association with HPV infection and P16 expression. Anticancer Res ;30(5):1605-12.

[21] Thariat J, Ahamad A, El-Naggar AK, Williams MD, Holsinger FC, Glisson BS, Allen PK, Morrison WH, Weber RS, Ang KK, Garden AS. Outcomes after radiotherapy for basaloid squamous cell carcinoma of the head and neck: a case-control study. Cancer 2008 Jun 15;112(12):2698-709.

[22] Hewan-Lowe, K., and I. Dardick.. Ultrastructural distinction of basaloid-squamous carcinoma and adenoid cystic carcinoma. Ultrastruct Pathol 1995; 19:371-81.

[23] Kim K H, Sung M W et al Adeniod cystic carcinoma of the head and neck.Arch Otolaryngol,Head Neck Surg 1994,120;721-726.

[24] Azorín D, López-Ríos F, Ballestín C, Barrientos N, Rodríguez-Peralto JL. Primary cutanous, adenosquamous carcinoma case report and review of the litreture .J Cutan Pathol. 2001 Nov; 28(10):542-5.

[25] Paulino A, Singh M, Shah A, Huvos A. Basaloid Squamous Cell Carcinoma of the Head and Neck. The Laryngoscope Volume 110, Issue 9, pages 1479–1482, September 2000.

Part 2

Adjuvant Therapeutic Strategies for Squamous Cell Carcinoma

5

Neoadjuvant Chemotherapy Using Platinum-Based Regimens for Stage Ib2-II Squamous Cell Carcinoma and Non-Squamous Cell Carcinoma of the Cervix

Tadahiro Shoji et al.*
Department of Obstetrics and Gynecology, Iwate Medical University School of Medicine Japan

1. Introduction

The methods used for treating stage Ib2-IIb cervical cancers, with a bulky mass, differ between Japan and Western countries. In Western countries, concurrent chemoradiation (CCRT) has been recommended as a standard therapy for such tumors based on the results of multiple large-scale randomized trials and meta-analyses (Morris et al., 1999; Rose et al., 1999; Whitney et al., 1999; Pearcey et al., 2002; Eifel et al. 2004; Green et al. 2001; Lukka et al., 2002). In Japan, Korea, Italy and some other countries, the neoadjuvant chemotherapy (NAC) approach has been extensively introduced to clinical practice (Sugiyama et al., 1999). NAC is considered to be clinically significant in 2 respects: it is expected to improve the radicality and safety of surgery by reducing tumor size; and it is expected to exert systemic effects, i.e., effects on lymph node occult micrometastases, etc. A disadvantage of NAC is delayed initiation of the primary treatment, suggesting the necessity of completing NAC as an auxiliary therapy within a short period of time. Therefore, we may find that NAC is valuable if it can exert efficacy rapidly with high platinum dose intensity (DI), assuring that subsequent primary surgical therapy can be performed as soon as possible. At our facility, a platinum-based regimen has been used for NAC in patients with cervical cancer. Herein, we review the efficacy and safety data on NAC for squamous cell carcinoma of the uterine cervix. We previously reported our interim data and now present the results of an ongoing pilot study on the efficacy and safety of NAC for non-squamous cell carcinoma of the uterine cervix.

2. Subjects and methods

2.1 Subjects

We studied 43 patients with locally advanced cancer of the uterine cervix (clinical stage Ib2 to IIb) who gave informed consent to participate in this study between January 2002 and

---

*Eriko Takatori, Hideo Omi, Masahiro Kagabu, Tastuya Honda, Yuichi Morohara, Seisuke Kumagai, Fumiharu Miura, Satoshi Takeuchi, Akira Yoshizaki and Toru Sugiyama
Department of Obstetrics and Gynecology, Iwate Medical University School of Medicine, Japan

September 2010. All 43 were scheduled to undergo a radical hysterectomy, including 23 with squamous cell carcinoma and 20 with non-squamous cell carcinoma.

2.2 Inclusion criteria

The following set of inclusion criteria was employed for selection of study subjects. (1) Histologically verified squamous cell carcinoma or non-squamous cell carcinoma of the uterine cervix; (2) locally advanced stage Ib2 to IIb; (3) age: 20 years upward and less than 70 years; (4) Eastern Cooperative Oncology Group (ECOG) performance status (PS): 0-2; (5) initially treated case; (6) the presence of an MRI-measurable bulky mass in the uterine cervix; (7) hematologic and blood biochemical findings meeting the following criteria [WBC count $\geq$ 4,000/mm^3 ; neutrophil count $\geq$ 2,000/mm^3 ; platelet count $\geq$ 100,000/mm^3 ; hemoglobin $\geq$10.0 g/dl ; AST and ALT levels $\leq$ 2 times the upper limit of normal reference range at study site ; serum total bilirubin level $\leq$1.5 mg/dl ; serum creatinine $\leq$1.5 mg/dl ; and creatinine clearance $\geq$60 ml/min]; (8)life expectancy $\geq$6 months; and (9) written informed consent personally given by the subject.

2.3 Exclusion criteria

Exclusion criteria were prescribed as follows. (1) Patients with overt infection; (2) patients with a serious complication(s) (e.g., cardiac disease, poorly controlled diabetes mellitus, malignant hypertension, bleeding tendency); (3) patients with active multiple cancer; (4) patients with interstitial pneumonia or pulmonary fibrosis; (5) patients with effusions; (6) patients with a history of unstable angina or myocardial infarction within 6 months after registration, or with a concurrent serious arrhythmia requiring treatment; (7) patients in whom treatment with cisplatin (CDDP), irinotecan (CPT-11), paclitaxel (PTX), docetaxel (DTX) and carboplatin (CBDCA) is contraindicated; (8) patients with (watery) diarrhea; (9) patients with intestinal paralysis or ileus; (10) pregnant women, nursing mothers or women wishing to become pregnant; (11) patients with a history of serious drug hypersensitivity or drug allergy; and (12) patients who were inadequate for safe conduct of this study as judged by the attending physician.

2.4 Administration method and criteria for modification

2.4.1 NAC for squamous cell carcinoma

One course of NAC consisted of 21 days, with a CDDP dose of 70 mg/m^2 on Day 1 and intravenous CPT-11 doses of 70 mg/m^2 on Days 1 and 8. As a rule, 2 courses of NAC were administered to each patient (Fig.1).

2.4.1.1 Criteria for skipping CPT-11

In cases in which hematological data within 2 days before Day 8 did not satisfy the following criteria, CPT-11 was skipped on Day 8: 1) neutrophil count $\geq$ 1,000/mm^3, 2) platelet count $\geq$ 75,000/mm^3.

2.4.1.2 Criteria for starting the next course of NAC

In cases in which hematological data within 2 days before the planned start of the next course of treatment did not satisfy the following criteria, starting the second course was postponed by 2 weeks at a maximum: 1) neutrophil count ≥ 1,500/mm³, 2) platelet count ≥ 75,000/mm³, 3) serum creatinine ≤ 1.5 mg/dl.

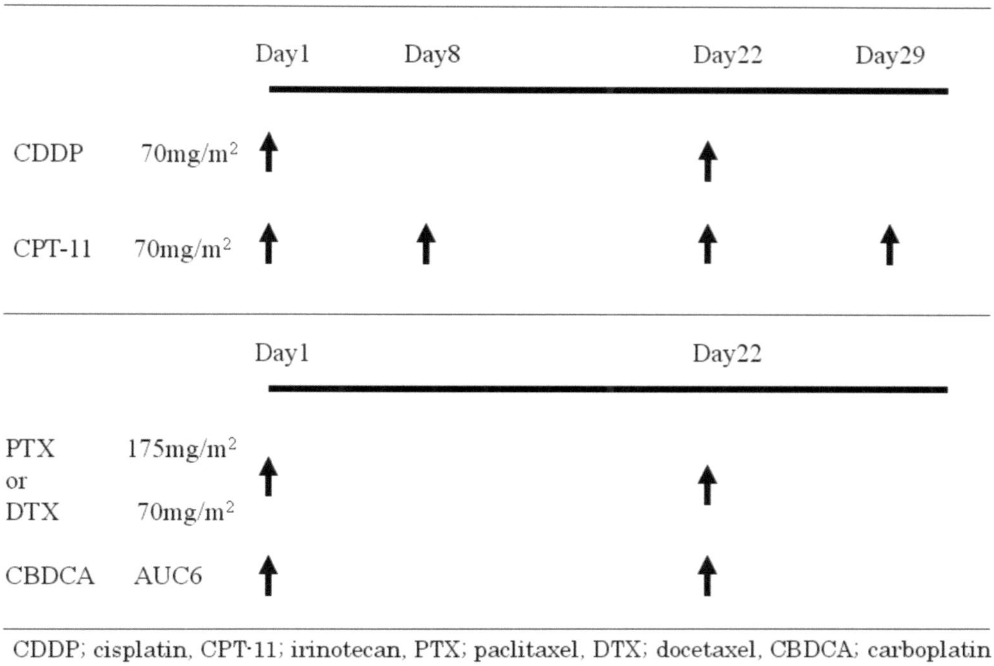

Fig. 1. Treatment protocol of NAC for cervical cancer

2.4.1.3 Dose reduction criteria

In cases exhibiting the following signs of toxicity during the first course of treatment, the CPT-11 and CDDP doses for the second course were reduced from 70 mg/m² to 60 mg/m²: Grade 4 neutropenia lasting 7 days or more; febrile neutropenia lasting 4 days or more; Grade 4 thrombocytopenia; Grade 3 thrombocytopenia accompanied by bleeding; and Grade 3 or more severe non-hematological signs of toxicity other than nausea and vomiting.

2.4.2 NAC for non-squamous cell carcinoma

One course of treatment was 21 days, with a PTX dose of 175 mg/m² or DTX dose of 70 mg/m² on Day 1 and intravenous CBDCA AUC 6 on Day 1. As a rule, 2 courses of treatment were administered to each patient (Fig.1) .

2.4.2.1 Criteria for starting the next course of treatment

In cases in which hematological data within 2 days before the planned start of the second course of treatment did not satisfy the following criteria, starting the second course was postponed by 2 weeks at a maximum: 1) neutrophil count ≥ 1,000/mm³, 2) platelet count ≥ 75,000/mm³.

2.4.2.2 CBDCA dose reduction criteria

In cases exhibiting the following signs of toxicity during the first course of treatment, the CBDCA dose for the second course was reduced from AUC 6 to 5. If signs of toxicity remained after this dose reduction, that for the third course of treatment was reduced from AUC 5 to 4: Grade 4 thrombocytopenia; and Grade 3 thrombocytopenia accompanied by bleeding.

2.4.2.3 PTX dose reduction criteria

In cases exhibiting signs of Grade 2 or more severe peripheral nerve toxicity during the first course, the PTX dose for the second course was reduced from 175 mg/m^2 to 135 mg/m^2. If Grade 2 or more severe peripheral nerve toxicity remained after dose reduction, the PTX dose for the third course was reduced from 135 mg/m^2 to 110 mg/m^2.

2.4.2.4 DTX dose reduction criteria

In cases exhibiting the following signs of toxicity during the first course, the DTX dose for the second course was reduced from 70 mg/m^2 to 60 mg/m^2. If signs of toxicity remained after this dose reduction, the DTX dose for the third course was reduced from 60 mg/m^2 to 50 mg/m^2: Grade 4 neutropenia lasting 7 days or more; and febrile neutropenia lasting 4 days or more.

2.5 Supportive therapy

A granulocyte-colony stimulating factor (G-CSF) preparation was administered in patients developing Grade 4 neutropenia during the first course of NAC. Administration of the G-CSF preparation was permitted for prophylactic purposes during the second and subsequent courses of NAC in cases exhibiting Grade 4 neutropenia during the first course. Anti-emetics were additionally used for prophylactic purposes.

2.6 Observations and tests

The primary endpoint was anti-tumor response. Secondary endpoints were adverse events, surgery completion rate, progression-free survival period, and overall survival period. Hematological tests and urinalysis were carried out before the start of treatment and once weekly, as a rule, after starting treatment. Electrocardiograms and chest X-rays were obtained before the start and at the end of treatment.

2.6.1 Evaluation of anti-tumor response

Anti-tumor response was evaluated using Response Evaluation Criteria in Solid Tumors (RECIST) by comparing the baseline findings (before the start of treatment) on magnetic resonance imaging (MRI) with the MRI findings at the end of treatment courses. Efficacy evaluation adopted the best rating, without incorporating the response period.

2.6.2 Evaluation of adverse events

Adverse events were evaluated employing the National Cancer Institute Common Toxicity Criteria (NCI-CTCAE) version 3.0.

2.7 Primary treatment

Patients with stage Ib2-IIb carcinoma underwent a radical hysterectomy unless the response of the tumor to preoperative treatment was progressive disease (PD) and the tumor was up-staged. In cases in which surgery was not possible, concurrent CCRT was adopted.

2.8 Postoperative therapy

Postoperative radiotherapy or chemotherapy was undertaken additionally in patients with positive vaginal stump, positive lymphadenopathy, positive invasion of the cardinal ligament, or evident invasion of the vasculature.

3. Results

3.1. Results of NAC for squamous cell carcinoma

3.1.1 Background variables

The median age of the 23 patients was 40 (range: 25-63) years. PS was 0 in 20 cases (87.0%) and 1 in 3 (13.0%). The clinical stage of the tumor was Ib5 in 5 cases (21.7%), IIa in 2 (8.7%), and IIb in 16 (69.6%). All patients received 2 courses of NAC (Table 1).

		SCC (N=23)		Non-SCC (N=20)
Age years [Median, Range]		40 [25-63]		52 [32-63]
Performance status at entry	0	19 (82.6%)		15 (75.0%)
	1	4 (17.4%)		5 (25.0%)
	2	0 (0%)		0 (0%)
FIGO Stage at initial diagnosis	Ib	5 (21.7%)		5 (25.0%)
	IIa	2 (8.7%)		0 (0%)
	IIb	16 (69.6%)		15 (75.0%)
Cell type	SCC	23 (100.0%)	Mucinous	9 (45.0%)
			Endometrioid	3 (15.0%)
			Clear cell	1 (5.0%)
			Adenosquamous	7 (35.0%)
Number of Cycles	1	0 (0%)		1 (5.0%)
	2	23 (100%)		16 (80.0%)
	3	0 (0%)		3 (15.0%)

SCC; Squamous cell carcinoma

Table 1. Patient characteristics

3.1.2 Anti-tumor response

The response of the tumor to treatment was assessed in all cases. Five (21.7%) showed a complete response (CR), 15 (65.2%) a partial response (PR), 2 (8.7%) stable disease (SD), and 1 (4.3%) PD. Thus, the response rate was 87.0% (Table 2). Among the cases rated as showing

CR or PR, none showed tumor growth between the end of the first course and the end of the second course of treatment.

	CR	PR	SD	PD	Overall Response
SCC	5 (21.7%)	15 (65.2%)	2 (8.7%)	1 (4.3%)	20 (87.0%)
Non-SCC	4 (20.0%)	11 (55.0%)	5 (25.0%)	0 (0%)	15 (75.0%)

	Surgery completion rate	Median PFS (range)	Median OS (range)
SCC	100%	30 (8-93)	34 (8-93)
Non-SCC	75%	10.5 (3-70)	20 (6-70)

CR,; complete response; PR; pertial response; SD; stable disease; PD; progressive disease
PFS; Progression-free survival, OS; Overall survival

Table 2. Response and clinical outcome

3.1.3 Adverse events

Grade 3 or more severe leukopenia and neutropenia were seen in 6 cases (26.1%) and 14 cases (60.9%), respectively. Grade 3 febrile neutropenia was seen in 1 case (4.3%). The G-CSF preparation was used in 11 (55.0%) of the 23 cases; during 17 (42.5%) of the 46 treatment cycles in total. The mean duration of G-CSF treatment during each course was 3.1 days. Grade 3 or more severe anemia was noted in 3 cases (15.0%), including one patient with Grade 1 anemia requiring blood transfusion. None of the patients developed Grade 3 or more severe thrombocytopenia. Signs of Grade 3 or more severe non-hematological toxicity included nausea in 2 cases (8.7%) and vomiting in 1 (4.3%) (Table 3). No treatment-associated deaths occurred. Chemotherapy was completed as scheduled in 21 (91.3%) of the 23 cases. In the remaining 2 cases, the CPT-11 dose on Day 2 of the second course was skipped. In these 2 cases, the dose was skipped at the discretion of the attending physician because of persistent Grade 3 nausea. There were 2 cases (8.7%) in which the start of the second course was postponed because the neutrophil count criterion was not satisfied. In both cases, the second course was started within 7 days. In one case (4.3%) showing febrile neutropenia lasting at least 4 days, the CDDP and CPT-11 doses for the second course were reduced from 70 mg/m^2 to 60 mg/m^2.

3.1.4 Surgery completion rate and survival period

The completion rate of radical hysterectomy after NAC was 100%. The median follow-up period was 35 months (range: 8-93 months). The median progression-free survival period was 30 months (8-93 months). The median overall survival period was 34 months (8-93 months) (Table 2).

	Grade				
	1	2	3	4	≥3 (%)
Leukopenia	2	15	5	1	6 (26.1)
Neutropenia	1	8	7	7	14(60.9)
Thrombocytopenia	5	2	0	0	0
Anemia	9	12	1	1	2 (8.7)
Nausea	15	6	2	0	2 (8.7)
Vomiting	12	7	1	0	1 (4.3)
Diarrhea	1	0	0	0	0
Neurotoxicity	0	0	0	0	0
Renaltoxicity	0	0	0	0	0
Fibrile neutropenia	0	0	1	0	1 (4.3)

CDDP; cisplatin, CPT-11; irinotecan

Table 3. Toxicity of CPT-11+CDDP therapy (n=23)

3.2 Results of NAC for non-squamous cell carcinoma

3.2.1 Background variables

The median age of the 20 patients was 51 (range: 30-63) years. PS was 0 in 15 cases (75.0%) and 1 in 5 (15.0%). The clinical stage was Ib2 in 5 cases (25.0%) and IIb in 15 (75.0%). The histological type was mucinous adenocarcinoma in 9 cases (45.0%), endometrioid adenocarcinoma in 3 (15.0%), clear cell adenocarcinoma in 1 (5.0%), and adenosquamous carcinoma in 7 (35.0%). One course of NAC was administered to 1 case (5.0%), 2 courses to 16 (80.0%), and 3 courses to 3 (15.0%) (Table 1).

3.2.2 Anti-tumor response

The response was rated as CR in 4 cases (20.0%), PR in 11 (55.0%), SD in 5 (10.0%), and PD in 1 (4.3%), with the response rate being 75.0% (Table 2).

3.2.3 Adverse events

Grade 3 or more severe leukopenia and neutropenia were seen in 10 (50.0%) and 19 (95.0%) cases, respectively. Grade 3 febrile neutropenia was noted in 2 cases (10.0%). The G-CSF preparation was used for 13 (65.0%) of the 20 cases; it was administered during 19 (45.2%) of the 42 cycles in total. The mean duration of G-CSF preparation treatment during each course was 3.0 days. None of the cases showed Grade 3 or more severe anemia or thrombocytopenia. The only sign of Grade 3 or more severe non-hematological toxicity was nausea, seen in one case (5.0%). None of the cases had signs of Grade 2 or more severe neurotoxicity (Table 4).

In 3 cases (15.0%), the start of the second course of treatment was postponed because the neutrophil count criterion was not satisfied. In all 3 of these cases, the second course was started within 7 days. Both cases (10.0%) with Grade 3 febrile neutropenia for 4 days or more had received DTX/CBDCA therapy prior to the development of neutropenia. In these 2 cases, DTX (from 70 mg/m2 to 60 mg/m2) and CBDCA (from AUC 6 to 5) doses were reduced for the second course of treatment.

3.2.4 Surgery completion rate and survival period

A radical hysterectomy after NAC was completed in 15 of the 20 cases, i.e., the surgery completion rate was 75.0%. The median follow-up period was 20 months (6-70 months). The median progression-free survival period was 10.5 months (3-70 months) and the median overall survival period was 20 months (6-70 months) (Table2).

	Grade				
	1	2	3	4	≥3 (%)
Leukopenia	2	8	9	1	10(50.0)
Neutropenia	1	0	6	13	19(95.0)
Thrombocytopenia	10	0	0	0	0
Anemia	10	10	0	0	0
Nausea	9	2	1	0	1 (5.0)
Vomiting	5	2	0	0	0
Diarrhea	2	0	0	0	0
Neurotoxicity	18	0	0	0	0
Renaltoxicity	0	0	0	0	0
Dyspnea	2	0	0	0	0
Fibrile neutropenia	0	0	2	0	2 (10.0)

TC; Paclitaxel+Carboplatin, DC; Docetaxel+Carboplatin

Table 4. Toxicity of TC or DC therapy (n=20)

4. Discussion

A meta-analysis of the results of NAC for squamous cell carcinoma of the uterine cervix ruled out the effectiveness of radiotherapy applied as the primary treatment but suggested the effectiveness of surgery employed as primary therapy. This analysis suggested the effectiveness of NAC, if: one cycle of treatment lasted no more than 14 days; and the DI of CDDP exceeded 25 $mg/m^2/week$ (Neoadjuvant Chemotherapy for Cervical Cancer Meta-analysis Collaboration., 2003). Sugiyama et al reported a CDDP/CPT-11 therapy schedule involving CPT-11 doses on Days 1, 8, and 15 (one course = 28 days) (Sugiyama et al., 1999). We evaluated the efficacy and safety of CDDP/CPT-11 therapy, reportedly an effective NAC regimen, using modified doses and administration schedules. In our study, a single dose was set at 70 mg/m^2 for both CDDP and CPT-11, and the therapy was administered for 2 cycles at an interval of 3 weeks, with CDDP administered on Day 1 and CPT-11 on Days 1 and 8. In this way, the DI of CDDP was raised to 23.3 mg/m^2/week, and this schedule was expected to reduce the need to skip treatments. Thus, it seems valuable to be able to reduce the time interval from NAC to surgery.

In an analysis of adverse events, Grade 3 or more severe neutropenia developed in 14 (60.9%) of the 23 cases, but subsided in response to short-term treatment with a G-CSF preparation. Severe diarrhea, specific to CPT-11, was not seen in any case when this agent was administered at a dose of 70 mg/m^2, suggesting that the quality of life (QOL) of patients was maintained during this therapy. The first course of treatment was administered as scheduled in all cases. The start of the second course was delayed, by no more than 7 days, in 3 cases. Furthermore, the CPT-11 dose on Day 8 was skipped in 2 cases. Dose reduction during the second course was necessary in only 2 cases, suggesting that this regimen does not increase the toxicity of these drugs as compared to the dosing regimen with 4-week intervals. Furthermore, the response rate (87.6%) and the surgery completion rate (100%) were satisfactory. Regarding the outcomes of patients treated with this regimen, further follow-up is needed.

Non-squamous cell carcinoma of the uterine cervix has been steadily rising in Japan, currently accounting for approximately 10% to 15% of all cervical cancer cases. Lymph node metastasis is more frequent in cases with invasive non-squamous cell carcinoma than in those with invasive squamous cell carcinoma (Aoki et al., 2002) and sensitivities to radiotherapy and chemotherapy are considered to be lower with non-squamous cell carcinoma (Landoni et al., 1997). Thus, squamous and non-squamous cell carcinomas must be analyzed separately. It is advisable to try new therapeutic strategies for non-squamous cell carcinoma, but the number of published studies involving cases with this type of cervical cancer is small, and the number of cases analyzed is also small. Thus, no high-level evidence has been obtained for this type of cervical cancer. The response rates of adenocarcinoma are reportedly 20% (Thigpen et al., 1986), 15% (Sutton et al., 1993), 14% (Look et al., 1997), and 12% (Rose et al., 2003) to uncombined therapies with CDDP, ifosmide, 5-FU, and oral etoposide, respectively, indicating that the response rates of adenocarcinoma to these therapies tend to be lower than those of squamous cell carcinoma. However, according to the report by Curtin et al, the response rate of adenocarcinoma was as high as 31% even when PTX was used independently (Curtin et al., 2001). DTX has also been attracting considerable interest. Nagao et al evaluated the efficacy of combined chemotherapy using DTX + CBDCA (DTX 60 mg/m^2 on Day 1, CBDCA AUC 6 on day 1 and then every 21 days) in 17 patients with advanced/recurrent cervical cancer, including 6 with adenocarcinoma and 1 with adenosquamous carcinoma, reporting that a PR was obtained in 6 of the 7 cases with adenocarcinoma (including the one with adenosquamous carcinoma) and that the response rate was thus 86% (Nagao et al., 2005). Following these findings, we conducted a pilot study involving standard regimens of PTX/CBDCA and DTX/CBDCA conventionally used for the treatment of ovarian cancer.

In the analysis of adverse events, Grade 3 or more severe neutropenia developed in 19 (95.0%) of the 20 cases, but subsided in response to short-term treatment with a G-CSF preparation (mean dosing period: 3.0 days/course). During the first course of DTX/CBDCA therapy, Grade 3 febrile neutropenia developed in 2 cases. In these 2 cases, the dose was reduced during the next course of treatment (DTX, from 70 mg/m^2 to 60 mg/m^2; CBDCA, from AUC 6 to 5). All signs of peripheral neuropathy specific to taxanes, observed during this study, were Grade 1 or less severe, allowing continuation of treatment while preserving the QOL of individual patients. No serious adverse events occurred, and the response rate was 75%, but the completion rate of surgery (radical hysterectomy) was 75%. Thus, the outcomes of treatment in this study were not satisfactory. Possible reasons are: rapid progression of non-squamous cell carcinoma, frequent invasion of tissues/organs surrounding the uterus, and frequent lymph node metastasis.

Numerous reports on phase II studies of NAC for cervical cancer have been published, demonstrating effectiveness in 70%-80% of all cases. Table 5 shows the results of the present study in comparison to those of previous reports (Sugiyama et al., 1999; Hwang et al., 2001; Dueñas-Gonzalez et al., 2001; D'Agostino et al., 2002; Di Vagno et al., 2003; Dueñas-Gonzalez et al., 2003; Umesaki et al., 2004; Shoji et al., 2010; Shoji et al., 2010) and this study.

Author	Year	N.P.	Stage	Histlogical type	Regimens	R.R.(%)
Sugiyama T, et al	1999	23	Ib2, IIb, IIIb	SCC	CDDP+CPT-11	78
Hwang YY, et al	2001	80	Ib2-IIb	SCC, Non-SCC	CDDP+VLB+BLM	94
Gonzalez DA, et al	2001	41	Ib2-IIIb	SCC, Non-SCC	CDDP+GEM	95
Agostino G, et al	2002	42	Ib2-IVa	SCC, Non-SCC	CDDP+EPI+PTX	79
Vagno G, et al	2003	58	Ib2-IIIb	SCC, Non-SCC	CDDP+VNR	85
Gonzalez DA, et al	2003	43	Ib2-IIIb	SCC, Non-SCC	CBDCA+PTX	95
Umesaki N, et al	2004	25	Ib2, IIb, IIIb	SCC	CPT-11+MMC	76
Shoji T, et al	2010	15	Ib2-IIb	SCC	CDDP+CPT-11	87
Shoji T, et al	2010	66	Ib2-IIb	SCC	NDP+CPT-11	76
Shoji T, et al	·	*23*	*Ib2-IIb*	*SCC*	*CDDP+CPT-11*	*87*
Shoji T, et al	·	*20*	*Ib2-IIb*	*Non-SCC*	*CBDCA+PTX or DTX*	*75*

N.P.: number of patients
R.R.: response rate
CDDP: cisplatin, CPT-11: irinotecan, VLB: vinblastine, BLM: bleomycin, GEM: gemcitabine, PTX: paclitaxel, EPI: epirubicin, VNR: vinorelbine, CBDCA: carboplatin, MMC: mitomycinC, NDP: nedaplatin, DTX: docetaxel

Table 5. Phase II study of NAC for cervical cancer

Most of the reports shown pertain to evaluation of both squamous cell carcinoma and non-squamous cell carcinoma. There is an urgent need to conduct clinical studies on each histological type of cervical cancer and to establish new methods of treatment specific to each type. Only a limited number of reports have demonstrated a high response rate to correlate with a better outcome. Thus, randomized controlled trials (RCT) designed to assess improvement of long-term outcomes are essential. As an RCT evaluating outcomes after NAC, Sardi et al reported a study involving comparisons among 4 groups (NAC + surgery + radiotherapy, surgery + radiotherapy, uncombined radiotherapy, NAC + radiotherapy). They found that the survival rate improved significantly with NAC + surgery +

radiotherapy (7-year survival rate: 41%) as compared to surgery + radiotherapy (41%) (Sardi et al., 1997). Serur et al retrospectively compared the outcomes of treating stage Ib cases between a NAC + surgery group and a surgery alone group, demonstrating a higher 5-year survival rate in the NAC + surgery group although the difference was not statistically significant (80% vs 69%) (Serur et al., 1997). Tierney et al reported the results of a meta-analysis, stating that there was no prognostic improvement (Neoadjuvant Chemotherapy for Cervical Cancer Metaanalysis Colloaboration, 2003). Thus, there is no consensus on this issue.

The JCOG0102 was a representative randomized study of NAC conducted in Japan, designed as an RCT comparing the outcomes of treatment for stage Ib2-IIb cases with bulky tumors between radical hysterectomy (+RT) and NAC + radical hysterectomy (+RT). The JCOG0102 used bleomycin/vincristine/mitomycinC/cisplatin (BOMP) as the NAC regimen. In that study, the response rate to BOMP therapy was low as 61%, and the interim results did not endorse the usefulness of this therapy, forcing the study to be discontinued prematurely (Katsumata et al., 2006). The JGOG1065 was a phase II clinical study on NAC + radical hysterectomy, using nedaplatin and CPT-11 for NAC, carried out in 66 patients with stage Ib2-IIb cervical cancer with a bulky tumor. In that study, the response rate was 75.8% and the 2-year recurrence-free survival period was 73.8% (Shoji et al., 2010). This therapy is expected to reduce nephrotoxicity and adverse events such as nausea and vomiting and appears to be a useful regimen for patients with renal dysfunction and elderly patients from the viewpoint of QOL. However, the response rate to this therapy has not exceeded that to CDDP + CPT-11. At present, there is no plan to launch a phase III clinical study on NAC (NDP/CPT-11) + radical hysterectomy vs. CCRT. There is no evidence supporting the view that NAC improves the outcomes of patients with cervical cancer, and NAC has not been recommended in any set of guidelines. Further studies on the indications for and efficacy of NAC are clearly needed.

5. Conclusions

Irinotecan/cisplatin therapy for squamous carcinoma of the uterine cervix and PTX/CBDCA and DTX/CBDCA therapies for non-squamous cell carcinoma of the uterine cervix showed high anti-tumor efficacy, and the adverse reactions to these therapies could be dealt with satisfactorily, thus allowing safe treatment. In cases with squamous cell carcinoma, outcomes are expected to be improved by NAC, but further evaluation of the outcomes of patients with non-squamous cell carcinoma is awaited.

6. References

Aoki, Y.; Sato, T. & Watanabe, M. et al. (2002). Neoadjuvant chemotherapy using low-dose consecutive intraarterial infusion of cisplatin combined with 5FU for locally advanced cervical adenocarcinoma. *Gynecologic Oncology*, 81, pp. 496-499, ISSN 0090-8258

Curtin, JP.; Blessing, JA. & Webster, KD. et al. (2001). Paclitaxel, an active agent in nonsquamous carcinomas of the uterine cervix: a Gynecologic Oncology Group Study. *Journal of Clinical Oncology*, 19, pp. 1275-1278, ISSN 0732-183X

D'Agostino, G.; Distefano, M. & Greggi, S. et al. (2003). Neoadjuvant treatment of locally advances carcinoma of the uterine cervix with epirubicin, paclitaxel and cisplatin. *Cancer Chemotherapy and Pharmacology*, 49, pp. 256-260, ISSN 0344-5704

Di Vagno, G.; Cormio, G. & Pignata, S. et al. (2003). Cisplatin and vinorelbine as neoadjuvant chemotherapy in locally advanced cervical cancer: a phase II study. *International Journal of Gynecological Cancer* , 13, pp. 308-312, ISSN 1048-891X.

Dueñas-Gonzalez, A.; Lopez-Graniel, C. & Gonzalez-Enciso, A. et al. (2001). A phase II study of gemcitabine and cisplatin combination as induction chemotherapy for untreated locally advanced cervical carcinoma. *Annals of Oncology*, 12, pp. 541-547, ISSN 0923-7534

Dueñas-Gonzalez, A.; López-Graniel, C. & González-Enciso, A. et al. (2003). A phase II study of multimodality treatment for locally advanced cervical cancer: neoadjuvant carboplatin and paclitaxel followed by radical hysterectomy and adjuvant cisplatin chemoradiation. *Annals of Oncology*, 14, pp.1278-1284, ISSN 0923-7534

Eifel, PJ.; Winter, K. & Morris, M. et al. (2004). Pelvic irradiation with concurrent chemotherapy versus pelvic and para-aortic irradiation for high-risk cervical cancer: an update of radiation therapy oncology group trial (RTOG) 90-01. *Journal of Clinical Oncology*, 22, pp. 872-880, ISSN 0732-183X

Green, JA.; Kirwan, JM. & Tierney, JF. et al. (2001). Survival and recurrence after concomitant chemotherapy and radiotherapy for cancer of the uterine cervix: a systematic review and meta-analysis. *Lancet*, 358, pp. 781-786, ISSN 0140-6736

Hwang, YY.; Moon, H. & Cho, SH. et al. (2001). Ten-year survival of patients with locally advanced, stage ib-iib cervical cancer after neoadjuvant chemotherapy and radical hysterectomy. *Gynecologic Oncology*, 83, pp. 88-93, ISSN 0090-8258

Katsumata, N.; Yoshikawa, H. & Hirakawa, T. et al. (2006). Phase III randomized trial of neoadjuvant chemotherapy (NAC) followed by radical hysterectomy (RH) versus RH for bulky stage I/II cervical cancer (JCOG0102). *American Society of Clinical Oncology Annual Meeting Proceedings*, #5013, 2006

Landoni, F.; Maneo, A. & Colombo, A. et al. (1997). Randomised study of radical surgery versus radiotherapy for stage Ib-IIa cervical cancer. *Lancet*, 350, pp. 535-540, ISSN 0140-6736

Look, KY.; Blessing, JA. & Valea, FA. (1997). Phase II trial of 5-fluorouracil and high-dose leucovorin in recurrent adenocarcinoma of the cervix: a Gynecologic Oncology Group study. *Gynecologic Oncology*, 67, pp. 255-258, ISSN 0090-8258

Lukka, H.; Hirte, H. & Fyles, A. et al. (2002). Concurrent cisplatin-based chemotherapy plus radiotherapy for cervical cancer-a meta analysis. *Journal of Clinical Oncology*, 14, pp.203-212, ISSN 0732-183X

Morris, M.; Eifel, PJ. & Lu, J. et al. (1999). Pelvic radiation with concurrent chemotherapy compared with pelvic and para-aortic radiation for high risk cervical cancer. *The New England journal of Medicine*, 340, pp.1137-1143, ISSN 0028-4793

Nagao, S. Fujiwara, K. & Oda, T. et al. (2005). Combination chemotherapy of docetaxel and carboplatin in advanced or recurrent cervix cancer. A pilot study. *Gynecologic Oncology,* 96, pp. 805-809, ISSN 0090-8258

Neoadjuvant Chemotherapy for Cervical Cancer Meta-analysis Collaboration. (2003). Neoadjuvant chemotherapy for locally advanced cervical cancer. a systematic review and meta-analysis of individual patient data from 21 randomised trials. *European Journal of Cancer,* 39, pp. 2470-2486, ISSN 0959-8049

Pearcey, R.; Brundage, M. & Drouin, P. et al. (2002). Phase III trial comparing radical radiotherapy with and without cisplatin chemotherapy in patients with advanced squamous cell cancer of the cervix. *Journal of Clinical Oncology,* 20, pp. 966-972, ISSN 0732-183X

Rose, PG.; Blessing, JA. & Buller, RE. et al. Prolonged oral etoposide in recurrent or advanced non-squamous cell carcinoma of the cervix: a Gynecologic Oncology Group study. *Gynecologic Oncology,* 89, pp. 267-270, ISSN 0090-8258

Rose, PG.; Bundy, BN. & Watkins, EB. et al. (1999). Concurrent cisplatin-based radiotherapy and chemotherapy for locally advanced cervical cancer. *The New England journal of Medicine,* 340, pp.1144-1153, ISSN 0028-4793

Sardi, JE.; Giaroli, A. & Sananes, C. et al. (1997). Long-term follow-up of the first randomised trial using neoadjuvant chemotherapy in stage Ib squamous carcinoma of the cervix: The final results. *Gynecologic Oncology,* 67, pp. 61-69, ISSN 0090-8258

Serur, E.; Mathews, RP. & Gates, J. et al. (1997). Neoadjuvant chemotherapy in stage IB2 squamous cell carcinoma of the cervix. *Gynecologic Oncology,* 65, pp. 348-356, ISSN 0090-8258

Shoji, T.; Takatori, E. & Hatayama, S. et al. (2010). Phase II Study of Tri-weekly Cisplatin and Irinotecan as Neoadjuvant Chemotherapy for Locally Advanced Cervical Cancer. *Oncology letters,* 1, pp. 515-519, ISSN1792-1074.

Shoji, T.; Sugiyama, T. & Yamaguchi, S. et al. (2010). Phase II Study of Neoadjuvant Chemotherapy with CPT-11 and Nedaplatin (CPT-11/NDP) for Stage Ib2/II Carcinoma of the Cervix (Japanese Gynecologic Oncology Group 1065 Study). *Proceedings of European Society of Medical Oncology,* #993 2010.

Sugiyama, T.; Nishida, T. & Kumagai, S. et al. (1999). Combination chemotherapy with irinotecan and cisplatin as neoadjuvant in locally advanced cervical cancer. *British Journal of Cancer,* 81, pp. 95-98, ISSN 0007-0920

Sutton, GP.; Blessing, JA. & DiSaia, PJ. et al. (1993). Phase II study of ifosfamide and mesna in nonsquamous carcinoma of the cervix: a Gynecologic Oncology Group study. *Gynecologic Oncology,* 49, pp. 48-50, ISSN 0090-8258

Thigpen, JT.; Blessing, JA. & Fowler, WC Jr. et al. (1986). Phase II trials of cisplatin and piperazinedione as single agents in the treatment of advanced or recurrent non-squamous cell carcinoma of the cervix: a Gynecologic Oncology Group Study. *Cancer Treatment Reports,* 70, pp. 1097-1100, ISSN 0361-5960

Umesaki, N.; Fujii, T. & Nishimura, R. et al. (2004). Phase II study of irinotecan combined with mitomycin-C for advanced or recurrent squamous cell carcinoma of the uterine cervix: the JGOG study. *Gynecologic Oncology,* 95, pp. 127-132, ISSN 0090-8258

Whitney, CW.; Sause, W. & Bundy, BN. et al. (1999). Randomized comparison of fluorouracil plus cisplatin versus hydroxyurea as an adjunct to radiation therapy in stage II B-IV A carcinoma of the cervix with negative para-aortic lymph nodes: a Gynecologic Oncology Group and Southwest Oncology Group study. *Journal of Clinical Oncology*, 17, pp.1339-1348, ISSN 0732-183X

6

Combined Therapy For Squamous Carcinoma Cells: Application of Porphyrin-Alkaloid Modified Gold Nanoparticles

Jarmila Králová[1], Kamil Záruba[2], Pavel Řezanka[1], Pavla Poučková[3], Lenka Veverková[1] and Vladimír Král[1,4]
[1]*Academy of Sciences of the Czech Republic,*
[2]*Institute of Chemical Technology Prague,*
[3]*Charles University in Prague,*
[4]*Zentiva Development (Part of Sanofi-Aventis Group)*
Czech Republic

1. Introduction

Photodynamic therapy (PDT) is an established and useful modality for the clinical non-invasive treatment of cancer. This therapy requires a photosensitizing agent (photosensitizer) selectively taken up by tumor cells, visible light, and molecular oxygen to generate highly reactive oxygen species (ROS), which ultimately cause tumor destruction. The specificity achieved from drug uptake selectivity combined with light targeting makes PDT an appealing approach.

PDT consists of three phases: excitation of photosensitizers (PS) by light, production of ROS, and induction of cell death (Triesscheijn et al., 2006). In the first phase, irradiated light of a suitable wavelength, typically visible or near-infrared, excites the PS molecules. The light is generally selected to correspond with the maximum absorption wavelength of the PS. The PS molecules then absorb light energy and change to an excited singlet state. These excited molecules can fall back to their native state with emission of fluorescence. Thus, all PS molecules are also examples of fluorescent molecules. On the other hand, the molecules also have the ability to undergo an electron spin conversion to their triplet state followed by the transfer of this energy to oxygen molecules or to other substrate molecules in the surroundings which then react with oxygen.

1.1 History of PDT

The fact that sunlight can be used to treat a variety of diseases such as rickets, psoriasis, and skin cancer is known from ancient civilizations, i.e. Egyptian, Chinese and Indian (Ackroyd et al., 2001; Daniell & Hill, 1991; Fitzpatrick & Pathak, 1959). At the beginning of the 20th century the term "photodynamic action" was used by Tappeiner et al. to explain the oxygen-consuming chemical reactions induced by photosensitization (Moan & Peng, 2003; Szeimies et al., 2001). Tappeiner, in cooperation with Jesionek, successfully treated patients suffering from stage II syphilis, lupus vulgaris, and superficial skin cancer with topical eosin red solution (Szeimies et al., 2001). In 1942, Auler and Banzer observed specific uptake and retention of hematoporphyrin in tumors followed by higher fluorescence in cancer cells as compared with the surrounding tissue, and induction of necrosis after irradiation (Szeimies et al., 2001). Afterwards, PDT had not been used until Dougherty initiated revitalization by treating a group of patients suffering from cutaneous and subcutaneous tumors with the injection of photosensitizer dihematoporphyrin and red light produced by laser. The majority of the treated tumors showed either complete or partial remission (Dougherty et al., 1975; Dougherty et al., 1978; Szeimies et al., 2001).

Particularly, PDT has grown in reputation in dermatology, mostly due to the simple accessibility of light exposure for the skin and the simplicity of topical use of photosensitizers. In the late 1970s, Thomas Dougherty initiated human clinical trials of PDT with hematoporphyrin derivative (HpD) for the treatment of cutaneous cancer metastases (Blume & Oseroff, 2007; Dougherty, 1996; Zeitouni, 2003). PDT has been revived and has become more applicable to common dermatology since 1990, when Kennedy et al. introduced 5-aminolevulinic acid (ALA) (Fig. 1), a topical porphyrin precursor causing local accumulation of the endogenous photosensitizer protoporphyrin IX (PpIX) (Fig. 2) with no significant prolonged phototoxicity (Kennedy, 1990). Nowadays, PDT is used to treat diseases in a variety of fields, including respiratory medicine (Ost, 2001; Sutedja & Postmus, 1996), urology (Jichlinski, 2006; Juarranz et al., 2008; Pinthus et al., 2006), ophthalmology (Mittra, 2002), and gastroenterology (Barr et al., 2001; Wiedmann & Caca, 2004), as well as dermatology. Mostly porphyrins or phthalocyanines have been studied (Marmur et al., 2004). On the other hand, for dermatological purposes, only hematoporphyrin derivatives such as porfimer sodium, or PpIX-inducing precursors such as ALA or methyl aminolevulinate (MAL) are of useful concern. As systemic photosensitizing drugs caused extended phototoxicity (Marmur et al., 2004), topical photosensitizers are preferred for the use in dermatology. Several drugs containing ALA or MAL are used for treating epithelial cancers and there is an increasing importance in the use of PDT (Braathen, 2001; Dragieva et al., 2004a; Dragieva et al., 2004b).

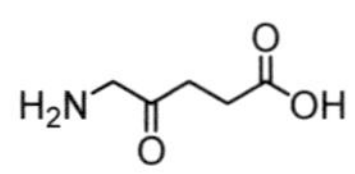

Fig. 1. Structure of 5-aminolevulinic acid

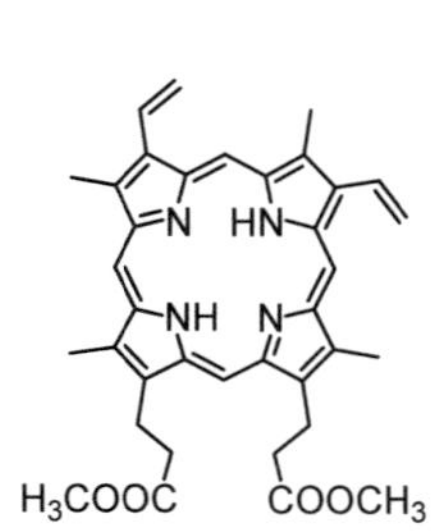

Fig. 2. Structure of protoporphyrin IX

1.2 Mechanism of PDT

PDT requires an interaction of three key elements: light, a photosensitizer, and oxygen. After exposure to particular wavelengths of light, the photosensitizer is excited from a ground state (S_0) to an excited singlet state (S_1) (Fig. 3) followed by intersystem crossing to a longer-living excited triplet state (T_1).

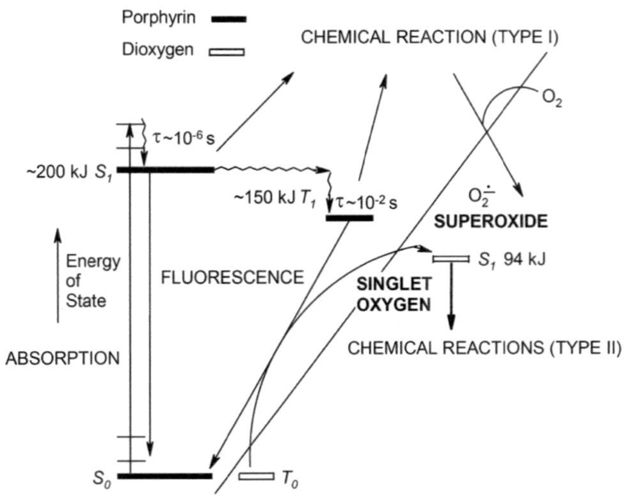

Fig. 3. Mechanism of PDT; State energies are represented by thick lines: ▬ porphyrin sensitizer, ▭ dioxygen; reactive dioxygen intermediates are in bold

After that, the photosensitizer at T_1 state is able to go through two types of reaction with nearby molecules: either a type I reaction through hydrogen or electron transfer generating free radicals, or a type II reaction through energy transfer to oxygen, creating molecular singlet oxygen ($^1O_2$). The type I reaction results in generation of reactive free radicals or radical ions, which then react with ground-state molecular oxygen to produce superoxide anion radicals, hydrogen peroxides and hydroxyl radicals (Foote, 1991). The type II reaction produces singlet oxygen which has an important role in the molecular processes initiated by PDT (Foote, 1991; Niedre et al., 2002).The singlet oxygen has a lifetime approx. 3 µs and can diffuse no more than 0.07 µm in cells (Moan, 1990; Hatz at al., 2007). Therefore, the initial damage is limited to the site of the PS molecule. This is usually the mitochondria, Golgi apparatus, plasma membrane, endosomes, lysosomes, and endoplasmic reticulum (Buytaert et al., 2007). Damage to the subcellular organelles and plasma membrane eventually leads to apoptotic, autophagic and/or necrotic cell death. Generally, PS molecules localized to the mitochondria or the endoplasmic reticulum cause apoptosis, while localization either in the plasma membrane or lysosomes is found to delay or block the apoptotic pathway. On the other hand, if the apoptotic route is blocked, damaged cells still die using the autophagic or necrotic pathways (Buytaert et al., 2007; Oleinick et al., 2002). Latest studies support apoptosis as probably the preferred path to cell death (Buytaert et al., 2007). Even though it is considered that $^1O_2$ is the main cytotoxic species and starts the pathway responsible for the damaging effects of PDT, free radicals formed by type I reactions significantly contribute to cell death as well (Foote, 1991).

1.3 Photosensitizers in PDT

The first generation of PS molecules was represented by HpD or its purified version porfimer sodium (Photofrin) (Fig. 4). Primarily, they were used as general PS and tested for cutaneous malignancies. On the other hand, general intravenous administration and the consequential prolonged phototoxicity, which can last 6–10 weeks, restricted their use (Dragieva et al., 2004; Fritsch et al., 1998).

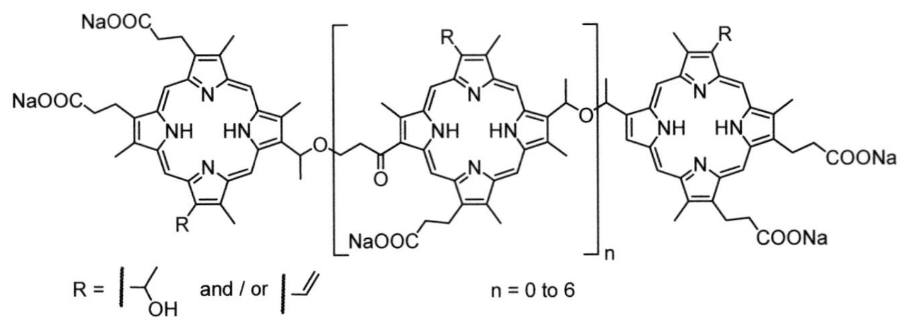

Fig. 4. Structure of Photofrin

Second generation PS molecules such as *m*-tetrahydroxyphenyl-chlorin, tin ethyl etiopurpurin, phthalocyanines, and chlorins (Fig. 5) are pure compounds that can be activated by light wavelengths in the range of 660–690 nm. Most significantly, they all have a lower tendency to cause prolonged photosensitivity compared with the first generation of photosensitizers (Moan & Berg, 1992).

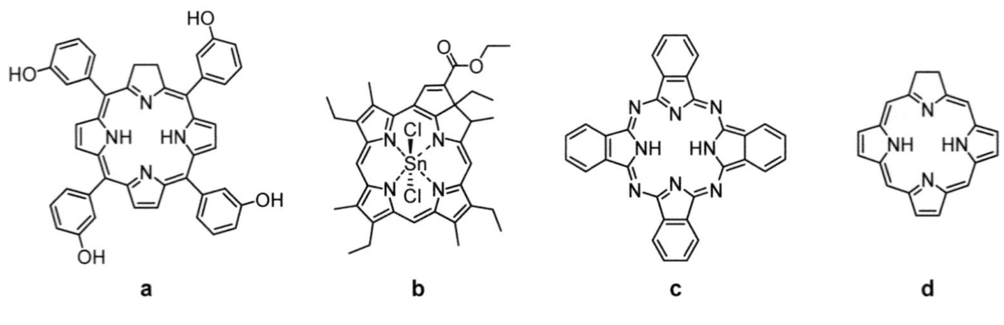

Fig. 5. Structure of *m*-tetrahydroxyphenyl-chlorin (a), tin ethyl etiopurpurin (b), phthalocyanines (c), and chlorins (d)

Third generation PS molecules (not yet approved) consist of antibody-conjugated PS (Josefsen & Boyle, 2008) and lutetium texaphyrin (Fig. 6) (Woodburn et al., 1998; Young et al., 1996). These drugs supporting deeper penetration into tissue with absorptions of 700–800 nm accumulate in tumor tissues with high selectivity.

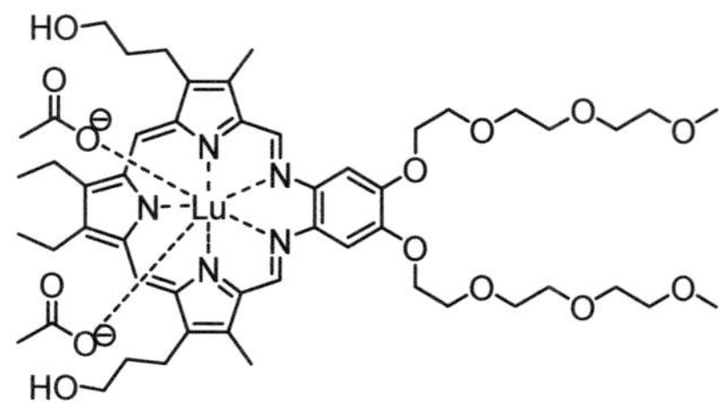

Fig. 6. Structure of lutetium texaphyrin

To avoid the prolonged photosensitivity caused by systemic administration, topically applied photosensitizers have been developed for the treatment of skin cancers. The most successful commercially accessible topical drugs are ALA and its methyl ester MAL. Levulan® using ALA and the Blu-U light source was accepted by the U. S. Food and Drug Administration for the treatment of nonhyperkeratotic actinic keratoses of the face and scalp in 1999 (Babilas et al., 2005; Kormeili et al., 2004). MAL was accepted in Europe for topical PDT of actinic keratosis (AK) and basal cell carcinoma (BCC) in 2001 (Morton, 2003; Morton et al., 2002) and for the treatment of AK in the USA in 2004 (Zeitouni et al., 2003; Garcia-Zuazaga et al., 2005). The endogenous photosensitizer PpIX generated from ALA or MAL can be fully metabolized to photodynamically inactive heme over 24–48 h (Blume & Oseroff, 2007; Morton, 2004), which radically decreases the unpleasant side effect of prolonged cutaneous phototoxicity.

1.4 Nanoparticles in PDT

In 2002 Konan et al. divided methods of PS molecules delivery into passive and active based on the presence or absence of a targeting molecule on the surface (Konan et al., 2002). The methods employed to bring the PS explicitly into diseased tissues using the target tissue receptors or antigens were designated active, whilst others that enable parenteral administration and passive targeting, such as PS conjugates of oil-dispersions, polymeric particles, liposomes, and hydrophilic polymers, were named passive. Active nanoparticles can be subclassified by their mechanism of activation and passive nanoparticles can be subclassified by material composition into (a) non-polymer-based nanoparticles, e.g. ceramic and metallic nanoparticles, and (b) biodegradable polymer-based nanoparticles.

1.4.1 Active nanoparticles

- Photosensitizer nanoparticles

Quantum dots (QDs) have great photostability, intensive fluorescent emission (high quantum yields) and possible use in specific pathological fields. They can be water soluble, and transfer energy to surrounding oxygen with resulting cellular toxicity. Many studies have been devoted to this field (Bakalova et al., 2004). The first report deals with cadmium selenide (CdSe) QDs and was published by Samia at al. in 2002. The authors presented the possibility to use semiconductor QDs alone to generate $^1O_2$ due to the intercalation of dissolved oxygen at the QD surface (Samia et al., 2003). They predicted a comparable interaction in water-soluble phospholipid-capped QDs. Moreover, they assumed that since the lowest excited state of CdSe QDs is a triplet state, the energy transfer was responsible for the generation of singlet oxygen ($^1O_2$) from triplet oxygen ($^3O_2$). On the other hand, the efficiency of generation of $^1O_2$ was about 5% (with 65% emission quantum yield of QDs) as compared to 43% for the PS only. It may be due to carrier trapping and nonradiative carrier recombinations occurring on the early picosecond time scale and the very small fraction of QD - $^3O_2$ pairs created at any moment (Samia et al., 2003). To avoid the ineffectiveness of QDs alone to produce singlet oxygen, several experiments have been carried out to covalently conjugate PSs to CdSe/ZnS via organic bridges (Hsieh et al., 2006; Samia et al., 2003). These experiments have a frequent problem with lower water solubility.

- Self-lighting nanoparticles

Scintillation or persistent luminescence nanoparticles with attached PS molecules such as porphyrins were applied as *in vivo* agents for PDT (Auzel, 2004). After exposure to ionizing radiation such as X-rays, scintillation luminescence is produced from the nanoparticles and stimulates the photosensitizers, followed by production of singlet oxygen that increases the destruction of cancer cells by ionizing radiation. Employment of common radiation therapy with PDT allows application of lower doses of radiation. Using $BaFBr:Eu^+,Mn^+$ nanoparticles displaying luminescence, short X-ray exposures could be applied followed by extended PS excitation. The period of phosphorescent decay is increased *in vivo* due to higher local temperatures (Chen et al., 2006).

- Upconversion nanoparticles

Upconversion and simultaneous two-photon absorption occurs in luminescent materials with triplet excitation states (Auzel, 2004). Upconverting nanoparticles are modified nanometer-sized composites that generate higher energy light from lower energy radiation typically near or middle infrared (anti-Stokes emission) using transition metal ions doped into a solid-state host (Boyer et al., 2006; Pires et al., 2006). For biological use, the desired nanocrystalline core should have morphological and optical features that are appropriate for conjugation with biological molecules and exhibit high intensity emission as well (Pires et al., 2006). Preparation of high-quality nanocrystals is needed, and the surface properties and growth dynamics must be precisely controlled (Wang et al., 2006). Upconversion nanoparticles can be prepared via numerous different ionic materials – typically rare earth ions such as lanthanides and actinides doped in a suitable crystalline matrix (Zijlmans et al., 1999). Micrometer-sized Er^{3+}/Yb^{3+} or Tm^{3+}/Yb^{3+} co-doped hexagonal $NaYF_4$ are examples of nanoparticles that exhibit the highest upconversion efficiencies (Heer et al., 2004) and are precursors of upconverting nanoparticles with biological applications (Zhang et al., 2006). In 2006, the $NaYF_4$ nanocrystals doped with Er and Yb and coated with organic polymers were prepared and strong emission upon activation with 980 nm NIR laser was shown (Feng et al., 2006). One year later, Zhang et al. used upconverting nanoparticles (nanoparticles of $NaYF_4:Yb^{3+},Er^{3+}$ coated with a porous thin layer of silica doped with merocyanine and functionalized with a tumor-targeting antibody) in PDT, but these nanoparticles were not activated in depth in animal tissue and the efficiency in killing cancer cells was very low (Zhang et al., 2007).

Another class of employed upconversion nanoparticles consists of zinc pthalocyanine (ZnPC) (Fig. 7) physically adsorbed to the surface of the nanoparticles with the encapsulation efficiency of 98 % (Ricci-Junior & Marchetti, 2006b). The fluorescence excitation spectrum of ZnPC exhibits an excitation maximum at 670 nm and greatly overlaps the red emission peak for the upconversion nanoparticles. Creation of $^1O_2$ by irradiation of the ZnPC-nanoparticle complex with 980 nm light was confirmed through the photobleaching of disodium 9,10-anthracenedipropionic acid (Wieder et al., 2006).

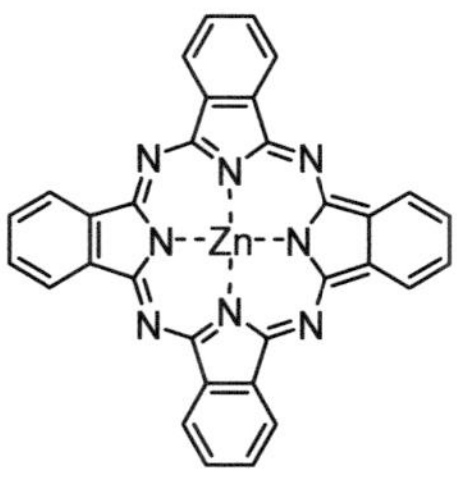

Fig. 7. Structure of zinc pthalocyanine

1.4.2 Passive nanoparticles

- Non-biodegradable nanoparticle carriers

In 2003 Roy et al. first reported ceramic-based nanoparticles used as a new drug-carrier system for PDT. It utilizes 30-nm silica-based spherical particles doped with the anticancer drug 2-devinyl-2-(1-hexyloxyethyl)pyropheophorbide (Fig. 8) (Roy et al., 2003).

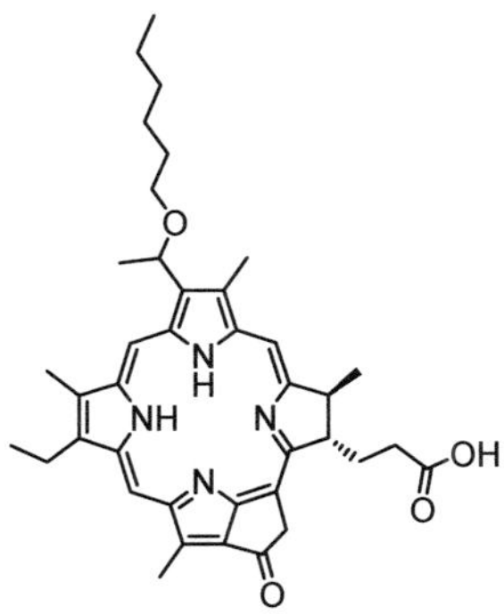

Fig. 8. Structure of 2-devinyl-2-(1-hexyloxyethyl)pyropheophorbide

Irradiation of the nanoparticles with light of appropriate wavelength led to efficient creation of singlet oxygen. On the other hand, noncovalent adsorption of PS into porous silica nanoparticles led to drug leakage. Covalent bonding of the PS into organically modified silica nanoparticles produced more stable material (Ohulchanskyy et al., 2007). Organically modified silica nanoparticles were also used for two-photon dye encapsulation (Kim et al., 2007). Cinteza et al. described a combination of magnetism and PDT using micellar polymeric diacylphospholipid-poly(ethylene glycol) capsules for encapsulation of the 2-devinyl-2-(1-hexyloxyethyl)pyropheophorbide PS and magnetic Fe_3O_4 nanoparticles (Cinteza et al., 2006). In contrast to the previous report (Kim et al., 2007), the magnetic nanoparticles were used for targeted delivery of PS to tumor cells and increased imaging (Cinteza et al., 2006). Wieder at el. described a delivery system consisting of gold nanoparticles modified with phthalocyanine (Wieder et al., 2006). Phthalocyanine derivative-modified gold nanaoparticles have 2-4 nm in diameter and have a maximum absorption peak at 695 nm. They generated $^1O_2$ catalytically with high efficiency. Upon irradiation of these nanoparticles, significant improvement in PDT efficiency was observed, probably thanks to 50% increase of $^1O_2$ quantum yields as compared to the free PS. In the same year El-Sayed reported efficient conversion of strongly absorbed light by plasmonic gold nanoparticles to heat energy. Easy bioconjugation of nanoparticles used suggests their application as selective photothermal agents in molecular cancer cell targeting (El-Sayed et al., 2006).

Two-photon dyes have received attention lately because of their ability to convert absorbed low-energy radiation to higher energy emissions. Dyes that can direct transfer of the higher energy to molecular oxygen for generation of $^1O_2$ can be very useful in PDT because they can be activated in deep tissues. The first use of two-photon dyes that are able to convert absorbed low-energy radiation to higher-energy emissions was recently reported using microemulsion to incorporate the two-photon dye porphyrin tetra(*p*-toluenesulfonate) into polyacrylamide nanoparticles (Gao et al., 2006).

- Biodegradable nanoparticle carriers

Biodegradable polymeric nanoparticles allow high drug loading and controlled drug release. They exist in a large variety of materials (Konan et al., 2002). Modifying the surface of nanoparticles with polymers such as poly(ethylene glycol) and poly(ethylene oxide) increases circulation times (McCarthy et al., 2005). Brasseur et al. described hematoporphyrin adsorbed in polyalkylcyanoacrylate nanoparticles (Brasseur et al., 1991), but the resulting materials showed poor carrier capacity and rapid drug release. Encapsulation of tetrasulfonated zinc phthalocyanine or aluminium naphthalocyanine into poly(isobutylcyanoacrylate) or poly(ethylbutylcyanoacrylate) nanocapsules or nanosphere was published in the same year (Labib et al., 1991). Then, second generation phthalocyanine derivatives were used in PEG-poly(lactic acid) nanoparticles (Allemann et al., 1995). The results showed that immobilization in the biodegradable nanoparticle improved PDT response of the tumor in contrast to conventional Cremophor EL emulsion by providing prolonged tumor sensitivity towards PDT (Allemann et al., 1995). After a few years, Konan et al. developed polyester poly(D,L-lactide-coglycolide) and poly(D,L-lactide) doped with PS with much higher loading than ever published before (Konan et al., 2003a; Konan et al., 2003b). In order to further investigate these nanoparticles, the efficacy of the encapsulated drug was assessed on the chick embryo chorioallantoic membrane model (Vargas et al., 2004). In another work the *in vitro* and *in vivo* photodynamic activities of verteporfin-loaded poly(D,L-lactide-coglycolide) nanoparticles were studied. The results showed improved photodynamic activity of PS (Konan-Kouakou et al., 2005).

The problem with side photosensitivity due to non-specific localization of the PS into healthy tissue or skin was studied by McCarthy et al., who developed a new nano-agent that has several desirable properties for use as photodynamic drug including no toxicity in extracellular spaces and time-dependent intracellular release of PS (McCarthy et al., 2005). They demonstrated in cell culture that the phototoxicity caused by non-internalized nanoparticles is minimal (9% cell death) in contrast to the effect of internalized nanoparticles (95% cell death under identical testing conditions) (Dougherty et al., 1978). In another study Ricci-Junior et al. reported the preparation, characterization, and results of the phototoxicity assay of poly(D,L-lactide-coglycolide) nanoparticles containing ZnPC for PDT use (Ricci-Junior & Marchetti, 2006a). Other photosensitizers that have been studied consist of Indocyanine green (Saxena et al., 2006) and Hypericin (Zeisser-Labouebe et al., 2006). These compounds have the potential to be used for both diagnostic and therapeutic purposes.

1.5 Combined therapy

Even if PDT has been used effectively for treating various tumors, it still has several restrictive factors for a target-specific response, such as an observed angiogenic effect and pronounced inflammatory reaction after PDT treatment (Pervaiz & Olivo, 2006). PDT in combination with other types of therapy is an attractive approach to suppress these problematic side effects.

PDT-induced hypoxia has been associated with an increase in the expression of many angiogenic growth factors, such as hypoxia-inducible factor 1 (HIF-1), fibroblast growth factor receptor-1(FGFR-1), cyclooxigenase-2 (COX-2), and vascular endothelial growth factor (VEGF). Combination therapy using antiangiogenic agents (e.g., COX-2 or VEGF inhibitors) with PDT led to a significant decrease of PDT-induced expression of prostaglandin E2 and VEGF, as well as a marked improvement in tumoricidal response (Akita et al., 2004; Ferrario et al., 2002; Zhou et al., 2005).

In contrast to radiotherapy, surgery or chemotherapy, PDT can lead to a strong acute inflammatory response, generally as tumor-localized edema. This PDT-induced immune activation makes it possible to positively reverse the tumor–host relationship from one that is tumor dominated to one that is oriented against the tumor. The combination with immunotherapy can reinforce the immune response triggered by PDT and thus significantly improve the anti-tumor immune response (Pervaiz & Olivo, 2006). Numerous recent clinical trials conclude that enhanced clinical outcomes can be achieved by a combination of ALA-PDT and immunomodulation therapy for the treatment of premalignant skin diseases, such as Bowen's disease (BD), BCC and AK (Wang et al., 2007; Wang et al., 2008).

In several cases, combination therapy can be done by linking the photosensitizer directly to an anticancer drug or to a specific antibody to target highly tumor-expressed receptors (Palumbo, 2007). It would also be easily accomplished by combining them using nanotechnology.

1.6 Light sources in PDT

A variety of light sources that are used in PDT consist of light-emitting diodes (LEDs), filtered xenon arc and metal halide lamps, fluorescent lamps, and lasers. Lasers and filtered broadband sources provide comparable efficacy in topical PDT (Clark et al., 2003). Non-laser light sources are also important in topical PDT, because in contrast to lasers they are stable, cheap, and offer broad-area illumination fields. Recently, LEDs showed significant progress in design, creating these low-cost sources suitable for broad-area irradiation, and were accepted for patient use. These LEDs are focused on the 630-to-635-nm activation peak of PpIX while excluding the inappropriate wavelengths present in broadband sources, thus allowing shorter irradiation times. Biophysical calculations show that LEDs with peak emission of 631 ± 2 nm can have a deeper PDT action in tissue than filtered halogen lamps with 560–740 nm emission, and hence LEDs may be more successful in treating the deeper parts of tumors (Juzeniene et al., 2004).

PpIX has its main absorption peak in the blue region at 410 nm (Soret band) with smaller absorption peaks at 505, 540, 580 and 630 nm. Most light sources for PDT seek to utilize the 630-nm absorption peak, in order to improve tissue penetration. On the other hand, a blue fluorescent lamp (peak emission 417 nm) is usually used. Nowadays, there are several reports that blue, green, and red light itself can be efficient in topical PDT of AK; however, the more deeply penetrating red light is better when treating BD and BCC (Morton et al., 2002).

The concept of ambulatory PDT to decrease hospital attendance for PDT was described by Moseley et al. (Moseley et al., 2006). In a study of five patients with BD, PDT was carried out with ALA and a portable LEDs device. Current studies have suggested that pulsed light therapy may be helpful for treatment in topical PDT of acne, AK and photorejuvenation. On the other hand, a recent controlled investigative study carried out in healthy human skin *in vivo* demonstrated that two pulsed light sources formerly reported in PDT brought evidence of minimal activation of photosensitizer, with a significantly smaller photodynamic reaction than observed with a conventional continuous wave broadband source (Strasswimmer & Grande, 2006). These sources deliver intense light in short periods (< 20 ms), which might suppress oxygen consumption (Kawauchi et al., 2004). Unplanned ambient light exposure may have considerably contributed to the clinical effect. However, three studies have recently addressed the possibility of using ambient light for ALA-PDT of AK (Batchelor et al., 2007; Marcus et al., 2007; Strasswimmer & Grande, 2006). Two of them report on therapeutic advantage. Nevertheless, the randomized ambient light-controlled study using ALA demonstrated no significant effect on lesion ablation. A randomized right/left intra-patient evaluation of conventional MAL-PDT combined with LEDs device *versus* daylight (for 2.5 h) for the treatment of AK of face and scalp demonstrated corresponding reduction in AK and significantly less pain with daylight (Wiegell et al., 2008).

Total effective light dosage is proposed as a concept for optimizing the accuracy of light dosimetry in PDT considering incident spectral irradiance and optical transmission through tissue and absorption by PS (Moseley, 1996). Actually, light dosimetry is explained as the irradiance rate (mW cm^{-2}) at the skin surface and the total dosage (J cm^{-2}) distributed to the surface, the second being a product of irradiance and time of exposure.

It has been suggested that lower fluence rates and fractionation of light exposure can improve lesional reaction by promotion of the photodynamic reaction (Henderson et al., 2004). A study of superficial BCC illuminated with 45 J cm^{-2} at 4 h and repeated at 6 h with 633-nm laser light at 50 mW cm^{-2} showed a total response of 84 % after a mean of 59 months (Star at el., 2006). Newer studies support advantages of the fractionation approach in BCC, although not in BD (Haas et al., 2006; Haas et al., 2007).

1.7 Synthetic *meso*-tetraphenylporphyrins in PDT

Extensive information about the application of various porphyrins and their derivatives in PDT has been published (Král et al., 2006). Accordingly, our laboratory synthesized porphyrin conjugates with glycol (Králová et al., 2008a), bile acid (Králová et al., 2008b), and cyclodextrins (Králová et al., 2006) and their *in vitro* and *in vivo* PDT activity has been tested. It was shown that these porphyrin conjugates are taken up preferentially by tumor cells and have the potential to be used for PDT to selectively ablate tumors (Králová et al., 2006; Králová et al., 2008a; Králová et al., 2008b).

Our contemporary strategy is to combine favorable features of gold nanoparticles mediating the photothermal effect with a photosensitizing compound mediating the photodynamic effect into one combined modality and thus introduce a therapeutic protocol efficient against SCC.

The key steps in our strategy are: i) generation of a synthetic ligand with photosensitizing properties, ii) ligand immobilization on the surface of modified gold nanoparticles to enable combination of PDT and thermo-effect, and iii) verification of the biological activity by *in vitro* and *in vivo* studies.

2. Experimental

2.1 Preparation of modified gold nanoparticles

Porphyrin–brucine conjugates **1** and **2** (Fig. 9) were prepared according to the procedure described previously (Král et al., 2005). Gold nanoparticles (14.7 nm) were prepared by citrate reduction of potassium tetrachloroaurate(III) (**Au-citr**). After modification with 3- mercaptopropanoic acid, derivatives **1** and **2** were immobilized as described elsewhere (Řezanka et al., 2008). Here, a solution of **1** or **2** (5 mg) in methanol was added to 50 ml of **Au-citr**. Modified nanoparticles (**Au-1** and **Au-2**, respectively) were isolated by centrifugation after three days of incubation. Using redispersion in methanol, methanol–water, water and dimethylsulfoxide, unbound porphyrin derivatives were removed and **Au-1** and **Au-2** molecules were concentrated to a volume of 1 ml. According to the spectral analysis of supernatants, 0.8 mg of **1** or **2** was present in the final 1 ml solution of **Au-1** and **Au-2** nanoparticles. The core of modified nanoparticles was characterized by transmission electron microscopy and photon cross-correlation spectroscopy (Nanophox). The chemical modification, ligand, was analyzed by absorption and fluorescence spectrometry. Fluorescence spectra were recorded using a Fluoromax spectrometer (Jobin-Yvon, Japan). A volume of 1 ml of sample was placed into 1 cm plastic cuvettes. The excitation wavelength was 520 nm.

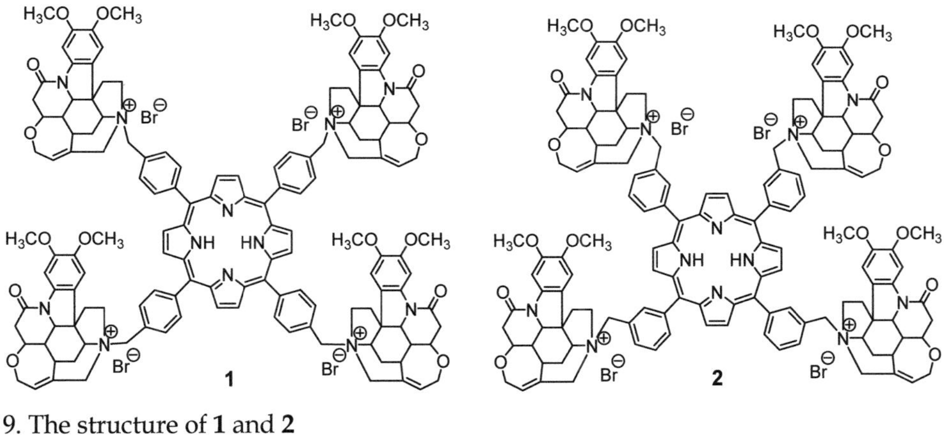

Fig. 9. The structure of **1** and **2**

2.2 Cell culture and *in vitro* experiments

4T1 (mouse mammary carcinoma) and A431 (epidermal squamous carcinoma) cells were purchased from ATCC and PE/CA-PJ34 (human basaloid squamous cell carcinoma) cells were purchased from ETCC. As described before (Králová et al., 2006), all cells were grown exponentially in RPMI 1640 medium with 10% fetal calf serum. For photodynamic experiments, 1–1.5 x 10^5 cells were seeded into 1.8 cm^{-2} wells and incubated overnight with the porphyrin–brucine conjugates or their counterparts immobilized on gold nanoparticles (1 and 2.5 μM). After incubation, cells were rinsed with PBS, cultured for 1 h in fresh medium without phenol red and illuminated with a 75 W halogen lamp with a band-pass filter (Andover, Salem, NH) that emitted light at wavelengths between 500–520 nm. The fluence rate at the level of the cell monolayer was 1 mW cm^{-2}, and the total light dose was 7.2 J cm^{-2}. Twenty-four hours post irradiation, the viability of PDT-treated cultures was determined by the Trypan blue exclusion method. In parallel, control "dark" experiments (without illumination) were performed.

2.3 Microscopic studies

Cells grown on coverslips in 35 mm Petri dishes were incubated with 2.5 μM porphyrin-brucine conjugates in culture medium for 16 h. After washing, porphyrin fluorescence was observed with a DM IRB Leica microscope equipped with a DFC 480 camera using a x63 oil immersion objective and Leica filter cube N2.1 (excitation filter BP 515–560 nm and long pass filter LP 590 nm for emission). To label lysosomes, 500 nM LysoTracker Green (Molecular Probes) was added to the culture media for 30 min. Cells were washed and examined by fluorescence microscopy using the Leica filter cube I3 (excitation filter BP 450–490 nm and long pass filter LP 515 nm for emission).

2.4 *In vivo* experiments

For *in vivo* experiments, the immuno-compromised nude mice with subcutaneously implanted human SCC tumors were used. When the tumor mass reached a volume of 100 mm^3 (10–14 days after injection), mice were intravenously injected with porphyrin-brucine conjugates (5 mg kg^{-1}) resuspended in a volume of 0.1 ml per 20 g mice and six hours later the tumor area (2 cm^2) was irradiated with a 500–700 nm xenon lamp ONL051 (maximum at 635 nm, Preciosa Crytur, Turnov, Czech Republic) with a total impact energy of 100 J cm^{-2} and fluence rate of 200 mW cm^{-2}. Each experimental group consisted of five or eight mice. The tumor size was measured repeatedly and the tumor volume was determined (Králová et al., 2006). All aspects of animal experimentation and husbandry were carried out in compliance with national and European regulations and were approved by the institutional committee.

3. Results and discussion

3.1 Modification by gold nanoparticles

Gold nanoparticles (14.7 nm) prepared by citrate reduction of potassium tetrachloroaurate(III) (**Au-citr**) were modified with 3-mercaptopropanoic acid, and the derivatives **1** and **2** were immobilized. Gold nanoparticles modified with **1** and **2** are designated **Au-1** and **Au-2**, respectively.

3.2 Fluorescence spectra

The fluorescence intensity of **1** and **2** was strongly dependent on the solvent used. The influence of additional compounds on the intensity of emitted fluorescence wavelengths was tested by measuring the emission spectra (excitation of the first Q-band of porphyrins at 520 nm) of **1** and **2** in water, an inorganic salt solution (corresponding to the cell culture media) supplemented with a 50 mg ml^{-1} solution of human serum albumin (HSA) (Fig. 10A). In comparison with water, the emission bands of **1** and **2** measured in the media were red-shifted (for **1**, from 638 and 700 nm to 644 and 709 nm, and for **2**, from 643 and 707 nm to 647 and 710 nm) and the fluorescence intensity of **1** increased slightly whilst that of **2** decreased. After immobilizing the porphyrin conjugates on nanoparticles, the intensity of fluorescence emission spectra significantly decreased (Fig. 10B) despite the concentration of porphyrins remained the same. The weak quantum yield may be attributed to that: (1) both porphyrins and nanoparticles absorb light at approximately 520 nm, (2) fluorescence quenching by porphyrin-to-metal energy transfer, (3) partial aggregation of the modified nanoparticles. In the case of **Au-1**, aggregation seems to be the cause (Fig. 10B, compare traces "**Au-1/water**" and "**Au-1/medium**"), as the intensity of emitted fluorescence was several times higher in cell culture medium compared to water only. These results demonstrate that both para- (**1**) and meta- (**2**) derivatives aggregate in a solution-dependent manner that is not affected by the presence of PS or immobilization on gold nanoparticles. Importantly, the presence of model plasma proteins present in the cell medium dramatically reduced the aggregation of modified nanoparticles. This observation led us to further test these compounds for *in vivo* PDT efficacy.

A

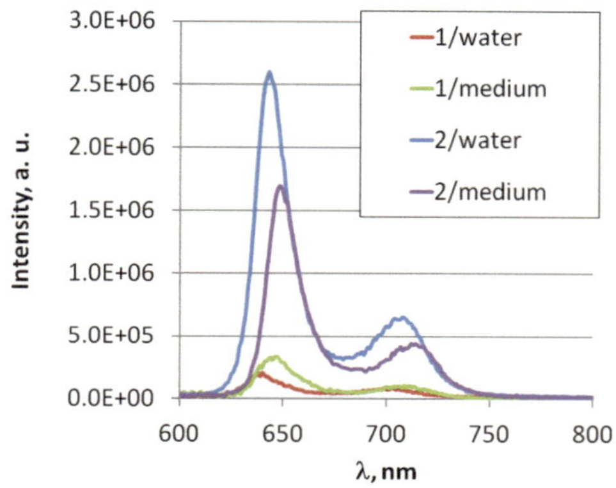

B

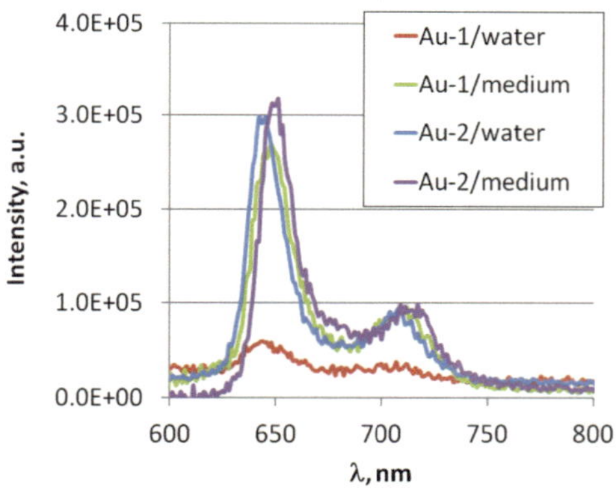

Fig. 10. The fluorescence emission spectra of porphyrins **1** and **2** (left) and porphyrin-modified nanoparticles **Au-1** and **Au-2** (right) in water and cell culture media. Excitation was performed at 520 nm. Porphyrin–brucine conjugates were used at a concentration of 3.5 μM. The concentration of human serum albumin used in growth medium was 50 mg ml^{-1}.

3.3 Intracellular localization

The porphyrin–brucine conjugates (**1** and **2**) were next analyzed for tumor cell uptake and intracellular distribution. The mammary carcinoma cell line, 4T1 was cultivated in the presence of the conjugates for 16 h, during which time the cells were well-dispersed and growing mostly as planar sheets, enabling focused images of fluorescence to be recorded. These cells exhibited punctate red fluorescence (Fig. 11).

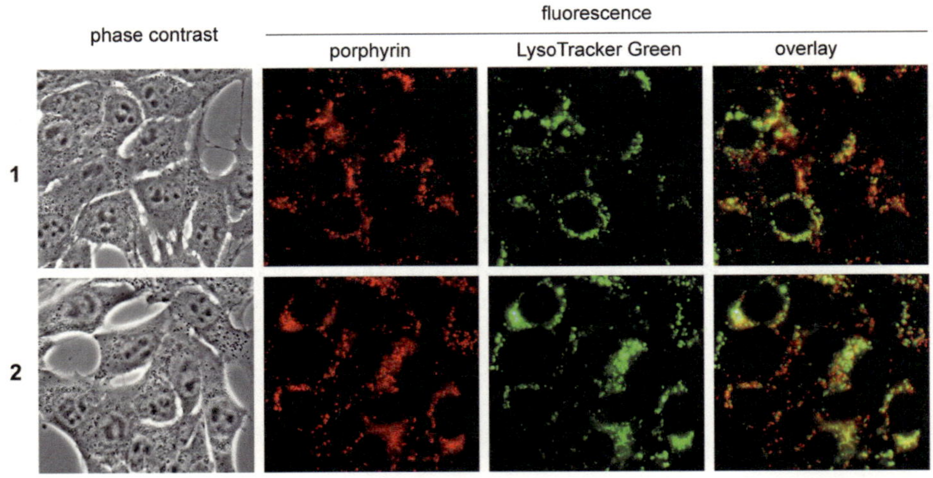

Fig. 11. The intracellular localization of porphyrin–brucine conjugates in 4T1 cells. The middle panels show the red fluorescence of **1** and **2** and co-staining with the lysosomal specific probe (LysoTracker Green); right panels represent an overlay of the green and red images and demonstrate co-localization (shown in orange/yellow). Porphyrin–brucine conjugates were used at a concentration of 2.5 μM.

To identify the intracellular compartment where **1** and **2** accumulate, co-staining with the LysoTracker Green fluorescence probe was performed. The merged images revealed that **1** and **2** colocalized to a subset of LysoTracker-stained structures that represent lysosomes. Similar localization was also observed in PE/CA-PJ34 basaloid squamous cell carcinoma cells and A431 epidermal squamous carcinoma, cell lines that were predominantly used in our study (data not shown). Upon addition of gold nanoparticle-conjugated **1** and **2** to cell culture media, aggregates formed, which were visible as a reddish precipitate that covered parts of the cell. These were particularly abundant in the case of **Au-1** (Fig. 12).

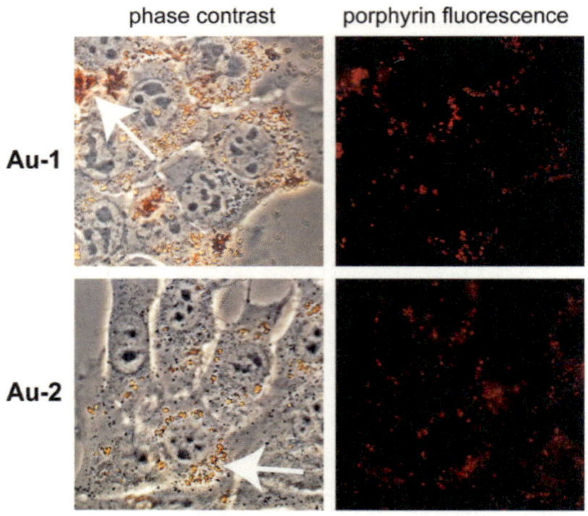

Fig. 12. Difference in aggregation behavior of porphyrin–brucine conjugates immobilized on gold nanoparticles (left panels). 4T1 cells were incubated with **Au-1** and **Au-2** at a concentration of 2.5 μM for 4 h before pictures were taken. Aggregates are highlighted by arrows.

3.4 *In vitro* phototoxicity

To investigate the photodynamic potential of the free porphyrin-brucine conjugates or those immobilized on gold nanoparticles, we incubated PE/CA-PJ34 cells in the presence of the conjugates for 16 h and subjected them to PDT. In parallel, cells were incubated with porphyrins without illumination to serve as dark controls. Twenty-four hours following the illumination of cells with filtered light, the mortality of post-PDT cultures was determined (Fig. 13).

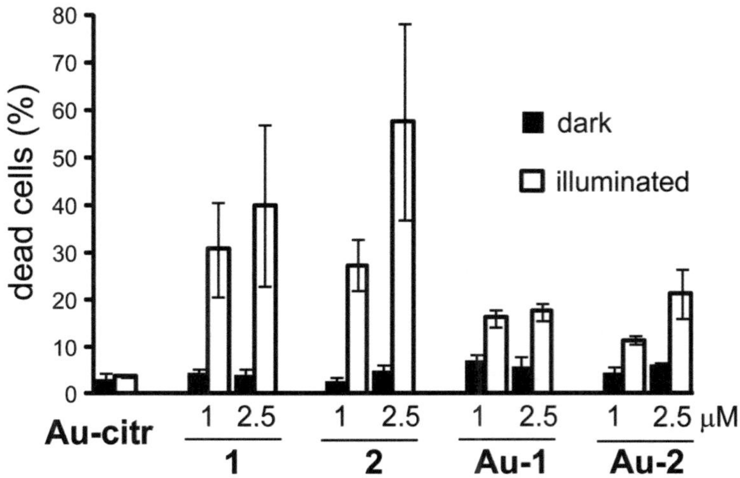

Fig. 13. The effect of free or immobilized porphyrin-brucine conjugates on the induction of cell death via PDT. PE/CA-PJ34 cells were incubated with either 1 or 2.5 μM of **1** and **2** or their modified Au-nanoparticles for 16 h. Cells were then illuminated with filtered light (500–520 nm, 7.2 J cm^{-2}). The percentage of dead cells was established the following day by using the Trypan blue exclusion method. The average and standard deviation for three independent experiments is shown.

Satisfyingly, the induction of cell death was both light and drug-dose dependent. Control cells incubated with unconjugated gold nanoparticles (**Au-citr**) did not display any increase in cell death after illumination. Thus, under these *in vitro* conditions we can exclude the possibility that any case of cell death is due to the photothermal activity of the gold nanoparticles. Interestingly, the phototoxicities of unbound porphyrin-brucine conjugates **1** and **2** were higher than those immobilized on gold nanoparticles. This reduction of photodynamic efficacy is likely to be a consequence of **Au-1** and **Au-2** aggregation that occurs in the aqueous cell growth media (Fig. 12).

3.5 In vivo PDT efficacy

Using an *in vivo* mouse cancer model, the PDT effectiveness of the unbound porphyrin-brucine conjugates **1** and **2** was compared with those immobilized on gold nanoparticles (**Au-1**, **Au-2**). Nude mice (NuNu) bearing basaloid squamous cell carcinoma PE/ CA-PJ34 cells received by intravenous injection either unmodified porphyrins or their gold nanoparticle-modified counterparts. Six hours post injection, tumors were illuminated with light at a dose of 100 J cm-2. Mice not injected with unmodified porphyrins or nanoparticles served as controls. Tumor size was measured after PDT at regular intervals (Fig. 14).

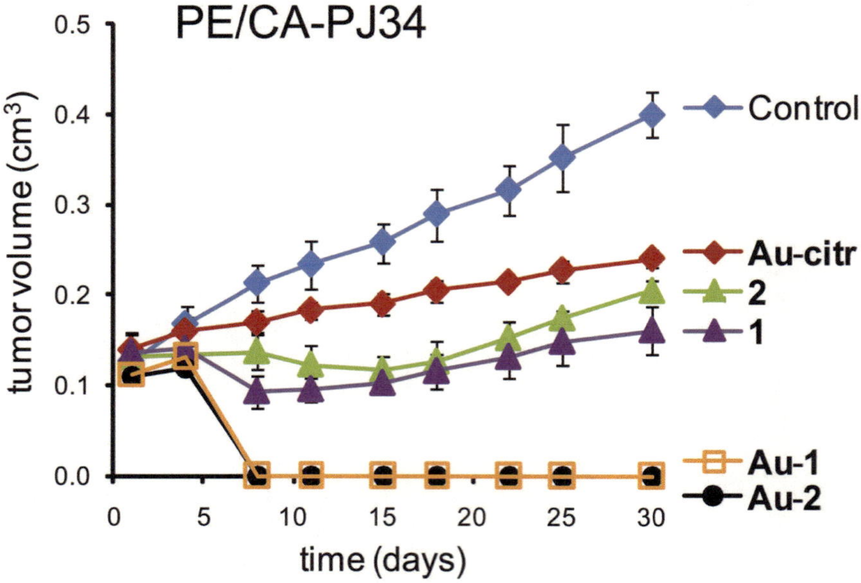

Fig. 14. The PDT effectiveness of **1** and **2** and their respective Au-immobilized nanoparticle counterparts to eradicate mouse tumors. Nude mice (NuNu) bearing subcutaneous PE/CA-PJ34 tumors (n = 8 per each group) received an intravenous dose of the drug (5 mg kg^{-1}). Tumors were illuminated with light (100 J cm^{-2}) six hours after injection. The tumor size was measured repeatedly and the tumor volume was determined. Control mice were exposed to illumination but did not receive the porphyrin drug. The **Au-citr** group represents mice injected with Au nanoparticles, **1** and **2** groups received porphyrin conjugates, **Au-1** and **Au-2** groups received porphyrin-modified Au nanoparticles.

We observed the greatest reduction in tumor growth in mice treated with **Au-1** and **Au-2**. All tumors were eliminated in animals that received these conjugated porphyrins and importantly, no detectable relapse of the primary tumor was observed. In contrast, animals treated with unbound **1** and **2** exhibited only a transient regression in tumor size that lasted until day 18, when the primary tumors began to gradually regrow. Presumably, this relapse in tumor growth comes from the small population of tumor cells that survived the PDT. Interestingly, mice treated with unconjugated gold nanoparticles exhibited slight tumor retardation in growth, which is most likely due to the photothermal effect described in other systems (Gamaleia et al., 2010; O'Neal et al., 2010; Řezanka et al., 2008).

These results clearly show that porphyrin alkaloid-modified gold nanoparticles are very effective against basaloid SCC *in vivo*. To verify more general applicability of porphyrin alkaloid-modified gold nanoparticles, the same approach was used against epidermal SCC tumors (Fig. 15). A431 cells formed fast progressing subcutaneous tumors, which were completely eradicated after **Au-2**-mediated PDT treatment in 60% mice or their growth was substantially reduced. These results demonstrate a high potential of porphyrin alkaloid-modified gold nanoparticles to fight SCC.

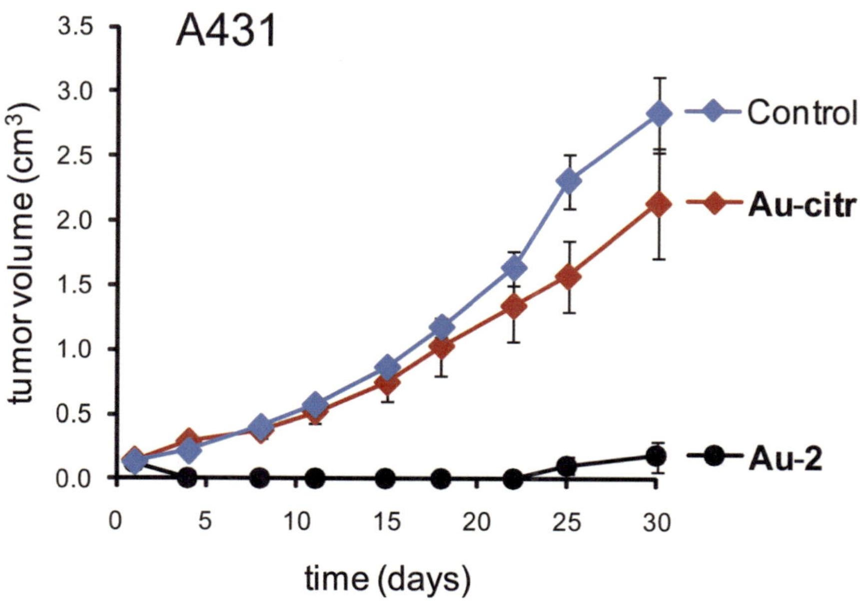

Fig. 15. The PDT effectiveness of Au-2 against fast progressing epidermal squamous carcinoma A431. Nude mice (NuNu) bearing subcutaneous A431 tumors ($n = 5$ per each group) received an intravenous dose of the drug (5 mg kg^{-1}). Tumors were illuminated with light (100 J cm^{-2}) six hours after injection. The tumor size was measured repeatedly and the tumor volume was determined. Control mice were exposed to illumination but did not receive the porphyrin drug. The **Au-citr** group represents mice injected with Au nanoparticles without porphyrin.

The apparent discrepancy in the *in vitro* and *in vivo* performance of unbound porphyrin-brucine conjugates **1** and **2** and those immobilized on gold nanoparticles (**Au-1** and **Au-2**) is likely to be due to the differing environmental conditions to which the porphyrin conjugates were exposed. The fluorescence data revealed that conjugates **1** and **2** were efficiently taken up by cells under the *in vitro* conditions tested. However, in culture media, **Au-1** and **Au-2** tended to aggregate, which resulted in their lower intracellular availability (Fig. 12) and lower PDT efficacy (Fig. 13). Under the *in vivo* conditions tested, the gold nanoparticle-immobilized conjugates were more effective than free conjugates alone. Both spectroscopic and ECD studies demonstrated that conjugated nanoparticles exhibited a strong interaction with plasma proteins (mainly HSA), which led to their self-assembly and to generation of supramolecular complexes. Subsequently, thanks to the enhanced permeability and retention (EPR) effect resulting in potent accumulation of **Au-1** and **Au-2** in the tumors, their PDT efficacy was increased. Moreover, the direct lethal effect of PDT on tumor cells combines well with the nanoscale size of gold-immobilized porphyrins that may limit the local blood supply (vascular impairment). This hypothesis of vascular damage after PDT with nanoparticles will be the subject of future work.

4. Conclusion

The spectroscopic studies demonstrated that fluorescence intensity of free and immobilized conjugates were strongly dependent on the solvent used. After immobilizing the porphyrin conjugates 1 and **2** on nanoparticles, the intensity of fluorescence emission spectra significantly decreased. The weak quantum yield may be attributed to that: (1) both porphyrins and nanoparticles absorb light at approximately 520 nm, (2) fluorescence quenching by porphyrin-to-metal energy transfer, (3) partial aggregation of the modified nanoparticles. Importantly, the presence of model plasma proteins in the cell medium dramatically reduced the aggregation of modified nanoparticles and prompted their use *in vivo*.

The evaluation of the biological activity of porphyrin-brucine conjugates, either free or immobilized to gold nanoparticles, started with determination of their intracellular uptake. It was shown that both forms were effectively taken into the cell, although a lower level was observed for immobilized forms. To investigate the photodynamic potential of the conjugates, SCC were exposed *in vitro* to photodynamic treatment and cell mortality of post-PDT cultures was determined. The phototoxicities of unbound porphyrin-brucine conjugates were higher than those of conjugates immobilized on gold nanoparticles. This reduction of photodynamic efficacy is likely to be a consequence of nanoparticle aggregation that occurs in the aqueous cell growth media.

In contrast, when the PDT effectiveness was tested *in vivo*, the greatest reduction in tumor growth was observed in mice treated with porphyrin conjugates immobilized on gold nanoparticles. All tumors were eliminated and no detectable relapse of the primary tumor was observed. When animals were treated with unbound conjugates, they exhibited only a transient regression in tumor size that lasted until day 18, and then the primary tumors began to gradually re-grow. Importantly, mice treated with gold nanoparticles without porphyrin exhibited slight tumor retardation in growth that is most likely attributed to the photothermal effect described in other systems. Thus, under the *in vivo* conditions tested, the gold nanoparticle-immobilized conjugates were more effective than free conjugates alone. In addition, both spectroscopic and ECD studies demonstrated that conjugated nanoparticles exhibited a strong interaction with plasma proteins (mainly serum albumin), which led to their self-assembly and generation of supramolecular complexes, and thereby to the enhanced permeability and retention effect. It further contributed to potent accumulation of immobilized conjugates in tumors leading to increased PDT efficacy. Moreover, the direct lethal effect of PDT on tumor cells combines well with the nanoscale size of gold-immobilized porphyrins that may limit the local blood supply (vascular impairment).

5. Acknowledgements

This work was funded by grants from the Grant Agency of the Czech Republic (Grant No. 203/09/1311 and P303/11/1291), supported in part by projects LC06077 and 512 awarded by the Ministry of Education of the Czech Republic, by project AV0Z50520514 awarded by the Academy of Sciences of the Czech Republic to J. Králová, and by projects MSM6046137307, BIOMEDREG CZ. 1.05./2.1.00/01.0030, and KAN2001008016.

6. References

Ackroyd, R; Kelty, C.; Brown, N. & Reed, M. (2001). The history of photodetection and photodynamic therapy. *Photochem. Photobiol.*, Vol.74, No.5, pp. 656–669, ISSN 1751-1097

Akita, Y.; Kozaki, K.; Nakagawa, A.; Saito, T.; Ito, S.; Tamada, Y.; Fujiwara, S.; Nishikawa, N.; Uchida, K.; Yoshikawa, K.; Noguchi, T.; Miyaishi, O.; Shimozato, K.; Saga S. & Matsumoto, Y. (2004). Cyclooxygenase-2 is a possible target of treatment approach in conjunction with photodynamic therapy for various disorders in skin and oral cavity. *Br. J. Dermatol.* Vol.151, No.2, pp. 472–480, ISSN 1365-2133

Allemann, E.; Brasseur, M.; Benrezzak, O.; Rousseau, J.; Kudrevich, S.V.; Boyle, R.W.; Leroux, J.C.; Gurny, R. & van Lier, J.E. (1995). PEG-coated poly(lactic acid) nanoparticles for the delivery of hexadecafluoro zinc phthalocyanine to EMT-6 mouse mammary tumours. *J. Pharm. Pharmacol.*, Vol.47, pp. 382–387, ISSN 0022-3573

Auzel, F. (2004). Upconversion and anti-Stokes processes with f and d ions in solids. *Chem. Rev.*, Vol.104, pp. 139–173, ISSN 1520-6890

Babilas, P.; Karrer, S.; Sidoroff, A.; Landthaler, M. & Szeimies, R.M. (2005). Photodynamic therapy in dermatology - an update. *Photodermatol. Photoimmunol. Photomed.*, Vol.21, No.3, pp. 142–149, ISSN 1600-0781

Bakalova, R.; Ohba, H.; Zhelev, Z.; Ishikawa, M. & Baba, Y. (2004). Quantum dots as photosensitizers? *Nat. Biotechnol.*, Vol.22, pp. 1360–1361, ISSN 1087-0156

Barr, H; Dix, A.J.; Kendall, C. & Stone, N. (2001). Review article: the potential role for photodynamic therapy in the management of upper gastrointestinal disease. *Aliment. Pharmacol. Ther.*, Vol.15, No.3, pp. 311–321, ISSN 1365-2036

Batchelor, R.J.; Stables, G.I. & Stringer, M.R. (2007). Successful treatment of scalp actinic keratoses with photodynamic therapy using ambient light. *Br. J. Dermatol.*, Vol. 156, No.4, pp 779–781, ISSN 1365-2133

Blume, J.E. & Oseroff, A.R. (2007). Aminolevulinic acid photodynamic therapy for skin cancers. *Dermatol. Clin.*, Vol.25, No.1, pp. 5–14, ISSN 1879-1131

Boyer, J.C.; Vetrone, F.; Cuccia, L.A. & Capobianco, J.A. (2006). Synthesis of colloidal upconverting $NaYF_4$ nanocrystals doped with Er^{3+}, Yb^{3+} and Tm^{3+}, Yb^{3+} via thermal decomposition of lanthanide trifluoroacetate precursors. *J. Am. Chem. Soc.*, Vol.128, pp. 7444–7445, ISSN 1520-5126

Braathen, L.R. (2001). Photodynamic therapy. *Tidsskr Nor Laegeforen*, Vol.121, pp. 2635–2636, ISSN 0807-7096

Brasseur, N.; Brault, D. & Couvreur, P. (1991). Adsorption of hematoporphyrin onto polyalkylcyanoacrylate nanoparticles: carrier capacity and drug release. *Int. J. Pharm.*, Vol.70, pp 129, ISSN 0378-5173

Britton, J.E.R.; Goulden, V.; Stables, G.; Stringer, M. & Sheehan-Dare, R. (2005). Investigation of the use of the pulsed dye laser in the treatment of Bowen's disease using 5-aminolaevulinic acid phototherapy. *Br. J. Dermatol.*, Vol.153, No.4, pp. 780–784, ISSN 1365-2133

Buytaert, E.; Dewaele, M. & Agostinis, P. (2007). Molecular effectors of multiple cell death pathways initiated by photodynamic therapy. Biochim. Biophys. Acta, Vol.1776, pp. 86–107, ISSN 0006-3002

Cinteza, L.O.; Ohulchanskyy, T.Y.; Sahoo, Y.; Bergey, E.J.; Pandey, R.K. & Prasad, P.N. (2006). Diacyllipid micelle-based nanocarrier for magnetically guided delivery of drugs in photodynamic therapy. *Mol. Pharmacol.*, Vol.3, pp. 415–423, ISSN 1521-0111

Clark, C.; Bryden, A.; Dawe, R.; Moseley, H.; Ferguson J. & Ibbotson, S.H. (2003). Topical 5-aminolaevulinic acid photodynamic therapy for cutaneous lesions: outcome and comparison of light sources. *Photodermatol. Photoimmunol. Photomed.*, Vol.19, No.3, pp. 134–141, ISSN 1600-0781

Daniell, M.D. & Hill, J.S. (1991). A history of photodynamic therapy. *ANZ J. Surg.*, Vol.61, No.5, pp. 340–348, ISSN 1445-2197

Dougherty, T.J. (1996). A brief history of clinical photodynamic therapy development at Roswell Park Cancer Institute. *J. Clin. Laser Med. Surg.*, Vol.14, No.5, pp. 219–221, ISSN 1044-5471

Dougherty, T.J.; Grindey, G.B.; Fiel, R.; Weishaupt, K.R. & Boyle, D.G. (1975). Photoradiation therapy. II. Cure of animal tumors with hematoporphyrin and light. *J. Natl. Cancer Inst.*, Vol.55, pp. 115–121, ISSN 1460-2105

Dougherty, T.J.; Kaufman, J.E.; Goldfarb, A.; Weishaupt, K.R.; Boyle, D. & Mittleman, A. (1978). Photoradiation therapy for the treatment of malignant tumors. *Cancer Res.*, Vol.38, pp. 2628–2635, ISSN 1538-7445

Dragieva, G.; Hafner, J.; Dummer. R; Schmid-Grendelmeier, P; Roos, M.; Prinz, B.M.; Burg, G.; Binswanger, U. & Kempf, W. (2004a). Topical photodynamic therapy in the treatment of actinic keratoses and Bowen's disease in transplant recipients. *Transplantation*, Vol.77, No.1, pp. 115–121, ISSN 1534-0608

Dragieva, G.; Prinz, B.M.; Hafner, J.; Dummer, R.; Burg, G.; Binswanger, U. & Kempf, W. (2004b). A randomized controlled clinical trial of topical photodynamic therapy with methyl aminolaevulinate in the treatment of actinic keratoses in transplant recipients. *Br. J. Dermatol.*, Vol.151, No.1, pp. 196–200, ISSN 1365-2133

Dragieva, G.; Scharer, L.; Dummer, R. & Kempf, W. (2004). Photodynamic therapy - a new treatment option for epithelial malignancies of the skin. *Onkologie*, Vol.27, No.4, pp. 407–411, ISSN 1423-0240

El-Sayed, I.H.; Huang, X. & El-Sayed, M.A. (2006). Selective laser photo-thermal therapy of epithelial carcinoma using anti-EGFR antibody conjugated gold nanoparticles. *Cancer Lett.*, Vol.239, pp. 129–135, ISSN 0304-3835

Feng, W.; Dev, K.C.; Zhengquan, L.; Yong, Z.; Xianping, F. & Minquan, W. (2006). Synthesis of polyethylenimine/NaYFbSUBN4b/SUBN nanoparticles with upconversion fluorescence. *Nanotechnology*, Vol.17, pp. 5786, ISSN 1361-6528

Ferrario, A.; von Tiehl, K.; Wong, S.; Luna, M. & Gomer, C.J. (2002). Cyclooxygenase-2 inhibitor treatment enhances photodynamic therapy-mediated tumor response. *Cancer Res.*, Vol.62, No.14, pp. 3956–3961, ISSN 1538-7445

Fitzpatrick, T.B. & Pathak, M.A. (1959). Historical aspects of methoxsalen and other furocoumarins. *J. Invest. Dermatol.*, Vol.32, No.2, pp. 229–231, ISSN 1523-1747

Foote, C.S. (1991). Definition of type I and type II photosensitized oxidation. *Photochem. Photobiol.*, Vol.54, pp. 659, ISSN 1751-1097

Fritsch, C.; Goerz, G. & Ruzicka, T. (1998). Photodynamic therapy in dermatology. *Arch. Dermatol.*, Vol.134, No.2, pp. 207–214, ISSN 0096-5359

Gamaleia, N.F.; Shishko, E.D.; Dolinsky, G.A.; Shcherbakov, A.B.; Usatenko A.V. & Kholin, V.V. (2010). Photodynamic activity of hematoporphyrin conjugates with gold nanoparticles: experiments in vitro. *Exp. Oncol.*, Vol.32, pp. 44–47, ISSN 1812-9269

Gao, D.; Agayan, R.R.; Xu, H.; Philbert, M.A. & Kopelman, R. (2006). Nanoparticles for twophoton photodynamic therapy in living cells. *Nano Lett.*, Vol.6, pp. 2383–2386, ISSN 1530-6984

Garcia-Zuazaga, J.; Cooper, K.D. & Baron, E.D. (2005). Photodynamic therapy in dermatology: current concepts in the treatment of skin cancer. *Expert Rev. Anticancer Ther.*, Vol.5, No.5, pp. 791–800, ISSN 1473-7140

de Haas, E.R.M.; Kruijt, B.; Sterenborg, H.J.C.M.; Neumann, H.A.M. & Robinson, D.J. (2006). Fractionated illumination significantly improves the response of superficial basal cell carcinoma to aminolevulinic acid photodynamic therapy. *J. Invest. Dermatol.*, Vol.126, No.12, pp. 2679–2686, ISSN 1523-1747

de Haas, E.R.M.; Sterenborg, H.J.C.M.; Neumann, H.A.M. & Robinson, D.J. (2007). Response of Bowen disease to ALA-PDT using a single and a 2-fold illumination scheme. *Arch. Dermatol.*, Vol.143, pp. 264–265, ISSN 0096-5359

Hatz, S.; Lambert, J.D. & Ogilby, P.R. (2007). Measuring the lifetime of singlet oxygen in a single cell: addressing the issue of cell viability. *Photochem. Photobiol. Sci.*, Vol.6, pp. 106–1116, ISSN 1474-905X

Heer, S.; Kompe, K.; Gudel, H.U.; Haase, M. (2004). Highly efficient multicolour upconversion emission in transparent colloids of lanthanide-doped $NaYF_4$ nanocrystals, *Adv. Mater.*, Vol.16, pp. 2102–2105, ISSN 1521-4095

Henderson, B.W.; Gollnick, S.O.; Snyder, J.W.; Busch, T.M.; Kousis, P.C.; Cheney, R.T. & Morgan, J. (2004). Choice of oxygenconserving treatment regimen determines the inflammatory response and outcome of photodynamic therapy of tumours. *Cancer Res.*, Vol.64, No.6, pp. 2120–2126, ISSN 1538-7445

Hsieh, J.M.; Ho, M.L.; Wu, P.W.; Chou, P.T.; Tsai, T.T. & Chi, Y. (2006). Iridium-complex modified CdSe/ZnS quantum dots; a conceptual design for bi-functional toward imaging and photosensitization. *Chem. Commun.*, No.6, pp. 615–617, ISSN 1359-7345

Chen, W. & Zhang, J. (2006). Using nanoparticles to enable simultaneous radiation and photodynamic therapies for cancer treatment. *J. Nanosci. Nanotech.*, Vol.6, pp. 1159–1166, ISSN 1533-4899

Jichlinski, P. (2006). Photodynamic applications in superficial bladder cancer: facts and hopes! *J. Environ. Pathol. Toxicol. Oncol.*, Vol.25, No.1–2, pp. 441–451, ISSN 0731-8898

Josefsen, L.B. & Boyle, R.W. (2008). Photodynamic therapy: novel third generation photosensitizers one step closer? *Br. J. Pharmacol.*, Vol.154, No.1, pp. 1–3, ISSN 1476-5381

Juarranz, A; Jaen, P.; Sanz-Rodriguez, F.; Cuevas, J. & Gonzalez, S. (2008). Photodynamic therapy of cancer. Basic principles and applications. *Clin. Transl. Oncol.*, Vol.10, No.3, pp. 148–154, ISSN 1699-048X

Juzeniene, A.; Juzenas, P.; Ma, L.W.; Iani, V. & Moan, J. (2004). Effectiveness of different light sources for 5-aminolevulinic acid photodynamic therapy. *Lasers Med. Sci.*, Vol.19, No.3, pp. 139–149, ISSN 1435-604X

Kawauchi, S.; Morimoto, Y.; Sato, S.; Arai, T.; Seguchi, K.; Asanuma, H. & Kikuchi, M. (2004). Differences between cytotoxicity in photodynamic therapy using a pulsed laser and a continuous wave laser: study of oxygen consumption and photobleaching. *Lasers Med. Sci.*, Vol.18, No. 4, pp. 179–83, ISSN 1435-604X

Kennedy, J.C.; Pottier, R.H. & Pross, D.C. (1990). Photodynamic therapy with endogenous protoporphyrin IX: basic principles and present clinical experience. *J. Photochem. Photobiol. B Biol.*, Vol.6, No.1–2, pp. 143–148, ISSN 1011-1344

Kim, S.; Ohulchanskyy, T.Y.; Pudavar, H.E.; Pandey, R.K. & Prasad, P.N. (2007). Organically modified silica nanoparticles co-encapsulating photosensitizing drug and aggregation- enhanced two-photon absorbing fluorescent dye aggregates for twophoton photodynamic therapy. *J. Am. Chem. Soc.*, Vol.129, pp. 2669–2675, ISSN 1520-5126

Konan, Y.N.; Gurny, R. & Allemann, E. (2002). State of the art in the delivery of photosensitizers for photodynamic therapy. *J. Photochem. Photobiol., B*, Vol.66, pp. 89–106, ISSN 1011-1344

Konan, Y.N.; Berton, M.; Gurny, R. & Allemann, E. (2003a). Enhanced photodynamic activity of meso-tetra(4-hydroxyphenyl)porphyrin by incorporation into sub-200 nm nanoparticles. *Eur. J. Pharm. Sci.*, Vol.18, pp. 241–249, ISSN 0928-0987

Konan, Y.N.; Cerny, R.; Favet, J.; Berton, M.; Gurny, R. & Allemann, E. (2003b). Preparation and characterization of sterile sub-200 nmmeso-tetra(4-hydroxylphenyl)porphyrin-loaded nanoparticles for photodynamic therapy. *Eur. J. Pharm. Biopharm.*, Vol.55, pp. 115–124, ISSN 0939-6411

Konan-Kouakou, Y.N.; Boch, R.; Gurny, R. & Allemann, E. (2005). In vitro and in vivo activities of verteporfin-loaded nanoparticles. *J. Control. Release*, Vol.103, pp. 83–91, ISSN 0168-3659

Kormeili, T; Yamauchi, P.S. & Lowe, N.J. (2004). Topical photodynamic therapy in clinical dermatology. *Br. J. Dermatol.*, Vol.150, No.6, pp. 1061–1069, ISSN 1365-2133

Král, V.; Pataridis, S.; Setnička, V.; Záruba, K.; Urbanová, M. & Volka, K. (2005). New chiral porphyrin–brucine gelator characterized by methods of circular dichroism. *Tetrahedron*, Vol.61, No.23, pp. 5499–5506, ISSN 0040-4020

Král V.; Králová, J.; Kaplánek, R.; Bříza, T. & Martásek, P. (2006). Quo vadis porphyrin chemistry? Physiol. Res., Vol.55 (Suppl. 2), pp. S3-S26, ISSN 1802-9973

Králová, J.; Synytsya, A.; Poučková, P.; Koc, M.; Dvořák, M. & Král, V. (2006). Novel porphyrin conjugates with a potent photodynamic antitumor effect: differential efficacy of mono- and bis-β-cyclodextrin derivatives in vitro and in vivo. *Photochem. Photobiol.*, Vol.82, No. 2, pp. 432–438, ISSN 1751-1097

Králová, J.; Bříza, T.; Moserová, I.; Dolenský, B.; Vašek, P.; Poučková, P.; Kejík, Z.; Kaplánek, R.; Martásek, P.; Dvořák, M. & Král, V. (2008a). Glycol Porphyrin Derivatives as Potent Photodynamic Inducers of Apoptosis in Tumor Cells. *J. Med. Chem.*, Vol.51, No.19, pp. 5964-5973, ISSN 1520-4804

Králová, J.; Koivukorpi, J.; Kejík, Z.; Poučková, P.; Sievänen, E.; Kolehmainen, E. & Král, V. (2008b). Porphyrin–bile acid conjugates: from saccharide recognition in the solution to the selective cancer cell fluorescence detection. *Org. Biomol. Chem.*, Vol.6, pp. 1548–1552, ISSN 1477-0539

Labib, A.; Lenaerts, V.; Chouinard, F.; Leroux, J.C.; Ouellet, R. & van Lier, J.E. (1991). Biodegradable nanospheres containing phthalocyanines and naphthalocyanines for targeted photodynamic tumor therapy. *Pharm. Res.*, Vol.8, pp. 1027–1031, ISSN 0724-8741

Marcus, S.L.; Houlihan, A.; Lundahl, S. & Ferdon, M.E. (2007). Does ambient light contribute to the therapeutic effects of topical photodynamic therapy (PDT) using aminolevulinic acid (ALA)? *Lasers Surg. Med.*, Vol.39, pp. 201–202, ISSN 1096-9101

Marmur, E.S.; Schmults, C.D. & Goldberg, D.J. (2004). A review of laser and photodynamic therapy for the treatment of nonmelanoma skin cancer. *Dermatol. Surg.*, Vol.30, pp. 264–271, ISSN 1524-4725

McCarthy, J.R.; Perez, J.M.; Bruckner, C. & Weissleder, R. (2005). Polymeric nanoparticle preparation that eradicates tumors. *Nano Lett.*, Vol.5, pp. 2552–2556, ISSN 1530-6984

Mittra, R.A. & Singerman, L.J. (2002). Recent advances in the management of age-related macular degeneration. *Optom. Vis. Sci.*, Vol.79, No.4, pp. 218–224, ISSN 1538-9235

Moan, J. (1990). On the diffusion length of singlet oxygen in cells and tissues. *J. Photochem. Photobiol. B Biol.*, Vol.6, No.3, pp. 343–347, ISSN 1011-1344

Moan, J. & Berg, K. (1992). Photochemotherapy of cancer: experimental research. *Photochem. Photobiol.*, Vol.55, No.6, pp. 931–948, ISSN 1751-1097

Moan, J. & Peng, Q. (2003). An outline of the hundred-year history of PDT. *Anticancer Res.*, Vol.23, No.5A, pp. 3591–3600, ISSN 1791- 7530

Morton, C.A.; Brown, S.B.; Collins, S.; Ibbotson, S.; Jenkinson, H.; Kurwa, H.; Langmack, K.; McKenna, K.; Moseley, H.; Pearse, A.D.; Stringer, M.; Taylor, D.K.; Wong, G. & Rhodes, L.E. (2002). Guidelines for topical photodynamic therapy: report of a workshop of the British Photodermatology Group. *Br. J. Dermatol.*, Vol.146, pp. 552–567, ISSN 1365-2133

Morton, C.A. (2003). Methyl aminolevulinate (Metvix) photodynamic therapy - practical pearls. *J. Dermatolog. Treat.*, Vol.14(Suppl. 3), pp. 23–26, ISSN 1471-1753

Morton, C.A. (2004). Photodynamic therapy for nonmelanoma skin cancer–and more? *Arch. Dermatol.*, Vol.140, pp. 116–120, ISSN 0096-5359

Moseley, H.; Allen, J.W.; Ibbotson, S.; Lesar, A.; McNeill, A.; Camacho-Lopez, M.A.; Samuel, I.D.W.; Sibbett, W. & Ferguson, J. (2006). Ambulatory photodynamic therapy: a new concept in delivering photodynamic therapy. *Br. J. Dermatol.*, Vol.154, No.4, pp. 747–750, ISSN 1365-2133

Moseley, H. (1996). Total effective fluence: a useful concept in photodynamic therapy. *Lasers Med. Sci.*, Vol.11, pp. 139–143, ISSN 1435-604X

Niedre, M.; Patterson, M.S. & Wilson, B.C. (2002) Direct near-infrared luminescence detection of singlet oxygen generated by photodynamic therapy in cells in vitro and tissues in vivo. *Photochem. Photobiol.*, Vol.75, pp. 382–391, ISSN 1751-1097

O'Neal, D.P.; Hirsch, L.R.; Halas, N.J.; Payne, J.D. & West, J.L. (2004). Photo-thermal tumor ablation in mice using near infrared-absorbing nanoparticles. *Cancer Lett.*, Vol.209, No.2, pp. 171–176, ISSN 0304-3835

Ohulchanskyy, T.Y.; Roy, I.; Goswami, L.N.; Chen, Y.; Bergey, E.J.; Pandey, R.K.; Oseroff, A.R. & Prasad, P.N. (2007). Organically modified silica nanoparticles with covalently incorporated photosensitizer for photodynamic therapy of cancer. *Nano Lett.*, Vol.7, pp. 2835–2842, ISSN 1530-6984

Oleinick, N.L.; Morris, R.L. & Belichenko, I. (2002). The role of apoptosis in response to photodynamic therapy: what, where, why, and how. *Photochem. Photobiol. Sci.*, Vol.1, pp. 1–21, ISSN 1474-905X

Ost, D. (2003). Photodynamic therapy in lung cancer. A review. *Methods Mol. Med.*, Vol.75, pp. 507–526, ISSN 1543-1894

Palumbo, G. (2007). Photodynamic therapy and cancer: a brief sightseeing tour. *Expert Opin. Drug. Deliv.*, Vol.4, No.2, pp. 131–148, ISSN 1744-7593

Pervaiz, S.; Olivo M. Art and science of photodynamic therapy. Clin. Exp. Pharmacol. Physiol. 33(5–6), 551–556 (2006).

Pinthus, J.H.; Bogaards, A.; Weersink, R.; Wilson, B.C. & Trachtenberg, J. (2006). Photodynamic therapy for urological malignancies: past to current approaches. *J. Urol.*, Vol.175, No.4, pp. 1201–1207, ISSN 0022-5347

Pires, A.M.; Heer, S.; Gudel, H.U. & Serra, O.A. (2006). Er, Yb doped yttrium based nanosized phosphors: particle size, "host lattice" and doping ion concentration effects on upconversion efficiency. *J. Fluoresc.*, Vol.16, pp. 461–468, ISSN 1573-4994

Ricci-Junior, E. & Marchetti, J.M. (2006a). Zinc(II) phthalocyanine loaded PLGA nanoparticles for photodynamic therapy use. *Int. J. Pharm.*, Vol.310, pp. 187–195, ISSN 0378-5173

Ricci-Junior, E. & Marchetti, J.M. (2006b). Preparation, characterization, photocytotoxicity assay of PLGA nanoparticles containing zinc (II) phthalocyanine for photodynamic therapy use. *J. Microencapsul.*, Vol.23, pp. 523–538, ISSN 1464-5246

Roy, I.; Ohulchanskyy, T.Y.; Pudavar, H.E.; Bergey, E.J.; Oseroff, A.R.; Morgan, J.; Dougherty, T.J. & Prasad, P.N. (2003). Ceramic-based nanoparticles entrapping water-insoluble photosensitizing anticancer drugs: a novel drug-carrier system for photodynamic therapy. *J. Am. Chem. Soc.*, Vol.125, pp. 7860–7865, ISSN 1520-5126

Řezanka, P.; Záruba, K. & Král, V. (2008). A change in nucleotide selectivity pattern of porphyrin derivatives after immobilization on gold nanoparticles. *Tetrahedron Lett.*, Vol.49, No.45, pp. 6448–6453, ISSN 0040-4039

Samia, A.C.; Chen, X. & Burda, C. (2003). Semiconductor quantum dots for photodynamic therapy. *J. Am. Chem. Soc.*, Vol.125, pp. 15736–15737, ISSN 1520-5126

Saxena, V.; Sadoqi, M. & Shao, J. (2006). Polymeric nanoparticulate delivery system for Indocyanine green: biodistribution in healthy mice. *Int. J. Pharm.*, Vol.308, pp. 200–204, ISSN 0378-5173

Shi, L.; Hernandez, B. & Selke, M. (2006). Singlet oxygen generation from water-soluble quantum dot-organic dye nanocomposites. *J. Am. Chem. Soc.*, Vol.128, No.19, pp. 6278–6279, ISSN 1520-5126

Star, W.M.; van't Veen, A.J.; Robinson, D.J.; Munte, K.; de Haas, E.R. & Sterenborg, H.J. (2006). Topical 5-aminolevulinic acid mediated photodynamic therapy of superficial basal cell carcinoma using two light fractions with a two-hour interval: long-term follow-up. *Acta Derm. Venereol.*, Vol.86, No.5, pp. 412–417, ISSN 0001-5555

Strasswimmer, J. & Grande, D.J. (2006). Do pulsed lasers produce an effective photodynamic therapy response? *Lasers Surg. Med.*, Vol.38, pp. 22–25, ISSN 1096-9101

Sutedja, T.G. & Postmus, P.E. (1996). Photodynamic therapy in lung cancer. A review. *J. Photochem. Photobiol. B Biol.*, Vol.36, No.2, pp. 199–204, ISSN 1011-1344

Szeimies, R.M.; Dräger, J.; Abels, C. & Landthaler, M. (2001). History of photodynamic therapy in dermatology. Photodynamic therapy and fluorescence diagnosis in dermatology. Amsterdam: Elsevier, pp. 3–16

Triesscheijn, M.; Baas, P. Schellens, J.H. & Stewart, F.A. (2006). Photodynamic therapy in oncology. *Oncologist*, Vol.11, pp. 1034–1044, ISSN 1083-7159

Vargas, A.; Pegaz, B.; Debefve, E.; Konan-Kouakou, Y.; Lange, N.; Ballini, J.P.; van den Bergh, H.; Gurny, R. & Delie, F. (2004). Improved photodynamic activity of porphyrin loaded into nanoparticles: an in vivo evaluation using chick embryos. *Int. J. Pharm.*, Vol.286, pp. 131–145, ISSN 0378-5173

Wang, X.; Zhuang, J.; Peng, Q. & Li, Y. (2006). Hydrothermal synthesis of rare-earth fluoride nanocrystals. *Inorg. Chem.*, Vol.45, pp. 6661–6665, ISSN 0020-1669

Wang, X.L.; Wang, H.W.; Guo, M.X. & Huang, Z. (2007). Combination of immunotherapy and photodynamic therapy in the treatment of Bowenoid papulosis. *Photodiagnosis Photodyn. Ther.*, Vol.4, No.2, pp. 88–93, ISSN 1873-1597

Wang, X.L.; Wang, H.W.; Guo, M.X. & Xu, S.Z. (2008). Treatment of skin cancer and pre-cancer using topical ALA-PDT - a single hospital experience. *Photodiagnosis Photodyn. Ther.*, Vol.5, No.2, pp. 127–133, ISSN 1873-1597

Wieder, M.E.; Hone, D.C.; Cook, M.J.; Handsley, M.M.; Gavrilovic, J. & Russell, D.A. (2006). Intracellular photodynamic therapy with photosensitizer-nanoparticle conjugates: cancer therapy using a 'Trojan horse'. *Photochem. Photobiol. Sci.*, Vol.5, pp. 727–734, ISSN 1474-905X

Wiedmann, M.W. & Caca, K. (2004). General principles of photodynamic therapy (PDT) and gastrointestinal applications. *Curr. Pharm. Biotechnol.*, Vol.5, No.4, pp. 397–408, ISSN 1873-4316

Wiegell, S.R.; Haedersdal, M.; Philipsen, P.A.; Eriksen, P.; Enk, C.D. & Wulf, H.C. (2008). Continuous activation of PpIX by daylight is as effective as and less painful than conventional photodynamic therapy for actinic keratoses; a randomized, controlled, single-blinded study. *Br. J. Dermatol.*, Vol.158, No.4, pp. 740–746, ISSN 1365-2133

Woodburn, K.W.; Fan, Q.; Kessel, D.; Luo, Y. & Young, S.W. (1998). Photodynamic therapy of B16F10 murine melanoma with lutecium texaphyrin. *J. Invest. Dermatol.*, Vol.110. No.5, pp. 746–751, ISSN 1523-1747

Young, S.W.; Woodburn, K.W.; Wright, M.; Mody, T.D.; Fan, Q.; Sessler, J.L.; Dow, W.C. & Miller, R.A. (1996). Lutetium texaphyrin (PCI-0123): a near-infrared, water-soluble photosensitizer. *Photochem. Photobiol.*, Vol.63, No.6, pp. 892–897, ISSN 1751-1097

Zeisser-Labouebe, M.; Lange, N.; Gurny, R. & Delie, F. (2003). Hypericin-loaded nanoparticles for the photodynamic treatment of ovarian cancer. *Int. J. Pharm.*, Vol.326, pp. 174–181, ISSN 0378-5173

Zeitouni, N.C.; Oseroff, A.R. & Shieh, S. (2003). Photodynamic therapy for nonmelanoma skin cancers. Current review and update. *Mol. Immunol.*, Vol.39, No.17–18, pp. 1133–1136, ISSN 1872-9142

Zhang, P.; Rogelj, S.; Nguyen, K. & Wheeler, D. (2006). Design of a highly sensitive and specific nucleotide sensor based on photon upconverting particles. *J. Am. Chem. Soc.*, Vol.128, pp. 12410–12411, ISSN 1520-5126

Zhang, P.; Steelant, W.; Kumar, M. & Scholfield, M. (2007). Versatile photosensitizers for photodynamic therapy at infrared excitation. *J. Am. Chem. Soc.*, Vol.129, pp. 4526–4527, ISSN 1520-5126

Zhou, Q.; Olivo, M.; Lye, K.Y.; Moore, S.; Sharma, A. & Chowbay, B. (2005). Enhancing the therapeutic responsiveness of photodynamic therapy with the antiangiogenic agents SU5416 and SU6668 in murine nasopharyngeal carcinoma models. *Cancer Chemother. Pharmacol.*, Vol.56, No.6, pp. 569–577, ISSN 1432-0843

Zijlmans, H.; Bonnet, J.; Burton, J.; Kardos, K.; Vail, T.; Niedbala, R.S. & Tanke, H.J. (1990). Detection of cell and tissue surface antigens using up-converting phosphors: a new reporter technology. *Anal. Biochem.*, Vol.267, pp. 30–36, ISSN 1096-0309

Part 3

Molecular Aspects of Tumor Invasion and Progression in Squamous Cell Carcinoma

7

Cadherin Expression and Progression of Squamous Cell Carcinomas of the Oral Cavity

Kazushi Imai, Genta Maeda and Tadashige Chiba
Department of Biochemistry, School of Life Dentistry at Tokyo,
The Nippon Dental University
Japan

1. Introduction

Cell-cell adhesion plays fundamental and dynamic roles in the development and maintenance of multi-cellular organisms. Epithelial sheet is a typical structure and composed of cells that work together and separate from a lumen or space from underlying tissue. It lines most internal surfaces, including gastrointestinal tract and kidney tubes, and external layer of the epithelium as the epidermis of skin. The oral cavity is covered with stratified squamous cell epithelium in which keratinizing epithelial cells strongly connect with each other and differentiate from basal cells at the bottom to keratinized surface cells. Epithelial cells are connected together by junctional complexes that have distinct order with respect to their ultra-structures; zonula occludens (tight junctions), gap junctions, zonula adherens (adherence junctions) and macula adherens (desmosomes). Adherence junctions in epithelial sheet are belt like junctions and composed of cadherins that bind with proteins at the cytoplasmic domain. In other cell types, adherence junctions display different morphology; spotty and discontinuous in fibroblastic cells and punctate in the synaptic junctions. Desmosome is a spot-like junction associated with desmosomal cadherins (desmogleins and desmocollins) and tightly associated with adjacent cell membranes compared to adherence junctions. Stratified squamous epithelial cells express large amount of cadherins and well organize adherence junctions and desmosomes. Disruption of desmosomes by autoantibodies against desmoglein causes pemphigus that are multiple and bullous diseases in the skin and oral mucosa. Cadherins are most characterized cell-cell adhesion molecules and implicated in the development and progression of carcinomas of the epithelial origin. In this chapter, we overview the regulation and role of cadherins in the pathology of oral squamous cell carcinomas (OSCCs).

2. The cadherin superfamily

Cadherins are calcium-dependent transmembrane proteins that are evolutionary conserved and have two or more extracellular domains (EC domains). Yoshida and Takeich (1992) cloned a transmembrane protein from the calcium-dependent junctions and termed cadherin. Since many related molecules were cloned, cadherins constitute a superfamily and the original cadherins are now called as "classic cadherins" (Fig. 1). Approximately twenty members of cadherins are included in the classic cadherin family depending on their domain structures. In vertebrate, they have five repetitive EC domains that contains calcium-binding sequences and highly conserved cytoplasmic domain that directly interacts with catenins. The binding of calcium ions with the EC domains is prerequisite for the conformation and adhesive function of the extracellular region, and the extracellular region undergoes interactions with apposed cells. The classic cadherins are subdivided into type I and type II. Type I cadherin contains a His-Arg-Val sequence in the N-terminal EC domain, and other classic cadherins that do not contain the sequence are grouped into type II cadherin. The type I cadherin includes epithelial-cadherin (E-cadherin, CDH1), neural-cadherin (N-cadherin, CDH2), placental-cadherin (P-cadherin, CDH3) and others, and vascular endothelial-cadherin (VE-cadherin, CDH5), osteoblast-cadherin (OB-cadherin, CDH11) and others belong to the type II cadherins. Although it is still controversial, the classic cadherin basically binds with the same-type cadherin but not with other types. This nature of homophilic binding is implicated in the sorting of different cell types. Besides to the classic cadherins, a number of nonclassic cadherins that conserve EC domains but have divergent cytoplasmic sequences has been identified. Desmosomal cadherins are most closed to the classic cadherins and required for desmosome formation in the epithelium. Other nonclassic cadherins, including protocadherins, Fat and Flamingo, appear not to organize specialized junctions, nor to be the essential adherence junction components (Meng & Takeichi, 2009; Gumbiner, 2005).

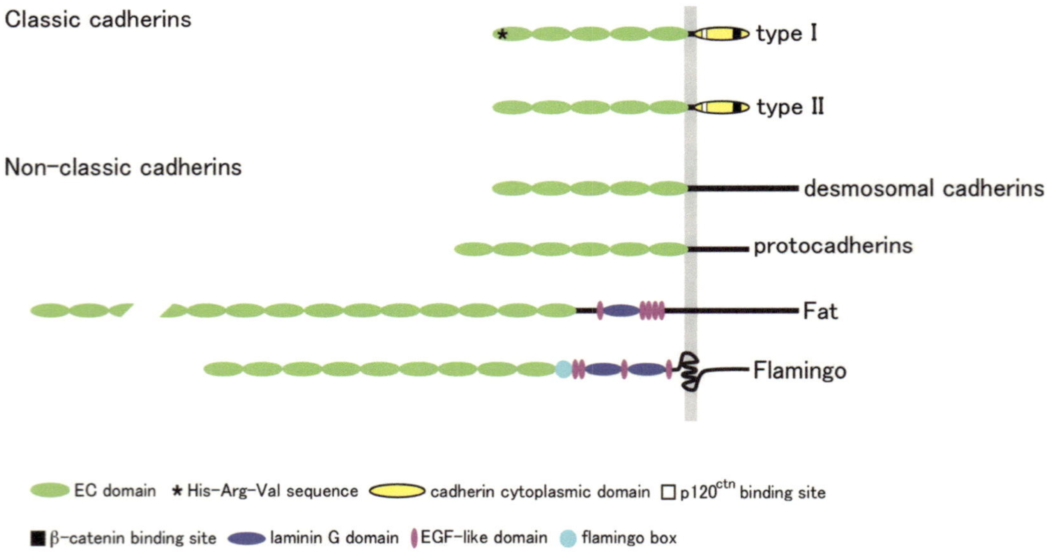

Fig. 1. Domain structures of cadherin superfamily. Molecules conserving EC domains in the extracellular region consist of the cadherin superfamily. The classic cadherins have five EC domains and the cytoplasmic domain possessing the binding sites for p120^{ctn} and β-catenin. They are subdivided into type I and type II groups according to the presence or absence of His-Arg-Val sequence in the N-terminal EC domain, respectively. Non-classic cadherins do not preserve the cytoplasmic domain and have unique cytoplasmic amino acid structures in each cadherin. Numbers of EC domains in each non-classic cadherin are different depending on members. For example, in desmosomal cadherins, desmoglein and desmocollin have four and five EC domains, respectively.

3. Cadherin functions at the adherence junction

The highly conserved cytoplasmic domains of the classic cadherins interact with catenins (Fig. 2). The juxtamembrane region of the cytoplasmic domain binds with p120-catenin

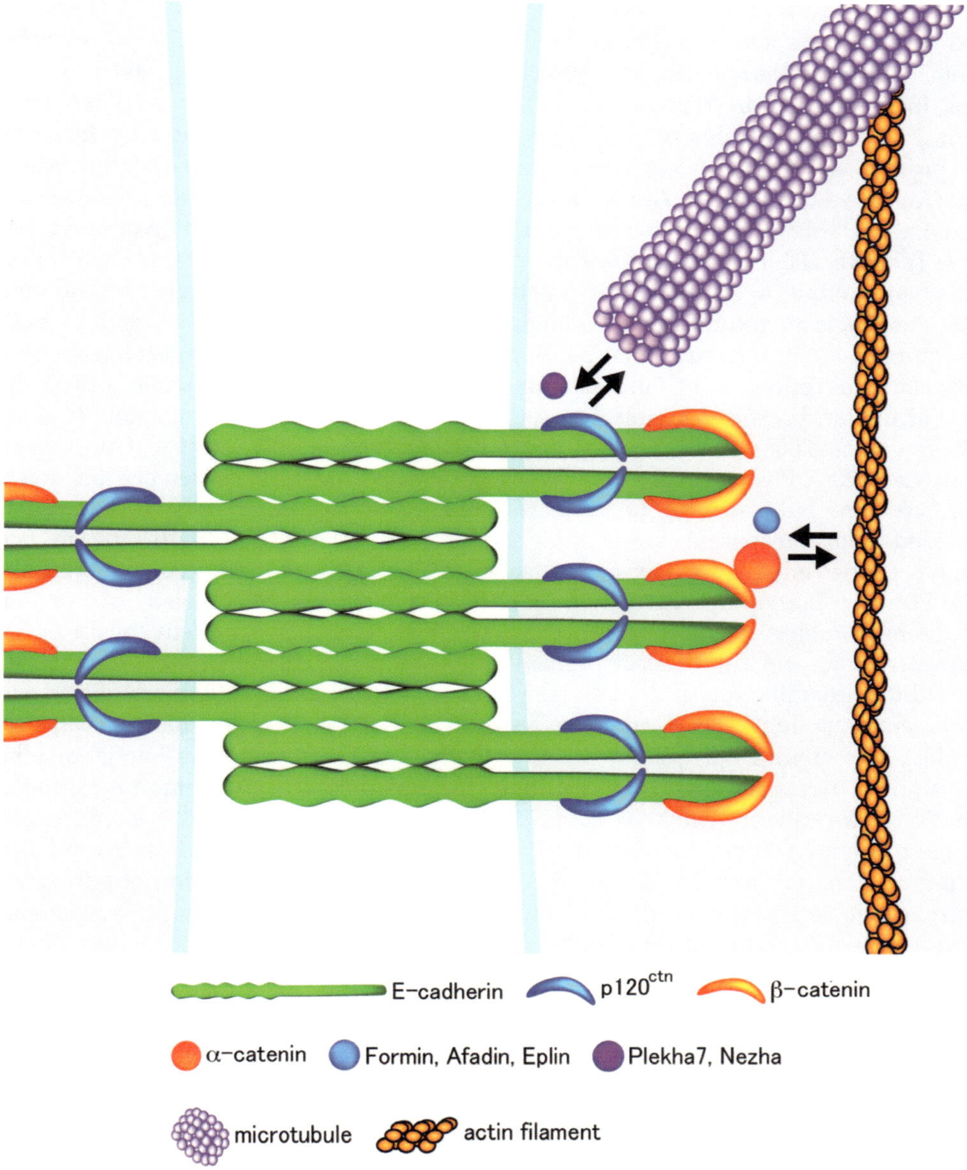

Fig. 2. Molecular structural organization of adherence junction containing E-cadherin. E-cadherins homotypically bind with adjacent cells by the EC domain interaction, and p12O^{ctn} and β-catenin interact with the cytoplasmic domain of E-cadherin. pl20^{ctn} directly associate with microtubules or indirectly mediated by Plekha 7 and Nezha. The β-catenin-α-catenin complex associates with actin filaments with or without linker proteins (Formin, Afadin and Eplin).

($p120^{ctn}$), and the carboxy-terminal half with β-catenin. The cytoplasmic domain indirectly binds with α-catenin through β-catenin, resulting in formation of the cadherin-β-catenin-α-catenin complex. The complex ligates with actin filaments that are essential for assembly and integrity of adherence junctions. Although early studies suggested that α-catenin acts as a linker protein which in turn interact with the complex and actin filament, recent studies showed that free α-catenin can bind the filament and promote the bundling of actin filaments, but not α-catenin in the complex (Drees et al., 2005; Yamada et al., 2005). Several proteins, including Formin (Kobielad et al., 2004), Afadin (Mandai, 1997) and Eplin (Abe & Takeichi, 2008), are suggested to work as a linker between α-catenin and actin filament. $p120^{ctn}$ protein also regulates actin reorganization and contractility by regulating RhoA activity (Anastasiadis et al., 2007). However, since the roles on the formation of adherence junction and the linkage with actin filament are appeared different depending on cell types (Meng & Takeichi, 2009), further studies are required to define the molecular mechanism for actin filament-binding to the adherence junction complex. Another cytoskeleton connected with the complex is microtubules. Microtubules extend to adherence junctions, and blocking the microtubules extension reduces accumulation of E-cadherin to the junctions (Stehbens et al., 2006; Harris & Tepass, 2010). Furthermore, depolymerization of microtubules disrupt the integrity of the junctions and inhibit disassembly of cell junctions (Waterman-Storer et al., 2000; Ivanov et al., 2006). Recent studies showed that microtubules interact with adherence junctions via $p120^{ctn}$, Plekha7 and Nezha (Meng & Takeichi, 2009). The adherence junction is a static structure but cadherin proteins are recycled in epithelial cells. E-cadherin is endocytosed and transported to recycling endosomes followed by trafficking in late endosomes to the cell surface (Meng & Takeichi, 2009). The surface-located cadherins are stabilized by their homophilic interactions at adherence junctions. $p120^{ctn}$ also has a pivotal role in the microtubule assembly at adherence junctions. The $p120^{ctn}$ protein consist of the N-terminal region, armadillo repeat domain and C-terminal tail region. The N-terminal region and the armadillo repeat domain are responsible for binding with microtubules and the juxtamembrane domain of E-cadherin, respectively (Ichii & Takeichi, 2007; Ishiyama et al., 2010). The binding of $p120^{ctn}$ to E-cadherin masks a dileucine motif on the juxtamembrane domain, which is sensitive to endocytosis and ubiquitin-mediated degradation of E-cadherin (Ishiyama et al., 2010). It is suggested that $p120^{ctn}$ stabilizes the microtubule polymerization independent of a mechanistic trait of E-cadherin-mediated cell-cell adhesion (Ichii & Takeichi, 2007). Thus, the assembly and the function of adherence junctions are regulated by multi-dimensional factors, including E-cadherin *per se*, catenins, the related molecules and association with actin filaments and microtubules.

4. Roles of E-cadherin in the epithelium

E-cadherin-null mutation is lethal and the conditional knockout mice in skin epithelium show hyperproliferation of basal cells with defects in terminal differentiation (Ohsugi et al., 1997; Tinkle et al., 2004). An animal model of pancreatic carcinomas demonstrated a direct role of E-cadherin in adenoma-to-carcinoma conversion (Perl et al., 1998). These studies indicate that E-cadherin plays a critical role in developmental and pathological events *in vivo*. Forced expression of E-cadherin in the intestinal epithelium represses migration of epithelial cells along with the crypt-villus axis and stimulates the apoptotic rate of epithelial cells (Hermiston et al., 1996). Recent studies implicate that cadherins regulate interaction of growth factor receptors with ligands and modulate their signaling. Cadherins bind to growth factor receptors, including transforming growth factor-β receptor (TGFBR), fibroblast growth factor receptor (FGFR), epidermal growth factor receptor (EGFR), vascular endothelial cell growth factor receptor (VEGFR) and platelet-derived growth factor receptor (PDGFR), and the cytoplasmic domain can suppress growth-promoting cell signaling, such as Src, phosphatidylinositol-3-kinase (PI3K)/AKT and extracellular signal-regulated kinase (ERK) pathways (Reddy et al., 2005; Suyama et al., 2002; Georgopoulos et al., 2010; Cavallaro & Dejana, 2011). Sensitivity to the EGFR inhibitor, cetuximab, requires intact E-cadherin expression and silencing of E-cadherin reduces responsiveness to the inhibitor (Black et al., 2008). Cadherins regulate the growth factor signaling by recruiting the receptors at the cell surface, stimulating the receptor dimerization, and modulating their activities (Cavallaro & Dejana, 2011). β-catenin is a leading player in WNT signaling, which has a predominant role in developmental and pathophysiological conditions. Binding of WNTs to the receptors protected β-catenin from the degradation by the ubiquitin-protease pathway and increases the cytoplasmic free pool (Maher et al., 2009). The cytoplasmic free-β-catenin translocates into the nucleus and modulates gene transcription by interacting with lymphoid enhancer factor (LEF) and T cell factor (TCF). Since the cadherin-β-catenin interaction is constitutive, cadherins interfere with the transcriptional activity of β-catenin. Therefore, unveiling the regulatory mechanisms of E-cadherin expression is a pivotal theme to understand the initiation and progression of carcinomas and develop a novel strategy for the treatment of carcinoma patients.

5. Regulation of E-cadherin expression

Loss or reduction of E-cadherin expression results from somatic mutations, chromosomal deletions, proteolytic cleavage, promoter hypermethylation and transcriptional repression. Germ-line mutation of the E-cadherin gene causing inactivation of one allele has been reported in several families from New Zealand and Europe, and is associated with hereditary diffuse-type high-grade gastric carcinomas (Guiford et al., 1998; Gayther et al., 1998). Although single nucleotide polymorphisms have been described to associate with the reduction of transcription efficiency of E-cadherin gene (Li et al., 2000), the mechanism of reduction awaits for future studies to establish. However, genomic deletion and germ-line mutation with loss of heterozygosity, referred to as Knudson's two-hit theory, are rare events in sporadic carcinomas (Brown, 1997). Loss of E-cadherin expression stimulates carcinoma progression and carcinoma cells in the metastatic loci frequently re-express E-cadherin (Cheng et al., 2001), indicating the genetic mutation and polymorphism are not a major cause in sporadic carcinomas. In mammalian genome, methylation emerges at a cytosine located 5′ to a guanosime in a CpG dinucleotide. CpG islands are found in promoter region of approximately half of the genes in human genome. In the development of cancers, epigenetic silencing of tumor-suppressive genes as a result of cytosine methylation in CpG islands has been documented as one of most important alterations. Increasing evidence highlight the fact that there are target genes for CpG island hypermethylation in many types of cancers, especially carcinomas of the epithelial origin (Fazzari & Greally, 2004; Jones & Baylin, 2002; Maeda et al., 2007a; Maeda et al., 2007b; Chiba et al., 2009). The hypermethylation at CpG islands determines the transcriptional status of a gene by blocking the access of certain transcription factors that are sensitive to cytosine methylation in their binding motifs, and by packaging chromatin into compacted nucleosomes with deacetylated histones and recruiting a methyl-cytosine-binding protein complex that represses transcription (Fazzari & Greally, 2004; Jones & Baylin, 2002). The transcription repressors, including Snail, Slug, Twist, zinc finger E-box binding homeobox

(ZEB)1, ZEB2, and E47, bind to the E-box (5′-CANNTG-3′) in the promoter and repress E-cadherin expression. After identification of Snail as a transcription repressor of E-cadherin in 2000 (Cano et al, 2000; Batlle et al, 2000), several other repressors were implicated in tumor progression and the epithelial-mesenchymal transition (EMT) induction. The EMT stimulates migration, earns the drug-resistance and the stem cell-like features of carcinoma cells and energizes carcinomas to an aggressive subset, and the loss of E-cadherin expression is the most prominent event (Hanahan & Weinberg, 2011). Expression of E-cadherin repressors is regulated by multiple pathways activated by growth factors. Among them, TGFβ signaling is frequently activated in aggressive carcinomas and induces the EMT of carcinoma cells at the invasive front. High mobility group protein A-2 (HMGA2), which is specifically expressed in undifferentiated mesenchymal cells, are strongly misexpressed in oral carcinoma cells at the invasive front in patients with poor prognosis (Fig. 3; Miyazawa

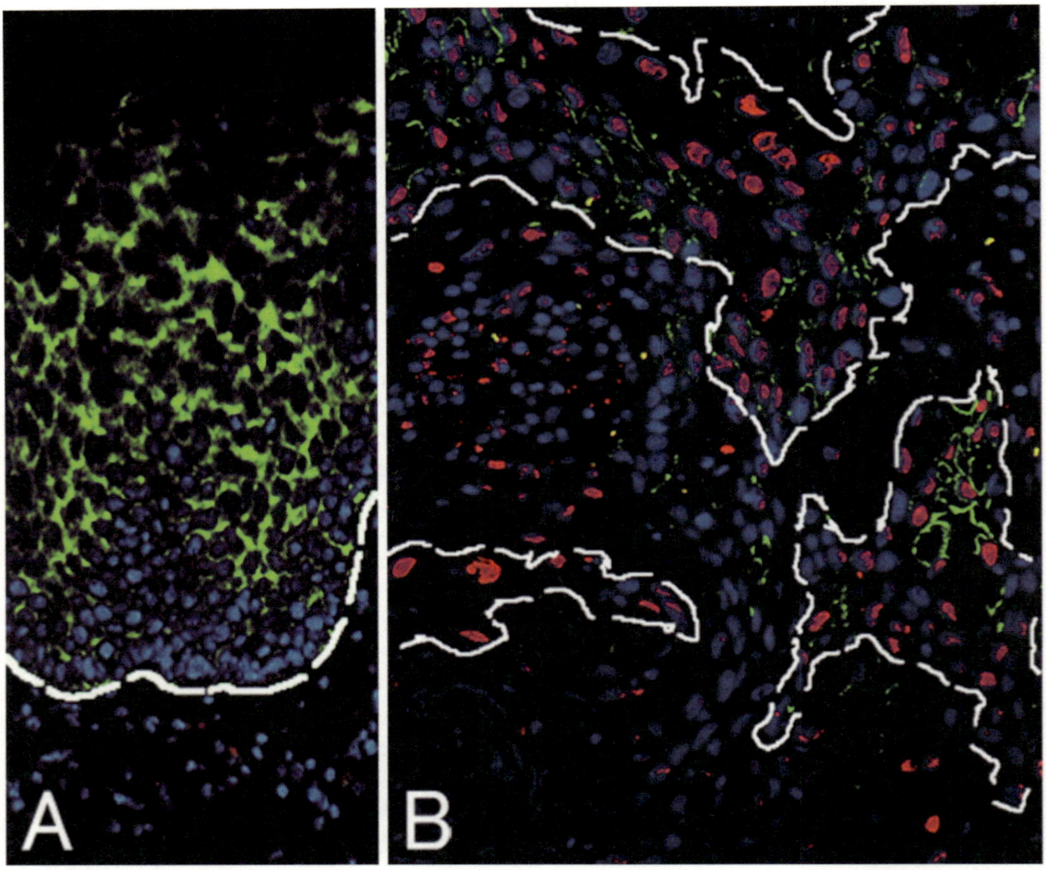

Fig. 3. Expression of E-cadherin and HMGA2 in oral epithelium and carcinomas. E-cadherin (green) expression is detected by iimmunofluorescent microscopy at the cell-cell boundaries of normal oral epithelium (A) while in carcinoma cells at the invasive dramatically lose the immunoreactivities (B). In contrast, the mesenchyme-specific HMGA2 expression (red) is localized in carcinoma cells that are negative for E-cadherin, and not detected in normal oral epithelial cells. The data in a panel B is reproduced from Miyazawa et al., [*Cancer Research*, Vol. 64, No.(6) pp.2024-2029, ISSN 1078-0432].

et al., 2004), and integrates the TGF-β-mediated EMT in carcinoma cell in combination with the induction of Snail, Slug and Twist (Thuault et al., 2006). In addition, inhibition of WNT signaling promotes degradation of Snail by the ubiquitin-proteasome pathway (Shou et al, 2004). Expression of E-cadherin is also post-transcriptionally regulated by the microenvironment of carcinoma cells. Furthermore, series of immunohistochemical studies suggest the differential roles of repressors; Snail in the induction of initial migratory phenotype of carcinoma cells followed by the maintenance of phenotype by Slug, Twist and ZEB1/2 (Peinado et al., 2007). The transcription repressors attenuate E-cadherin expression while they are negatively regulated by micoRNAs (miRNAs). Expression of miR-200, which binds to ZEB1 and ZEB2 mRNAs and abrogates their translation into proteins, is inhibited by TGF-β signaling but stimulated a tumor suppressor gene p53 (Kim et al., 2011; Gregory et al., 2011). The miR-92, which directly targets E-cadherin mRNA, downregulates p53 expression (Neveu et al., 2010; Chen et al., 2011). TGF-β also upregulates expression of matrix metalloproteinases (MMPs), which liberate TGF-β from surrounding tissues to cells after degradation of extracellular matrix proteins (Imai et al., 1997). Since MMPs shed the extracellular region of E-cadherin (Zheng et al., 2009; Imai & Okada, 2009), the TGFβ-MMP loop enhances disruption of E-cadherin-mediated adherence junctions of carcinoma cells. Therefore, the state of E-cadherin comprehensively regulated by the intrinsic and extrinsic factors of carcinoma cells (Fig. 4).

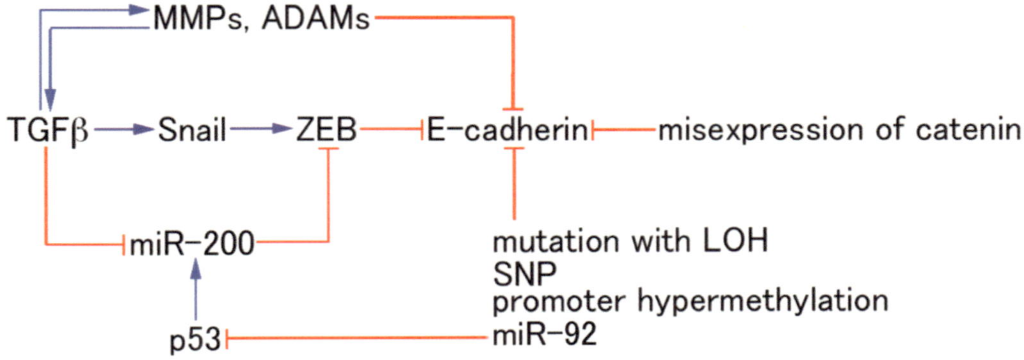

Fig. 4. A schematic representation for the E-cadherin expression and repression machineries. In carcinoma cells of epithelial origin, expression of E-cadherin is regulated by several pathways that directly or indirectly control the expression. Blue lines indicate stimulation and red lines indicate suppression.

6. Loss of E-cadherin expression in oral squamous cell carcinomas

As mentioned above, multi-factors may regulate the E-cadherin repression in oral carcinoma cells. Although germ-line mutation with the loss of heterozygosity is rare (Saito et al., 1998), epigenetic aberrations, including the promoter hypermethylation and expression of transcription repressors, are commonly observed in an aggressive subset of OSCCs. The hypermethylation is detected in 35-85% of OSCCs (Viswanathan et al., 2003; Yeh et al., 2002) and prompts carcinoma cells to develop invasive tumors (Nakayama et al., 2001). Kudo et al. (2004) reported that the hypermehtylation was observed in oral carcinoma cells at the invasive front but not in non-invasive areas. Although increasing number of investigations revealed the presence of E-cadherin transcription repressors, their expression is largely dependent on cell and tissue types (Peinado et al., 2004). Snail is a most studied molecule that is responsible for repression of E-cadherin gene expression in many types of carcinomas including OSCCs (Yokoyama et al., 2001).

Snail expression is observed at the invasive front oral carcinoma cells of patients with poor prognosis (Yu et al., 2011). Although we could not find a reverse correlation between expression of Snail and E-cadherin in oral carcinoma cells, ZEB2 expression was upregualted in the E-cadherin-low cells and detected in carcinoma cells at the invasive front of OSCC patients with poor prognosis (Maeda et al., 2005). Upregulation of Twist in OSCCs is reported while its significance to E-cadherin expression is uncertain (Vered et al., 2010; Liang et al., 2011). In addition to the loss of E-cadherin expression, the involvement of catenins is also documented. The role of $p120^{ctn}$ in E-cadherin expression and carcinoma progression has been attracting a lot of attention. Loss of $p120^{ctn}$ expression in the oral epithelium in mice spontaneously develops invasive OSCCs, induces the EMT of carcinoma cells, and recruits chronic inflammatory reactions within carcinoma tissues (Stairs et al., 2011). Cell membrane-associated E-cadherin become endocytosis upon the loss of $p120^{ctn}$, leading to the reduction of cell-cell adhesion (Liu et al., 2007). The loss or mislocalization of $p120^{ctn}$ correlates with poor patient prognoses of carcinomas of the colon, bladder, stomach, breast, prostate, lung and pancreas (Thoreson & Reynolds, 2002). Cytoplasmic mislocation of $p120^{ctn}$ in oral carcinoma cell lines, while it is localized at the cell membrane of normal oral keratinocytes, was reported previously (Lo Muzio et al., 2002). However, the loss of expression in the epidermis does not have an obvious effect on cell-cell adhesion but reduces expression level of E-cadherin. The mice show epidermal inflammation due to activation of nuclear factor-kappa B (NF-κB) signaling (Perez-Moreno et al., 2006). Chronic inflammation increases production of inflammatory cytokines and reactive oxygen species and DNA damage, and results in development and progression of carcinomas (Meira et al., 2008). Oral carcinoma cells upregulate the E-cadherin-targeting miR-92 (Scapoli et al., 2010). Although expression of miR-200 in OSCCs is not known at present, nasopharyngeal carcinomas downregulate it which destabilizes ZEB1/2 mRNA (Chen et al., 2009). Regardless of the cause, loss of E-cadherin results in the liberation of β-catenin from adherence junctions and the increase of the cytoplasmic free-pool, which synergistically acts with the canonical WNT signaling. In fact, carcinoma cells at the invasive front, where loss of E-cadherin and expression of WNTs are observed, exhibit the cytoplasmic and/or nuclear staining of β-catenin (Uraguchi et al., 2004; Miyazawa et al., 2004). Silencing of β-catenin by RNA interference reduces proliferation of oral carcinoma cells (Duan & Fan, 2011). A recent study suggests that the loss of E-cadherin-mediated cell-cell adhesion and sequestering the β-catenin from E-cadherin have a differential role establishing metastatic properties of carcinoma cells (Onder et al., 2008). Although a precise mechanism is under debate, loss of E-cadherin expression and the gain of WNT expression may synergistically increase the cytoplasmic β-catenin and preserve it from degradation, allowing the nuclear translocation and transcriptional control of target genes toward the tumor progression. The WNT signaling represses transcription of E-cadherin gene but stimulates WNT protein expressions *per se*. The WNTs also upregulate E-cadherin suppressors, including Snail and Twist, and downregulate miR-200 (Saydam et al., 2009). E-cadherin suppresses activation of NF-κB, which strongly enhances aggressive behaviors of oral carcinoma cells and is upregulated in patients with poor outcome (Solanas et al., 2008). A mouse EMT model demonstrated the essential contribution of NF-κB to the induction of EMT, maintenance of the mesenchymal phenotype, and metastasis (Huber et al., 2004). NF-κB suppresses E-cadherin expression through ZEB1 and ZEB2 induction (Chua et al., 2007). Therefore, reduction and loss of E-cadherin expression in OSCCs is under the control of multiple factors and pathways including the gene transcription, catenins and growth factor signaling.

7. Cadherin switch and oral carcinoma progression

E-cadherin and N-cadherin are the most prominent members of the classic cadherins, and a numbers of studies have been reported about their roles in carcinoma progression. During the progression of many human gastrointestinal tumors, gradual loss of E-cadherin expression at the invasive front accompanies a *de novo* N-cadherin expression (Wheelock et al., 2008). Replacing the member of cadherins, usually E-cadherin-to-N-cadherin in carcinoma cells, is referred as the cadherin switch. Followed by the cadherin switch, carcinoma cells acquire motile, invasive and metastatic abilities. Although functional implications are unknown at present, expression pattern of N-cadherin in a belt-like structure in low-grade prostate carcinomas becomes a dotted pattern at the interface of interaction with stromal fibroblasts in parallel with loss of E-cadherin expression (Tomita et al., 2000). Inhibition of N-cadherin expression or function blocks motility and invasion of carcinoma cells (De Wever et al., 2004). The cadherin switch is initiated by the internal and microenvironmental programs of carcinoma cells. Carcinoma cell adhesion on extracellular matrix proteins, including laminin (Kim et al., 2011), type I collagen (Shintani et al., 2008) and fibronectin (Lefort et al., 2011), induces N-cadherin expression. Another key regulator of N-cadherin is TGF-β, which can act to carcinoma cells after the extracellular matrix degradation and promotes invasion of oral carcinomas (Imai et al., 1997; Lu et al., 2004).

In OSCCs, TGF-β and N-cadherin is predominantly expressed at the invasive front and stimulates the motility of cells (Franz et al., 2007). The TGF-β signaling promotes oral carcinoma cells to express N-cadherin without affecting E-cadherin expression and regulate the motility (Diamond et al., 2008). Li et al. (2009) reported that N-cadherin was positively stained in 92.4% of tongue carcinomas while E-cadherin in 11.3%. A previous study reported that N-cadherin was upregulated in OSCCs with reduced expression of E-cadherin, and that N-cadherin expressing OSCCs had a tendency to be less histologically differentiated, more invasive and metastatic to lymph nodes (Pyo et al., 2007). However, from a stand of view that the carcinoma cell EMT is a representative event at the invasive front, there is no clear experimental study to investigate the role of the EMT in OSCC progression so far.

8. Conclusion

Investigators have reported numerous molecules related to the stimulation and the suppression of OSCC progression. Among the molecules, E-cadherin is one of most well-studied and powerful suppressor of carcinoma progression. It is frequently downregulated in aggressive OSCCs at the invasive front. Its expression is negatively regulated by many factors, including genetic and epigenetic factors, transcriptional repressors, miRNAs, growth factor signaling, shedding and catenin expression. In addition to loss of E-cadherin expression, carcinoma cells become to express N-cadherin referred as the cadherin switch.

The cadherin switch takes an important part in the EMT, which strongly stimulate aggressive behaviors of carcinoma cells. Since E-cadherin expression is negatively regulated by multi-dimension, re-activation of E-cadherin in carcinoma cells may not be a straightforward strategy to treat OSCC patients. However, unveiling the regulatory mechanism and roles of E-cadherin downregulation and cadherin switch will greatly improve our knowledge on the pathology of OSCCs and contribute to establish the future direction for the patient treatment.

9. References

Abe, K. & Takeichi, M. (2008). EPLIN mediates linkage of the cadherin catenin complex to F-actin and stabilizes the circumferential actin belt. *Proceedings of the National Academy of Science of the U.S.A.*, Vol.105, No.(1) pp.13-19, ISSN 1091-6490

Anastasiadis, P.Z. (2007). p120-ctn: A nexus for contextual signaling via Rho GTPases. *Biochimica et Biophysca Acta*, Vol.1173, No.(1) pp.34-46, ISSN 0006-3002

Batlle, E., Sancho, E., Francí, C., Domínguez, D., Monfar, M., Baulida, J. & Gariía de Herreros, A. (2000). The transcription factor Snail is a repressor of *E-cadherin* gene expression in epithelial tumor cells. *Nature Cell Biology*, Vol.2, No.(2) pp84-89, ISSN 1465-7392

Black, P.C., Brown, G.A., Inamoto, T., Shrader, A., Arora, A. Siefker-Radtke, A.O., Adam, L., Theodorescu, D., Wu, X., Munsell, M.F., Bar-Eli, M.B., McConkey, D.J. & Dinney, C.P.N. (2008). Sensitivity to epidermal growth factor receptor inhibitor requires E-cadherin expression in urothelial carcinoma cells. *Clinical Cancer Research*, Vol.14, No.(5) pp.1478-1486, ISSN 1078-0432

Brown, M.A. (1997). Tumor suppressor genes and human cancer. *Advances in Genetics*, Vol.36, No.(1) pp.45-135, ISSN 0065-2660

Cano, A., Pérez-Moreno, M.A., Rodrigo, I., Locascio, A., Blanco, M.J., del Barrio, M.G., Portillo, F. & Nieto, A. (2000). The transcription factor Snail controls epithelial-mesenchymal transitions by repressing E-cadherin expression. *Nature Cell Biology*, Vol.2, No.(2) pp.76-83, ISSN 1465-7392

Cavallaro, U. & Dejana, E. (2011). Adhesion molecules signalling: Not always a sticky business. *Nature Reviews Molecular Cell Biology*, Vol.12, No.(3) pp.189-197, ISSN 1471-0072

Chen, H.C., Chen, G.H., Chen, Y.H., Liao, W.L., Liu, C.Y., Cheng, K.P., Chang, Y.S. & Chen, S.J. (2009). MicroRNA deregulation and pathway alterations in nasopharyngeal carcinoma. *British Journal of Cancer*, Vol.100, No.(6) pp.1002-1011, ISSN 0007-0920

Chen, Z.L., Zhao, X.H., Wang, J.W., Li, B.Z., Wang, Z., Sun, J., Tan, F.W., Ding, D.P., Xu, X.H., Zhou, F., Tan, X.G., Hang, J., Shi, S.S., Feng, X.L. & He, J. (2011). MicroRNA-92a promotes lymph node metastasis of human esophageal squamous cell carcinoma via E-cadherin. *The Journal of Biological Chemistry*, Vol.286, No.(12) pp.10725-10734

Cheng, C.W., Wu, P.E., Yu, J.C., Huang, C.S., Yue, C.T., Wu, C.W. & Shen, C.Y. (2001). Mechanisms of inactivation of E-cadherin in breast carcinoma: Modification of the two-hit hypothesis of tumor suppressor gene. *Oncogene*, Vol.20, No.(29) pp.3814-3823, ISSN 5532-5542

Chiba, T., Maeda, G., Kawashiri, S., Kato, K. & Imai, K. (2009). Epigenetic loss of mucosa-associated lymphoid tissue 1 expression in patients with oral carcinomas. *Cancer Research*, Vol.69, No.(18) pp.7216-7223, ISSN 0008-5472

Chua, H.L., Bhat-Nakshatri, P., Clare, S.E., Morimiya, A., Badve, S. & Nakshatri, H. (2007). NF-kappaB represses E-cadherin expression and enhances epithelial to mesenchymal transition of mammary epithelial cells: Potential involvement of ZEB-1 and ZEB-2. *Oncogene*, Vol.26, No.(5) pp.711-724, ISSN 5532-5542

De Wever, O., Westbroek, W., Verloes, A., Bloemen, N., Bracke, M., Gespach, C., Bruyneel, E. & Mareel, M. (2004). Critical role of N-cadherin in myofibroblast invasion and migration in vitro stimulated by colon-cancer-cell derived TGF-beta or wounding. *Journal of Cell Science*, Vol.117, No.(20) pp.4619-4703, ISSN 0021-9533

Diamond, M.E., Sun, L., Ottaviano, A.J., Joseph, M.J. & Munshi, HG. (2008). Differential growth factor regulation of N-cadherin expression and motility in normal and malignant oral epithelium. *Journal of Cell Science*, Vol.121, No.(13) pp.2197-2207, ISSN 0021-0533

Drees, F., Pokutta, S., Yamada, S., Nelson, W.J. & Weis, W.I. (2005). α-catenin is a molecular switch that binds E-cadherin-β-catenin and regulates actin-filament assembly. *Cell*, Vol.123, No.(5) pp.903-915, ISSN 0092-8674

Duan, Y. & Fan, M. (2011). Lentivirus-mediated gene silencing of beta-catenin inhibits growth of human tongue cancer cells. *Journal of Oral Pathology and Medicine*, early publication ahead of print. ISSN 1600-0714

Fazzari, M.J. & Greally, J.M. (2004). Epigenomics: Beyond CpG islads. *Nature Reviews Genetics*, Vol.5, No.(6) pp.446-455, ISSN 1471-0056

Gayther, S.A., Gorringe, K.L., Ramus, S.J., Huntsman, D., Roviello, F., Grehan, N., Machado, J.C., Pinto, E., Seruca, R., Halling, K., MacLeod, P., Powell, S.M., Jackson, C.E., Ponder, B.A. & Calds, C. (1998). Identification of germ-line E-cadherin mutations in gastric cancer families of European origin. *Cancer Research*, Vol.58, No.(18) pp.4086-4089, ISSN 0008-5472

Georgopoulos, N.T., Kirkwood, L.A., Walker, D.C. & Southgate, J. (2010). Differential regulation of growth-promoting signalling pathways by E-cadherin. *PLoS One*, Vol.5, No.(10) pp.e13621. ISSN 1932-6203

Gregory, P.A., Bracken, C.P., Smith, E., Wright, J.A., Roslan, S., Morris, M., Wyatt, L., Farshid, G., Lim, Y.Y., Lindeman, G.L., Shannon, M.F., Drew, P.A., Khew-Goodall, Y. & Goodall, G.J. (2011). An autocrine TGF-β/ZEB/miR-200 signaling network regulates establishment and maintenance of epithelial-mesenchymal transition. *Molecular Biology of Cells*, Vol.22, No.(10) pp.1686-1698, ISSN 1059-1524

Guiford, P., Hopkins, J., Harraway, J., McLeod, M., McLeod, N., Harawira, P., Taite, H., Scoular, R., Miller, A. & Reeve, A.E. (1998). E-cadherin germline mutations in familial gastric cancer. *Nature*, Vol.392, No.(6674) pp.402-405, ISSN 0028-0836

Gumbiner, B.M. (2005). Regulation of cadherin-mediated adhesion in morphogenesis. *Nature Reviews Molecular Cell Biology*, Vol.6, No.(8) pp.622-634, ISSN 1471-0072

Hanahan, D. & Weinberg, R.A. (2011). Hallmarks of cancer: The next generation. *Cell*, Vol.144, No.(5) pp. 646-674, ISSN 0092-8674

Harris, T.J.C. & Tepass, U. (2010). Adhesion junctions: From molecules to morphogenesis. *Nature Reviews Molecular Cell Biology*, Vol.11, No.(7) pp502-512, ISSN 1471-0072

Hermiston, M.L., Wong, M.H. & Gordon, J.I. (1996). Forced expression of E-cadherin in the mouse intestinal epithelium shows cell migration and provides evidence for nonautonomous regulation of cell fate in a self-renewing system. *Genes and Development*, Vol.10, No.(8) pp.985-996, ISSN 0890-9369

Huber, M.A., Azoitei, N., Baumann, B., Grunert, S., Sommer, A., Pehamberger, H., Kraut, N., Beug, H. & Wirth, T. (2004). NF-kappaB is essential for epithelial-mesenchymal transition and metastasis in a model of breast cancer progression. *The Journal of Clinical Investigation*, Vol.114, No.(4) pp.569-581, ISSN 0021-9738

Ichii, T. & Takeichi, M. (2007). p120-catenin regulates microtubules dynamics and cell migration in a cadherin-independent manner. *Genes to Cells*, Vol.12, No.(7) pp.827-839, ISSN 1356-9597

Imai, K., Hiramatsu, A., Fukushima, D., Pierschbacher, M.D. & Okada, Y. (1997). Degradation of decorin by matrix metalloproteinases: Identification of the cleavage sites, kinetics and transforming growth factor-β1 release. *The Biochemical Journal*, Vol.332, No.(3) pp.809-814, ISSN 0264-6021

Imai, K. & Okada, Y. (2009). Purification of matrix metalloproteinases by column chromatography. *Nature Protocol*, Vol.3, No.(7) pp.1111-1124, ISSN 1750-2799

Ishiyama, N., Lee, S.H., Liu, S., Li, G.Y., Smith, M.J., Reichardt, L.F. & Ikura, M. (2010). Dynamic and static interactions between p120 catenin and E-cadherin regulate the stability of cell-cell adhesion. *Cell*, Vol.141, No.(1) pp117-128, ISSN 0092-8674

Ivanov, A.I., McCall, I.C., Babbin, B., Samarin, S.N., Nusrat, A. & Parkos, C.A. (2006). Microtubules regulate disassembly of epithelial apical junctions. *BMC Cell Biol.*, Vol.7 No. (1) pp.12. ISSN 1471-2121

Jones, P.A. & Baylin, S.B. (2002). The fundamental role of epigenetic events in cancer. *Nature Reviews Genetics*, Vol.3, No.(6) pp.415-428, ISSN 1471-0056

Kim, B.G., An, H.J., Kang, S., Choi, Y.P., Gao, M.Q., Park, H. & Cho, N.H. (2011). Laminin-233-rich tumor microenvironment for tumor invasion in the interface zone of breast cancer. *American Journal of Pathology*, Vol.178, No.(1) pp.373-381, ISSN 0002-9440

Kim, T., Veronese, A., Pichiorri, F., Lee, T.J., Jeon, Y.J., Volinia, S., Pineau, P., Marchio, A., Palatini, J., Suh, S.S., Alder, H., Liu, C.G., Dejean, A. & Croce, C.M. (2011). p53 regulates epithelial-mesenchymal transition through microRNAs targeting ZEB1 and ZEB2. *Journal of Experimental Medicine*, Vol.208, No.(5) pp.875-883, ISSN 0022-1007

Kobielak, A., Pasolli, H.A. & Fuchs, E. (2004). Mammalian formin-1 participates in adherens junctions and polymerization of linear actin cables. *Nature Cell Biology*, Vol.6, No.(1) pp.21-31, ISSN 1465-7392

Kudo, Y., Kitajima, S., Ogawa, I., Hiraoka, M., Sargolzaei, S. Keikhaee, M.R., Sato, S., Miyauchi, M. & Takata, T. (2004). Invasion and metastasis of oral cancer cells require methylation of E-cadherin and/or degradation of membranous β-catenin. *Clinical Cancer Research*, Vol.10, No.(16) pp.5455-5463, ISSN 1078-0432

Lee, S.H., Lee, N.H., Jin, S.M., Rho, Y.S. & Jo, S.J. (2011). Loss of heterozygosity of tumor suppressor genes (p16, Rb, E-cadherin, p53) in hypophrynx squamous cell carcinoma. *Otolaryngology Head and Neck Surgery*, early publication ahead of print, ISSN 0194-5998

Lefort, C.T., Wojciechowski, K. & Hocking, D. (2011). N-cadherin cell-cell adhesion complexes are regulated by fibronectin matrix assembly. *The Journal of Biological Chemistry*, Vol.286, No.(4) pp.3149-3160, ISSN 0021-9258

Li, L.C., Chui, R.M., Sasaki, M., Nakajima, K., Perinchery, G., Au, H.C., Nojima, D., Carroll, P. & Dahiya, R. (2000). A single nucleotide polymorphism in the *E-cadherin* gene promoter alters transcriptional activities. *Cancer Research*, Vol.6, No.(4) pp.873-876, ISSN 1538-7445

Li, S., Jiao, J., Lu, Z. & Zhang, M. (2009). An essential role for N-cadherin and β-catenin for progression in tongue squamous cell carcinoma and their effect on invasion and metastasis of Tca8113 tongue cancer cells. *Oncology Reports*, Vol.21, No.(5) pp.1223-1233, ISSN 1021-335X

Liang, X., Zheng, M., Jiang, J., Zhu, G., Yang, J. & Tang, Y. (2011). Hypoxia-inducible factor-1 alpha, in association with TWIST2 and SNIP1, is a critical prognostic factor in patients with tongue squamous cell carcinoma. *Oral Oncology*, Vol.47, No.(2) pp.92-97, ISSN 1368-8375

Libusova, L., Stemmler, M.P., Hierholzer, A., Schwarz, H. & Kemler, R (2010). N-cadherin can structurally substitute for E-cadherin during intestinal development but leads to polyp formation. *Development*, Vol.137, No.(14) pp.2297-2305, ISSN 0950-1991

Liu, H., Komiya, S., Shimizu, M., Fukunaga, Y. & Nagafuchi, A. (2007). Involvement of p120 carboxy-terminal domain in cadherin trafficking. *Cell Structure and Function*, Vol.32, No.(2) pp.127-137, ISSN 0386-7196

Lo Muzio, L., Pannone, G., Staibano, S., Mignogna, M.D., Serpico, R., Fanali, S., De Rosa, G., Piattelli, A. & Mariggió, M.A. (2002). $p120^{cat}$ delocalization in cell lines of oral cancer. *Oral Oncology*, Vol.38, No.(1) pp.64-72, ISSN 1368-8375

Lu, S. L., Reh, D., Li, A.G., Woods, J., Corless, C.L., Kulesz-Martin, M. & Wang, X.J. (2004). Overexpression of transforming growth factor beta1 in head and neck epithelia results in inflammation, angiogenesis, and epithelial hyperproliferation. *Cancer Research*, Vol.64, No.(13) pp.4405-4410, ISSN 1078-0432

Maeda, G., Chiba, T., Okazaki, M., Satoh, T., Taya, Y., Aoba, T., Kato, K., Kawashiri, S. & Imai, K. (2005). Expression of SIP1 in oral squamous cell carcinomas: Implications for E-cadherin expression and tumor progression. *International Journal of Oncology*, Vol.27, No.(6) pp.1535-1541, ISSN 1019-6439

Maeda, G., Chiba, T., Aoba, T. & Imai, K. (2007a). Epigenetic inactivation of *E-cadherin* by promoter hypermethylation in oral carcinoma cells. *Odontology*, Vol.95, No.(1) pp.24-29, ISSN 1618-1247

Maeda, G., Chiba, T., Kawashiri, S., Sato, T. & Imai, K. (2007b). Epigenetic inactivation of IκB kinase-α in oral carcinomas and tumor progression. *Clinical Cancer Research*, Vol.13, No.(17) pp.5041-5047, ISSN 1078-0432

Maher, M.T., Flozak, A.S., Stocker, A.M., Chenn, A. & Gottardi, C.J. (2009). Activity of the beta-catenin phosphodestruction complex at cell-cell contact is enhanced by cadherin-based adhesion. *The Journal of Cell Biology*, Vol.186, No.(2) pp.219-228, ISSN 0021-9525

Mandai, K., Nakanishi, H., Satoh, A., Obaishi, H., Wada, M., Nishioka, H., Itoh, M., Mizoguchi, A., Aoki, T., Fujimoto, T., Matsuda, Y., Tsukita, S. & Takai, Y (1997). Afadin: A novel actin filament-binding protein with one PDZ domain localized at cadherin-based cell-to-cell adherence junction. *The Journal of Cell Biology*, Vol.139, No.(2) pp.517-528, ISSN 0021-9525

Meira, L.B., Bugni, J.M., Green, S.L., Lee, C.W., Pang, B., Borenshtein, D., Rickman, B.H., Rogers, A.B., Moroski-Erkul, C.A., McFaline, J.L., Schauer, D.B., Dedon, P.C., Fox, J.G. & Samson, L.D. (2008). DNA damage induced by chronic inflammation contributes to colon carcinogenesis in mice. *Journal of Clinical Investigation*, Vol.118, No.(7) pp.2516-2525, ISSN 0021-9738

Meng, W. & Takeichi, M (2009). Adherence junction: Molecular architecture and regulation. *Cold Spring Harbor Perspectives in Biology*, Vol.1, No.(6) a002899, ISSN 1943-0264

Miyazawa, J., Mitoro, A., Kawashiri, S., Chada, K.K. & Imai, K. (2004). Expression of mesenchyme-specific gene HMGA2 in squamous cell carcinomas of the oral cavity. *Cancer Research*, Vol.64, No.(6) pp.2024-2029, ISSN 1078-0432

Nakayama, S., Sasaki, A., Mese, H., Alcalde, R.E. Tsuji, T. & Matsumura, T. (2001). E-cadherin gene is silenced by CpG methylation in human oral squamous cell carcinomas. *International Journal of Cancer*, Vol.93, No.(5) pp.667-673, ISSN 0020-7136

Neveu, P., Kye, M.J., Qi, S., Buchholz, D.E., Clegg, D.O., Sahin, M., Park, I.H., Kim, K.S., Daley, G.Q., Kornblum, H.I., Shraiman, B.I. & Kosik, K.S. (2010). MicroRNA profiling reveals two distinct p53-related human pluripotent stem cell states. *Cell Stem Cell*, Vol.7, No.(3) pp.671-681, ISSN 1934-5909

Ohusugi, M., Laure, L., Schwarz, H. & Kemler, R. (1997). Cell-junctional and cytoskeletal organization in mouse blastocysts lacking E-cadherin. *Developmental Biology*, Vol.185, No.(2) pp.261-271, ISSN 0021-1606

Peinado, H., Portillo, F. & Cano, A. (2004). Transcriptional regulation of cadherin during development and carcinogenesis. *The International Journal of Developmental Biology*, Vol.48, No.(5-6) pp.365-375, ISSN 0214-6282

Peinado, H., Olmeda, D. & Cano, A. (2007). Snail, ZEB and bHLH factors in tumour progression: An alliance against the epithelial phenotype? *Nature Review Cancer*, Vol.7, No.(6) pp.415-428, ISSN 1474-175X

Perez-Moreno, M., Dacia, M.A., Wong, E., Pasolli, H.A., Reynolds, A.B.& Fuchs, E. (2006). p120-catenin mediates inflammatory responses in the skin. *Cell*, Vol.124, No.(3) pp.631-644, ISSN 0092-8674

Perl, A.K., Wilgenbus, P., Dahl, U., Semb, H. & Christofori, G. (1998). A causal role for E-cadherin in the transition from adenoma to carcinoma. *Nature*, Vol.392, No.(6672) pp.190-193, ISSN 0028-0836

Pyo, S.W., Hashimoto, M., Kim, Y.S., Kim, C.H., Lee, S.H., Johnson, K.R., Wheelock, M.J. & Park, J.U. (2007). Expression of E-cadherin, P-cadherin and N-cadherin in oral squamous cell carcinoma: Correlation with the clinicopathologic features and patient outcome. *Journal of Cranio-Maxillofacial Surgery*, Vol.35, No.(1) pp.1-9, ISSN 1010-5182

Reddy, P., Liu, L, Ren, C., Lindgren, P., Boman, K., Shen, Y., Ludin, E., Ottander, U., Rytinki, M. & Liu, K. (2005). Formation of E-cadherin-mediated cell-cell adhesion activates Akt and mitogen activated protein kinase via phosphatidylinositol 3 kinase and ligand-independent activation of epidermal growth factor receptor in ovarian cancer cells. *Molecular Endocrinology*, Vol.19, No.(10) pp.2564-2578, ISSN 0888-8809

Saito, Y., Takazawa, H., Uzawa, K., Tanzawa, H. & Sato, K. (1998). Reduced expression of E-cadherin in oral squamous cell carcinoma: Relationship with DNA methylation of 5′ CpG island. *International Journal of Oncology*, Vol.12, No.(2) pp.293-298, ISSN 1019-6439

Saydam, O., Shen, Y., Würdinger, T., Senol, O., Boke, E., James, M.F., Tannous, B A., Stemmer-Rachamimov, A.O., Yi, M., Stephens, R.M., Fraefel, C., Gusella, J.F., Krichevsky, A.M. & Breakefield, X.O. (2009). Downregulated micoRNA-200a in meningiomas promotes tumor growth by reducing E-cadherin and activating the Wnt/beta-catenin signaling pathway. *Molecular and Cellular Biology*, Vol.29, No.(21) pp. 5932-5940, ISSN 0270-7306

Scapoli, L., Palmieri, A., Lo Muzio, L., Pazzetti, F., Rubini, C., Girardi, A., Farinella, F., Mazzotta, M. & Carnci, F. (2010). MicroRNA expression profiling of oral carcinoma identifies new markers of tumor progression. *International Journal of Immunotherapy and Pharmacology*, Vol.23, No.(4) pp.1229-1234, ISSN 0394-6320

Shintani, Y., Fukumoto, Y., Chaika, N., Svoboda, R., Wheelock, M.J. & Johnson, K.R. (2008). Collagen I-mediated up-regulation of N-cadherin requires cooperative signals from integrins and discoidin domain receptor 1. *The Journal of Cell Biology*, Vol.180, No.(6) pp.1277-1289, ISSN 0021-9525

Solanas, G., Porta-de-la-Riva, M., Agusti, C., Casagolda, D, Sánchez-Aguilera, F., Larriva, M.J., Pons, F., Peiró, S., Escriva, M., Muñoz, A., Duñach, M., de Herreros, A.G. & Baulida, J. (2008). E-cadherin controls β-catenin and NF-κB transcriptional activity in mesenchymal gene expression. *Journal of Cell Science*, Vol.121, No.(13) pp.2224-2234, ISSN 0021-0533

Stehbens, S.J., Paterson, A.D., Crampton, M.S., Shewan, A.M., Ferguson, C., Akmanova, A., Parton, R.G. & Yap, A.S. (2006). Dynamic microtubules regulated the local concentration of E-cadherin at cell-cell contacts. *Journal of Cell Science*, Vol.119 No.(9) pp.1801-1811, ISSN 0021-0533

Suyama, K., Shapiro, I., Guttman, M. & Hazan, R.B. (2002). A signaling pathway leading to metastasis is controlled by N-cadherin and the FGF receptor. *Cancer Cell*, Vol.2, No.(4) pp.301-314. ISSN 1535-6108

Thoreson, M.A. & Reynolds, A.B. (2002). Altered expression of the catenin p120 in human cancer: Implications for tumor progression. *Differentiation*, Vol.70, No.(9-10) pp.583-589, ISSN 0301-4681

Thuault, S., Valcourt, U., Petersen, M., Manfioletti, G., Heldin, C.H. & Moustakas, A. (2006). Transforming growth factor-beta employs HMGA2 to elicit epithelial-mesenchymal transition. *The Journal of Cell Biology*, Vol.174, No.(2) pp.175-183, ISSN 0021-9525

Tinkle, C.L., Lechler, T., Pasolli, H.A. & Fuchs, E. (2004). Conditional targeting of E-cadherin in skin: Insights into hyperproliferative and degenerative responses. *Proceeding of the National Academy of Science of the U.S.A.*, Vol.101, No.(2) pp.552-557, ISSN 1091-6490

Tomita, K., van Bokhoven, A., van Leenders, G.J.L.H., Ruijter, E.T.G., Jansen, C.F.J., Bussemakers, M.J.B. & Schalken, J.A. (2000). Cadherin switch in human prostate cancer progression. *Cancer Research*, Vol.60, No.(13) pp.3650-3654, ISSN 1078-0432

Uraguchi, M., Morikawa, M., Shirakawa, M., Sanada, K. & Imai, K. (2004). Activation of WNT family expression and signaling in squamous cell carcinomas of the oral cavity. *Journal of Dental Research*, Vol.83, No.(4) pp.327-332, ISSN 0022-0345

Vered, M., Dayan, D., Yahalom, R., Dobriyan, A., Barshack, I., Bello, I.O., Kantola, S. & Salo, T. (2011). Cancer-associated fibroblasts and epithelial-mesenchymal transition in metastatic oral tongue squamous cell carcinoma. *International Journal of Cancer*, Vol.127, No.(6) pp.1356-1362, ISSN 0020-7136

Viswanathan, M., Tsuchica, N. & Shanmugam, G. (2003). Promoter hypermethylation profile of tumor-associated genes p16, p15, MGMT and E-cadherin in oral squamous cell carcinoma. *International Journal of Cancer*, Vol.105, No.(1) pp.41-46, ISSN 0020-7136

Waterman-Storer, C.M., Salmon, W.C. & Salmon, E.D. (2000). Feedback interactions between cell-cell adherence junctions and cytoskeletal dynamics in newt lung epithelial cells. *Molecular Biology of the Cell*, Vol.11 No.(7) pp.2471-2483, ISSN 1059-1524

Wheelock, M.J., Shintani, Y., Maeda, M., Fukumoto, Y. and Johnson, K.R. (2008). Cadherin switching. *Journal of Cell Science*, Vol.121 No.(6) pp.727-735, ISSN 0021-0533

Yamada, S., Pokutta, S., Drees, F., Weis, W.I. & Nelson, W.J. (2005). Deconstructing the cadherin-catenin-actin complex. *Cell*, Vol.123 No.(5) pp.889-901, ISSN 0092-8674

Yeh, K.T., Shih, M.C., Lin, T.H., Chen, J.C., Chang, J.Y., Kao, C.F., Lin, K.L. & Chang, J.G. (2002). The correlation between CpG methylation on promoter and protein expression of E-cadherin in oral squamous cell carcinoma. *Anticancer Research*, Vol.22, No.(6C) pp.3971-3975, ISSN 0250-7005

Yokoyama, K., Kamata, N., Hayashi, E., Hoteiya, T., Ueda, N., Fujimoto, R. & Nagayama, M. (2001). Reverse correlation of E-cadherin and snail expression in oral squamous cell carcinoma cells *in vitro*. *Oral Oncol*ogy, Vol.37, No.(1) pp.65-71, ISSN 1368-8375

Yoshida, C. & Takeichi, M. (1982). Teratocarcinoma cell adhesion: Identification of a cell-surface protein involved in calcium-dependent cell aggregation. *Cell*, Vol.28, No.(2) pp.217-224, ISSN 0092-8674

Yu, C.C., Lo, W.L., Chen, Y.W., Huang, P.I., Hsu, H.S., Tseng, L.M., Hung, S.C., Kao, S.Y., Chang, C.J. & Chiou, S.H. (2011). Bmi-1 regulates Snail expression and promotes metastasis ability in head and neck squamous cancer-derived ALDH1 positive cells. *Journal of Oncology*, early publication ahead of print, ISSN 1687-8450

Zheng, G., Lyons, J.G., Tan, T.K., Wang, Y., Hsu, T.T., Min, D., Succar, L., Rangan, G.K., Hu, M., Henderson, B.R., Alexander, S.I. & Harris, D.C.H. (2009). Disruption of E-cadherin by matrix metalloproteinase directly mediates epithelial-mesenchymal transition downstream of transforming growth factor-β1 in renal tubular epithelial cells. *American Journal of Pathology*, Vol.175, No.(2) pp.580-591, ISSN 0002-9440

Zhou, B.P., Deng, J., Xia, W., Xu, J., Li, Y.M., Gunduz, M. & Hung, M.C. (2004). Dual regulation of Snail by GSK-3β-mediated phosphorylation in control of epithelial-mesenchymal transition. *Nature Cell Biology*, Vol.6, No.(10) pp.931-940, ISSN 1465-7392

8

The Role of EphB4 and EphrinB2 in Head and Neck Squamous Cell Carcinoma

Eric J. Yavrouian, Uttam K. Sinha and Rizwan Masood
Department of Otolaryngology – Head and Neck Surgery Keck School of Medicine of the University of Southern California, Los Angeles USA

1. Introduction

Head and neck squamous cell carcinoma (HNSCC) is the most common cancer arising in the upper aerodigestive tract. It is an epithelial tumor most commonly affecting the oral cavity, hypopharynx, and larynx. HNSCC is the fifth most common cancer worldwide with approximately 900,000 cases yearly worldwide. In the United States, there were approximately 36,000 cases in 2010 and 8,000 deaths. Men are at significantly greater risk with tobacco and alcohol consumption the most important etiologic risk factors.

The main treatment modality for HNSCC has traditionally been surgery and postoperative radiotherapy. However, over the past 30 years, no significant change has been made in treatment strategy with minimal improvement in survival. Overall survival at five years ranges from 70-85% for patients presenting with early-stage disease (stage I and II) to 30-40% for advanced-stage disease (stage III and IV).

2. Pathogenesis of head and neck cancer

Mutations in specific genes and alteration of their expression lead to neoplasia in the head and neck. The development of HNSCC is a multi-step process with sequential mutations in genes responsible for tumor surveillance. A microsatellite analysis of allelic alterations showed that with the accumulation of genetic mutations, one can follow the transformation of cells from simple squamous hyperplasia to severe dysplasia, and, ultimately, invasive squamous cell carcinoma. These changes include mutation of the p53 tumor suppressor, overexpression of epidermal growth factor receptor (EGFR), and inactivation of the cyclin dependent kinase inhibitor p16. Other changes such as Rb mutation, ras activation, cyclin D amplification, and myc overexpression are less frequent in HNSCC. There is also an alteration in those genes which control DNA repair, proliferation, immortalization, apoptosis, invasion, and angiogenesis in HNSCC.

The p53 gene is believed to be the most frequently mutated tumor suppressor in human cancer. p53 has been implicated in the early pathogenesis of HNSCC, as it controls cell growth through regulation of the cell-cycle and apoptosis. The p53 null keratinocytes possessing an activated ras oncogene proliferate at a higher rate than those expressing the tumor suppressor.

In a study by Kashiwazaki et al in HNSCC, 79% of cancers and 36% of dysplastic lesions were shown to have p53 mutations. Hyperplastic lesions were negative for p53 mutations in this study. A higher incidence of p53 mutations have been detected in invasive carcinomas (75%) than in non-invasive cancers (35%). p53 mutations were not detected in normal mucosal cells. This study also detected sequential mutations of different exons which suggested accumulation of alterations during neoplastic transformation. The incidence of p53 mutations correlated with the degree of dysplasia with significantly higher numbers found in smokers. In agreement with these studies, dysplastic lesions in non-smokers infrequently contained p53 mutations. These results indicate that p53 mutation and inactivation is an early event in head and neck tumorigenesis.

In addition to p53, alterations in the retinoblastoma (Rb) gene are involved in the pathogenesis of HNSCC. The Rb protein is also a tumor suppressor pathway. $p16^{INK4A}$, a major target of the Rb pathway is inhibited through a variety of pathways including loss of heterozygosity (LOH) of chromosome 9p21, where it is located. LOH of 9p21 is seen in 80% of malignant lesions.

In addition to the p53 and Rb genes, sphingosine kinase (SphK) has been implicated in HNSCC. SphK regulates levels of ceramide, sphingosine, and sphingosine-1-phosphate, influencing cells to enter proliferative states. SphK1, a SphK isozyme is upregulated in HNSCC with overexpression in recurrent and advanced stage tumors. Use of small molecular inhibitors or siRNA's targeting SphK1 sensitizes cells both in in vitro and in vivo studies leads to radiation induced cell death. As a cell cycle regulator overexpressed in HNSCC patients, SphK1 plays a significant role in the pathogenesis of HNSCC.

The Epidermal Growth Factor Receptor (EGFR) is of the most studied biomarkers in HNSCC. EFGR is a receptor tyrosine kinase that effects cell growth, angiogenesis, and invasion. The epidermal growth factor receptor gene encodes a transmembrane receptor for EGF and transforming growth factor (TGF)-α. Ligand binding to the extracellular domain induces receptor dimerization and activation of the cytoplasmic tyrosine kinase. Many epithelial cancers including that of the head and neck overexpress EGFR, its ligands, or both. EGFR has been detected in the basal layer of normal oropharyngeal mucosa. All cells from dysplastic head and neck lesions stain for EGFR as do the majority of carcinomas. Almost all cells in poorly differentiated head and neck tumors were positive for the receptor. Amplification of the EGFR gene has been demonstrated in cultured cells and tissues.

EGFR overexpression may result in constitutive activity of the kinase domain and consequently increase downstream signaling such as that of the mitogen activated protein kinase pathway. The tyrosine kinase activity of the receptor results in autophosphorylation and recruitment of a variety of intracellular signaling proteins containing Src homology 2 (SH2) or phosphotyrosine binding (PTB) domains. This recruitment provides a means of assembling the complexes required for receptor signaling. Proteins such as Grb2 and Shc, which contain SH2 and SH3 domains, mediate interactions with signal transduction proteins linking EGFR with the ras/mitogen activated protein kinase (MAPK) pathway. Ras also interacts with many proteins such as raf and phosphatidylinositol 3-kinase (PI3-K) to simulate downstream effectors such as MEK and ERK. These MAPKs are translocated to the nucleus where they activate a number of transcription factors which control cellular proliferation, migration, and differentiation.

With devastating effects on communication, swallowing, and most importantly, survival, new biomarkers and targeted therapies are needed to improve detection, treatment, and survival. Potential targeted therapies may be found in factors that regulate angiogenesis. Angiogenesis plays an important role in both tumor growth and metastasis. Tumors are unlikely to grow beyond 3mm without the growth of new vessels. Receptor tyrosine kinases (RTKs) have emerged as important molecules in the regulation of angiogenesis.

Abnormal RTK expression is characteristic of most human cancers. There are three families of receptor tyrosine kinases and their ligands important in vascular development, including the vascular endothelial growth factor receptor (VEGF) family, the angiopoietin family, and the ephrins and the Eph receptors. Of the three receptor tyrosine kinase families above, VEGF is the most extensively studied. VEGF has been shown to be overexppressed in tumor compared to normal cells. VEGF overexpression is associated with a 1.88 fold increased risk of death and is also shown to be associated with lymph node metastasis. This chapter focuses on the expression of EphB4 and EphrinB2 in HNSCC and possible therapeutic applications to reduce tumor burden and improve survival.

3. The Eph receptors and their ligands the ephrins

The Eph receptors (erythropoietin-producing human hepatocellcular carcinoma) form the largest family of RTKs. In this group of proteins, there are 15 members divided into EphA and EphB classes. The EphA subclass is tethered to the cell membrane by glycosyl phosphatidylinositol, and the EphB subclass has a transmembrane domain that is followed by a short cytoplasmic region.

Eph receptors have an extracellular domain composed of the ligand-binding globular domain, a cysteine rich region followed by a pair of fibronectin type III repeats. The cytoplasmic domain consists of a juxtamembrane region containing two conserved tyrosine residues, a protein tyrosine kinase domain, a sterile α-motif (SAM), and a PDZ-domain binding motif.

The ephrins (Eph family receptor interacting proteins) are the ligands for the Eph receptors, with 13 members, also divided into classes A and B. Class B Ephrins have a transmembrane domain and cytoplasmic region with five conserved tyrosine residues and a PDZ domain. EphrinB2 is the exclusive ligand for EphB4. EphB4 is normally expressed on venous endothelial cells while EphrinB2 on arterial endothelial cells. In contrast, the A class ligands have a glycosylphosphatidylinositol membrane anchor.

Eph receptors are activated by binding of clustered, membrane attached ephrins indicating that contact between cells expressing the receptors and cells expressing the ligands is required for Eph activation. A corollary of this is that soluble ligands would act as inhibitors of Eph activation. Ligand binding to the Eph receptor autophosphorylates the juxtamembrane tyrosine residues to acquire full activation. Specificity of the ligand to its receptor is mediated by the N-terminal domain of the receptor. The interactions between the Eph receptors and their ligands form a bi-directional signaling pathway with forward Eph receptor signaling and reverse ephrin signaling (Figure 1).

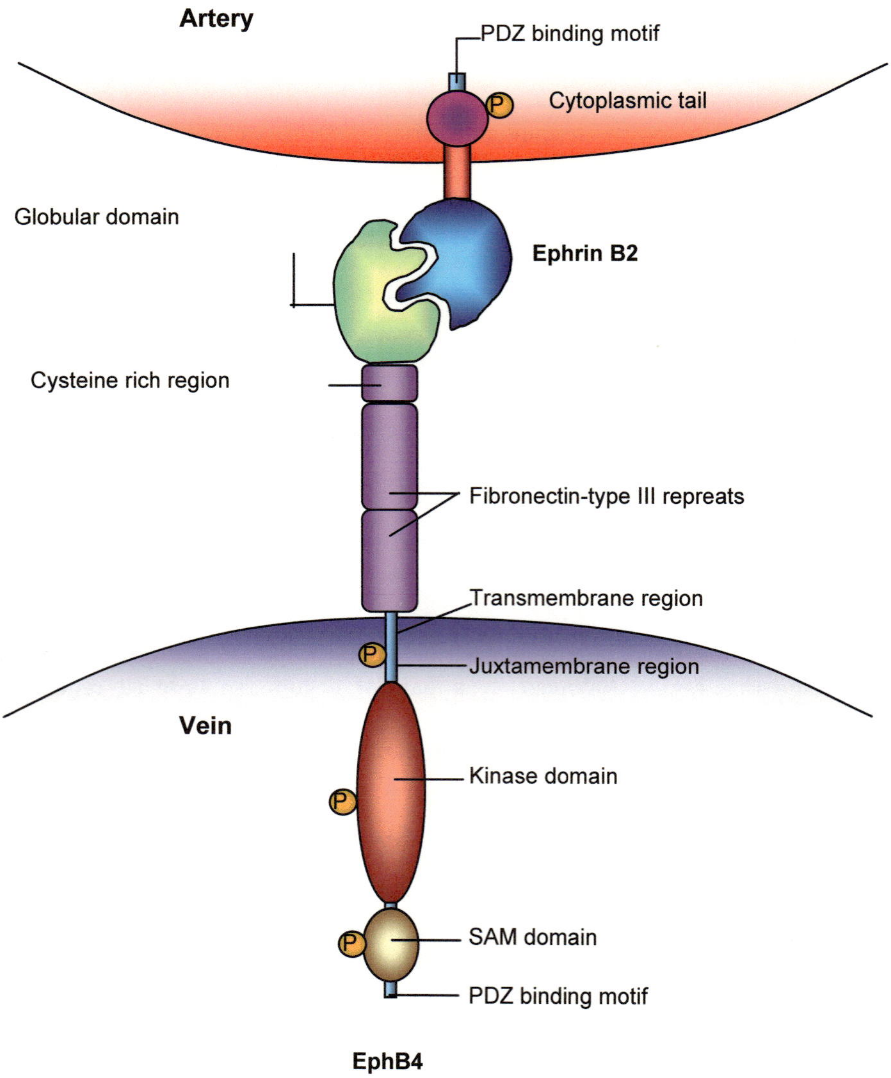

Fig. 1. Bidirectional signaling between EphB4 and EphrinB2.

When activated, EphB4 and EphrinB2 become phosphorylated, forming complexes with other proteins, and affect downstream signaling. Reverse signaling is initiated through recruitment of Src-family kinases followed by phosphorylation of ephrin B proteins. Evidence suggests that the Eph/ephrin interaction influences and is influenced in turn by other signaling pathways. The endothelial-specific receptor Tie-2 can directly phosphorylate ephrin cytoplasmic domains while EphrinB1 is phosphorylated by the PDGF receptor, and inhibits PDGF induced focus formation. Similarly, EphrinB2 inhibits VEGF signaling and the proliferation and migration of endothelial cells. The ephrins have also been shown to couple to GPCRs, such as the chemokine receptor CXCR4, via the PDZ linking proteins and a ternary complex involving the extracellular domains of EphrinB1, EphB2, and the 7-transmembrane GPCR subunit of the NMDA glutamate receptor has also been demonstrated.

The Eph receptor/ephrin system has been shown to play a role in several biologic processes. These processes include embryonic development, cell migration and aggregation, segmentation, pattern recognition, neural development, angiogenesis, vascular network development, and immune regulation. Recently, a role for these proteins has emerged in cancer.

Several studies have demonstrated that the Eph receptor/ephrin system plays a role in tumorigenesis. Dodolet et al and Wimmer-Kleikamp et al have shown involvement of the Eph receptor/ephrin system in angiogenesis, invasion, and tumor metastasis. There is also evidence that elevated expression of the Eph/Ephrin system correlates with increased invasiveness in tumors including malignant melanoma, ovarian carcinoma, breast cancer, kidney carcinoma, neuroblastoma, and prostate cancer. More specifically, elevated EphB4 expression has been shown in hematologic, breast, endometrial, prostate, bladder, ovarian, and colon cancers as well as malignant mesothelioma.

EphB4 activation has been shown to increase proliferation and survival of microvascular endothelial cells through increased phosphatidylinositol 3-kinase activity and phosphorylation of mitogen-activated protein kinase (MAPK) and protein kinase B (Akt). EphB4's involvement in cell migration and invasion is associated with EphB4 induction of MMP2 and MMP9, thus demonstrating a role for EphB4 in tumor metastasis.

4. Expression of EphB4 and EphrinB2 in HNSCC

As demonstrated in many other tumors, EphB4 is overexpressed in HNSCC. Through *in situ* hybridization, western blot analysis, and immunofluorescence of HNSCC tumor samples, EphB4 expression was found to be elevated in tumor tissue compared to normal adjacent tissue. In addition, EphB4 was overexpressed in metastatic lymph nodes (Figure 2). Furthermore, EphB4 overexpression correlated with advanced tumor stage (stage III or IV) and lymph node metastasis with stage III and IV tumors having 2.8 and 5.5-fold overexpression respectively compared to adjacent normal tissue.

Lymph nodes positive with tumor had 7.8-fold higher expression compared to normal adjacent tissue. In contrast, in patients with early-stage disease (stage I or II), EphB4 overexpression was 2.1-fold greater in tumor compared to adjacent normal tissue. Using

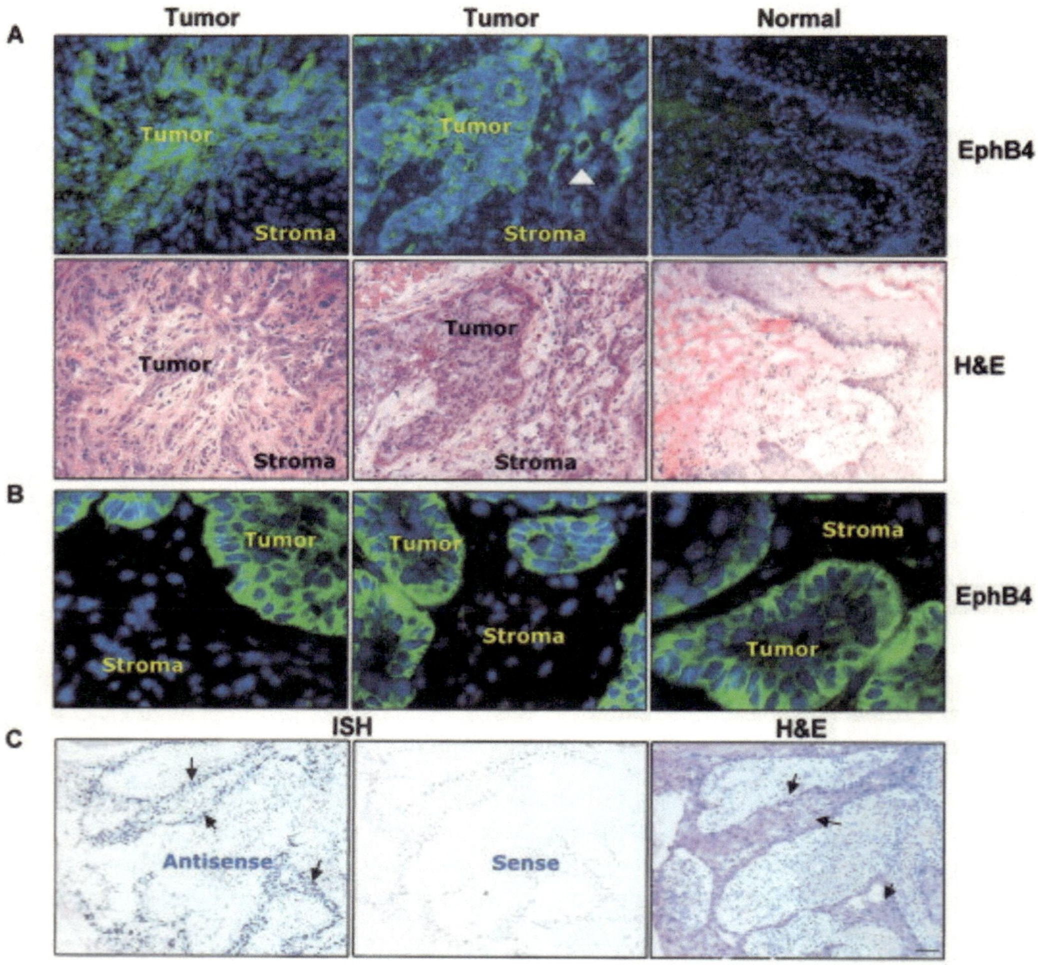

Fig. 2. EphB4 is expressed in HNSCC primary tissues and metastases. (*a*) Top panel: Immunofluorescence of representative fresh frozen sections of tumors (left and middle panels) or adjacent normal tissue (right panel) stained with EphB4-specific monoclonal antibody and visualized with FITC (green color). Sections were counter-stained with DAPI to identify cell nuclei. Bottom panel: Hematoxylin and Eosin (H&E) staining of the next serial section. Arrowhead in middle panel shows a vessel staining positive for EphB4. (*b*) Representative high power photomicrographs of tumor sections stained for EphB4 to document tumor cell membrane-specific expression. (*c*) *In situ* hybridization (ISH) of representative tumor sections with EphB4-specific antisense or sense probe. Arrows show positive signal for mRNA. H&E stain of the next section is shown in the right panel. Arrows indicate regions of the tumor.

quantitative PCR at the EphB4 gene locus, 30% of patients were found to have gene amplification of EphB4 with at least four copies of the gene locus. In a study of 42 patients with HNSCC, EphrinB2 expression was also analyzed with western blot analysis. EphrinB2 was found to be overexpressed in HNSCC tumor samples with an average overexpression of 2.2-fold greater when compared to normal adjacent tissue. Therefore, both EphB4 and EphrinB2 have been shown to be overexpressed in HNSCC.

5. HNSCC risk factors and EphB4 expression

The two main risk factors for HNSCC are alcohol and smoking. Studies have shown that tobacco use can lead to a 20-fold increased risk of HNSCC. Tobacco related substances can alter the genes and growth factors associated with HNSCC and can affect the genomic stability and extracellular environment in HNSCC. The expression of EphB4 in the oral mucosa of smokers without HNSCC was analyzed and results showed no expression of EphB4. However, in patients with HNSCC, EphB4 expression in tumor specimens in nonsmokers was compared to that of patients with a smoking history. There was a significantly increased expression of EphB4 in tumor samples from patients with a smoking history compared to nonsmokers, with a 3.8-fold overexpression of EphB4 in smokers compared to a 2.1 fold overexpression in nonsmokers. Therefore, tobacco-related substances may induce signaling changes that increase and activate EphB4 leading to changes in angiogenesis and tumor growth.

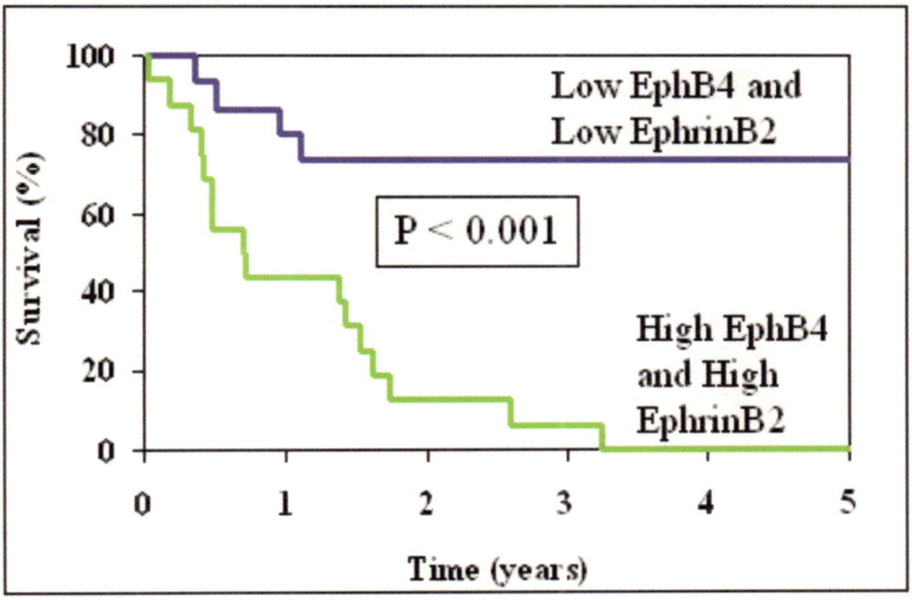

Fig. 3. Kaplan-Meier Curve for Overall Survival in Patients with Elevated Expression of EphB4 and EphrinB2.

In addition to smoking status, the effect of alcohol intake on EphB4 expression was also assessed in patients with HNSCC. Unlike with smoking status, EphB4 expression was not altered by a history of alcohol consumption. This is likely related to differing mechanisms of toxin induced carcinogenesis between alcohol and smoking.

6. EphB4 and EphrinB2 expression and survival

As increasing EphB4/EphrinB2 system expression is associated with advanced tumor stage and lymph node metastasis, the effect of EphB4 and EphrinB2 overexpression on survival was also studied. Patients who had high expression of EphB4 and EphrinB2 were compared to patients with low expression of EphB4 and EphrinB2. Those with high expression of EphB4 had a 5 year survival of 15% compared to 64% in patients with low EphB4 expression. Patients with elevated EphrinB2 expression had a 5 year survival of 9% compared to 79% in patients with low EphrinB2 expression.

In patients with elevated EphB4 and EphrinB2 expression, 5 year survival was 0% compared to 73% in patients with low EphB4 and low EphrinB2 expression (Figure 3). Therefore, elevated EphB4 and EphrinB2 expression is a significant predictor of poorer overall survival, even after adjusting for confounders including age, sex, race, stage, site of tumor, and mode of treatment. As all patients with high EphB4 and EphrinB2 expression died; this suggests a synergistic role between EphB4 and EphrinB2 in HNSCC.

7. Inhibition of EphB4 and tumor cell survival

EphB4 overexpression is associated with a worse overall survival in HNSCC; therefore, its inhibition in tumor cells is an important step to understanding possible therapeutic opportunities. Using small interfering RNA (siRNA) against the EphB4 sequence, which ablates EphB4 expression, results in a significant decrease in HNSCC tumor cells. In the presence of epidermal growth factor (EGF), which has been shown to induce EphB4 expression, inhibition with siRNA against EphB4 also led to a decrease in tumor cells (Figure 4). The population of cells exposed to the siRNA against EphB4 was found to accumulate in the sub-G0 phase, suggestive of apoptosis. EphB4 was shown to provide a survival advantage to cells by inhibition of apoptotic pathways. Inhibition of EphB4 in a murine HNSCC model showed a reduction in tumor growth. Its knockdown leads to an activation of capase-8 and subsequent cell death by apoptosis. Therefore, EphB4 expression in HNSCC provides a survival advantage to tumors cells and is an important potential biomarker whose inhibition may improve survival.

8. Therapeutic applications

Tumor biomarkers provide an opportunity with which one can improve early detection of tumor, monitoring, and treatment, and ultimately improve survival. Recently, several new biomarkers have emerged and are currently being studied for their effectiveness in HNSCC detection, prognosis, and treatment. One such molecule is cetuximab, a monoclonal antibody against the epidermal growth factor receptor. It is one of the most successful targeted therapies in HNSCC with a phase III clinical trial showing cetuximab in

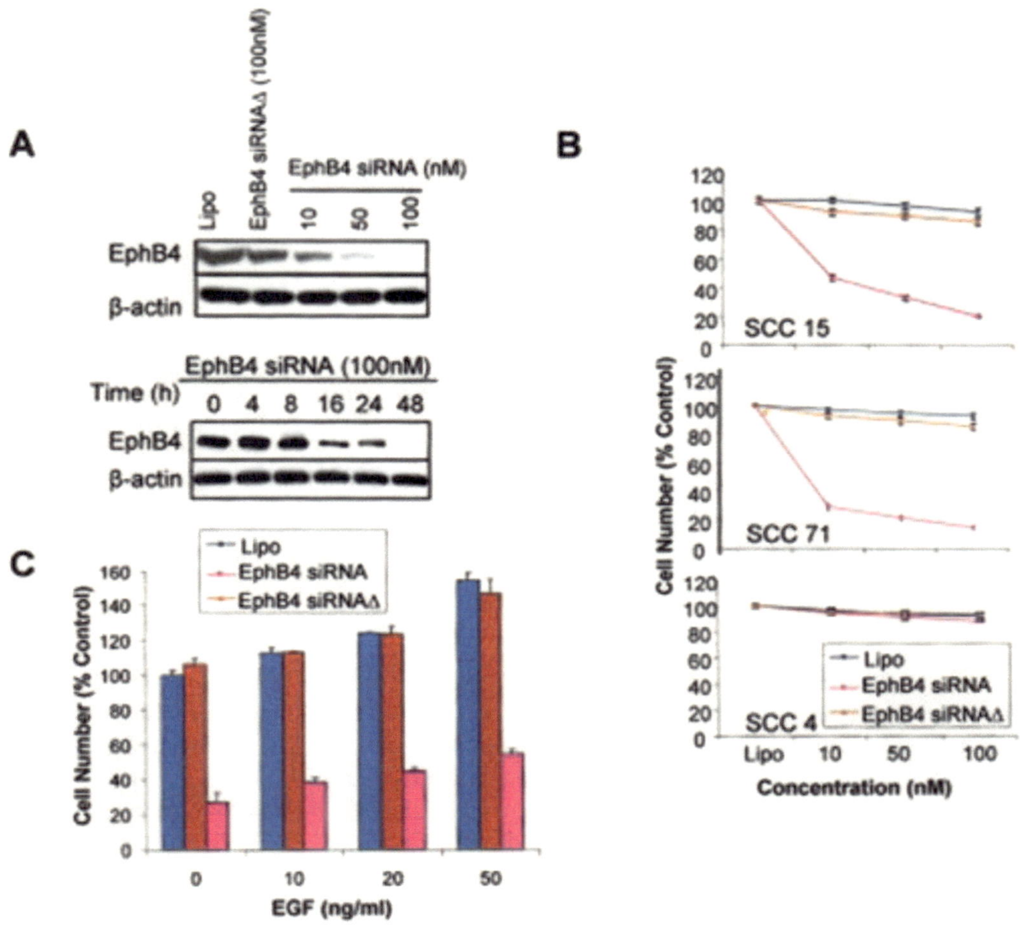

Fig. 4. Ablation of EphB4 in HNSCC cells lines results in reduction in cell numbers and inhibition of tumor cell migration/invasion. (*a*) Potent EphB4-specific siRNA chosen from their ability to block EphB4 was transfected at various concentrations into SCC-15 cells. A mutant siRNA (EphB4 siRNAΔ) with three base substitutions was used as negative control. Extracts of treated cells were analyzed by Western blotting to detect EphB4 and β-actin (upper panel). SCC-15 cells were transfected with 100 nM EphB4 siRNA and EphB4 expression analyzed at various time points (lower panel). (*b*) MTT cell number assays of EphB4-positive SCC cell lines (SCC-15 and -71) and an EphB4-negative cell line (SCC-4). Cell number was tested 48 hr following treatment with lipofectamine alone (Lipo), EphB4-specific siRNA (EphB4 siRNA) or mutant siRNA (EphB4 siRNAΔ). Data shown is mean ± SEM of triplicate samples. (*c*) MTT cell number assays of SCC-15 cells following treatment with increasing doses of EGF and lipofectamine alone (Lipo), EphB4-specific siRNA (EphB4 siRNA) or mutant siRNA (EphB4 siRNAΔ). Data shown is mean ± SEM of triplicate samples.

combination with radiotherapy provided an overall survival benefit of an additional 20 months compared to radiation alone. Downstream EGFR signaling activates the MAPK pathway as well as the PI3-K/Akt pathway. Signaling through the PI3-K/Akt pathway ultimately leads to inhibition of the tumor suppressor gene p53. EGFR has been shown to regulate EphB4 expression (Figure 5). EGFR signaling through the Akt pathway induces EphB4. Inhibition of EGFR through antibodies such as cetuximab may also downregulate EphB4 through Akt. Potentially, some of the survival benefit of cetuximab is achieved through EphB4 inhibition.

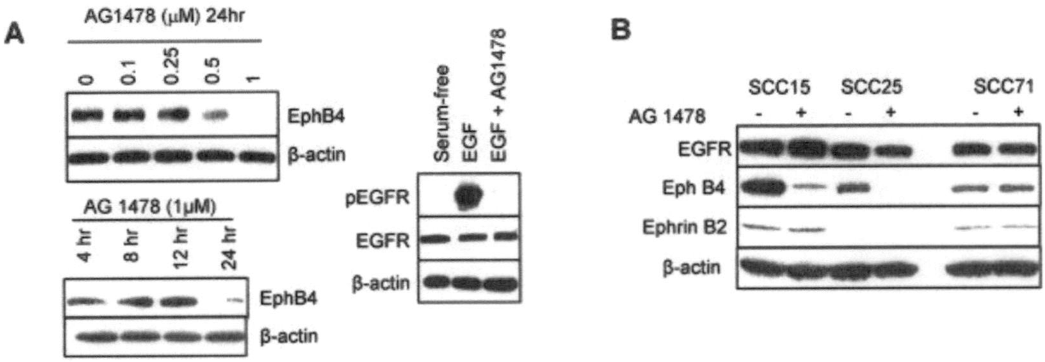

Fig. 5. Regulation of EphB4 expression by EGFR signaling pathway. (*a*) EGFR kinase inhibitor AG1478 was tested in SCC-15 for optimal dose (left upper panel) and time (left lower panel) for inhibition of EphB4 expression by Western blot of whole cell lysates. Equal loading of protein in each lane is shown by β-actin levels. Inhibition of EGFR activation by EGF in the presence of AG1478 (1 μM) is shown in right panel. (*b*) Western blot analysis of SCC-15, -25, and -71 cell lines for regulation of EphB4, EGFR and EphrinB2 in response to AG1478. Serial stripping and probing for various proteins was performed from the same blot.

Monoclonal antibodies to EphB4 have not been applied clinically as of yet, however, their development is crucial to improve survival in HNSCC. Xu et al have developed a humanized version of a mouse monoclonal antibody to EphB4 that binds the human EphB4 receptor. Krasnoperov et al have also developed two anti-ephB4 monoclonal antibodies targeting different EphB4 domains. These antibodies have yet to be tested in humans. Bardelle el al have demonstrated a non-benxodioxole inhibitor of EphB4 that may have applications in vivo but is also yet to be studied further.

In addition to the direct inhibition of the EphB4, several receptor tyrosine kinase inhibitors are being studied. These may also inhibit EphB4 function. Sunitinib, sorafenib, vandetanib, semaxanib, and foretinib are small molecule tyrosine kinase inhibitors currently being studied in phase II clinical trials. Machiels et al reviewed Sunitinib in a phase II clinical trial of 38 HNSCC patients in which it was given as a palliative treatment achieving a disease control rate of 50%. Due to several complications that occurred including bleeding, skin ulceration, and fistulas, they recommended further study of the drug to assess which patients would benefit. In recurrent/metastatic HNSCC and nasopharyngeal carcinoma,

Sorafenib's effect was studied and a response rate of 3.7% was achieved. As a multikinase inhibitor, its effect cannot be attributed only to its anti-angiogenic activity. As a single agent, Semaxanib was also studied in HNSCC, but was discontinued due to several adverse affects and its difficulty with administration. Given the potential improvement in survival with EphB4 inhibition in HNSCC, new therapies targeting EphB4 are essential and further investigation is necessary.

9. Conclusion

Head and neck squamous cell carcinoma is the most common cancer of the head and neck with devastating effects on communication, swallowing, quality of life, and, most importantly, survival. The Eph receptor family and its ligands, the ephrins, specifically EphB4 and EphrinB2, have an important role in many physiologic processes including cell aggregation and migration, angiogenesis, and vascular network development.

EphB4 and its sole ligand EphrinB2 are overexpressed in all HNSCC patients, with EphB4 overexpression correlating with advanced stage disease and lymph node metastasis. In vivo, EphB4 has also been demonstrated to provide a survival advantage to tumor cells, and, its inhibition has been shown to decrease the survival of the HNSCC tumor cells. Furthermore, EphB4/EphrinB2 overexpression is associated with a significantly poorer overall survival. Given that EphB4 and EphrinB2 are overexpressed in HNSCC and that this is associated with worse overall survival, EphB4 and EphrinB2 are potentially useful biomarkers that may provide another target for HNSCC treatment. While there are several investigators examining the therapeutic role of EphB4 inhibition in cancer, there is still a great deal of progress to be made to apply EphB4 and EphrinB2 inhibition in head and neck squamous cell carcinoma treatment.

10. References

[1] Adams RH, Wilkinson GA, Weiss C, et al. Roles of ephrinB ligands and EphB receptors in cardiovascular development: demarcation of arterial/venous domains, vascular morphogenesis, and sprouting angiogenesis. *Genes Dev.* 1999;13:295-306.

[2] Bardelle C, Barlaam B, Brooks N, et al. Inhibitors of the tyrosine kinase EphB4. Part 3: identification of non-benzodioxole-based kinase inhibitors. *Bioorg Med Chem Lett.* 2010 Nov 1;20(21):6242-5.

[3] Binns KL, Taylor PP, Sicheri F, et al. Phosphorylation of tyrosine residues in the kinase domain and juxtamembrane region regulates the biological and catalytic activities of Eph receptors. *Mol Cell Biol* 2000;20:4791-4805.

[4] Blume-Jensen P, Hunter T. Oncogenickinase signalling. *Nature* 2001;411:355–65.

[5] Bonner JA, Harari PM, Giralt J, et al. Radiotherapy plus cetuximab for squamous-cell carcinoma of the head and neck. *N Engl J Med.* 2006;354(6):567-78.

[6] Brachman DG. Molecular biology of head and neck cancer. *Semin Oncol.* 1994 ;21:320-329.

[7] Bruckner K, Pasquale EB, Klein R: Tyrosine phosphorylation of transmembrane ligands for Eph receptors. *Science* 1997;275:1640-1643.

[8] Califano J, Westra WH, Meininger G, et al. Genetic progression and clonal relationship of recurrent premalignant head and neck lesions. *Clin Cancer Res.* 2000 Feb;6(2):347-52.
[9] Cowan CA, Henkemeyer M. Ephrins in reverse, park and drive. *Trends Cell Biol.* 2002;12:339–46.
[10] Christensen ME. The EGF receptor system in head and neck carcinomas and normal tissues. Immunohistochemical and quantitative studies. *Dan Med Bull.* 199845:121-134.
[11] Cuvillier O, Pirianov G, Kleuser B, et al. Suppression of ceramide-mediated programmed cell death by sphingosine-1-phosphate. *Nature.* 1996; 381: 800–803.
[12] Dalva MB, Takasu MA, Lin MZ, et al. EphB receptors interact with NMDA receptors and regulate excitatory synapse formation. *Cell.* 2000;103:945-956.
[13] Davie JR, Spencer VA. Signal transduction pathways and the modification of chromatin structure. *Prog Nucleic Acid Res Mol Biol.* 2001;65:299-340.
[14] Davis S, Gale NW, Aldrich TH, Maisonpierre PC, et al. Ligands for EPH-related receptor tyrosine kinases that require membrane attachment or clustering for activity. *Science* 1994;266:816-819.
[15] Dodelet, V.C. and Pasquale, E.B. (2000). Eph receptors and ephrin ligands: embryogenesis to tumourigenesis. *Oncogene* 19, 5614-5619.
[16] Eisbruch A, Blick M, Lee JS, Sacks PG, Gutterman J. Analysis of the epidermal growth factor receptor gene in fresh human head and neck tumors. *Cancer Res.* 1987;47:3603-3605.
[17] Elser C, Siu LL, Winquist E, et al. Phase II trial of sorafenib in patients with recurrent or metastatic squamous cell carcinoma of the head and neck or nasopharyngeal carcinoma. *J Clin Oncol.* 2007;25(24):3766-73.
[18] Evan GI, Vousden KH. Proliferation, cell cycle and apoptosis in cancer. *Nature.* 2001;411:342-348.
[19] Folkman J. What is the evidence that tumors are angiogenesis dependent? *J Natl Cancer Inst.* 1990;82:4-6.
[20] Folkman J. Angiogenesis in cancer, vascular, rheumatoid and other disease. *Nat Med.* 1995;1:27-31.
[21] Folkman J. Clinical applications of research on angiogenesis. *N Engl J Med.* 1995;333:1757-63.
[22] Forastiere A, Koch W, Trotti A, Sidransky D. Medical progress: head and neck cancer. *N Engl J Med.* 2001;345(26):1890-1900.
[23] Folkman J, Hanahan D. Switch to the angiogenic phenotype during tumorigenesis. *Princess Takamatsu Symp.* 1991;22:339-47.
[24] Fury MG, Zahalsky A, Wong R, et al. A Phase II study of SU5416 in patients with advanced or recurrent head and neck cancers. *Invest New Drugs.* 2007;25(2):165-72.
[25] Gale NW, Yancopouloa GD. Growth factors acting via endothelial cell-specific receptor tyrosine kinases: VEGFs, angiopoietins, and ephrins in vascular development. *Genes Dev.* 1999;13:1055-1066.
[26] Gerety SS, Wang HU, Chen ZF, Anderson DJ. Symmetrical mutant phenotypes of the receptor EphB4 and its specific transmembrane ligand ephrin-B2 in cardiovascular development. *Mol Cell.* 1999;4(3):403-413.

[27] González MV, Pello MF, López-Larrea C, et al. Loss of heterozygosity and mutation analysis of the p16 (9p21) and p53 (17p13) genes in squamous cell carcinoma of the head and neck. *Clin Cancer Res.* 1995;1(9):1043-9.

[28] Greenblatt MS, Bennett WP, Hollstein M, Harris CC. Mutations in the p53 tumor suppressor gene: clues to cancer etiology and molecular pathogenesis. *Cancer Res.* 1994;54:4855-4878.

[29] Heroult, M., Schaffner, F., and Augustin, H.G. (2006).Eph receptor and ephrin ligand-mediated interactions during angiogenesis and tumour progression. *Exper.Cell Res.* 312, 642-650.

[30] Holder N, Klein R. Eph receptors and ephrins: effectors of morphogenesis. *Development.* 1999;126(10):2033-2044.

[31] Holland SJ, Peles E, Pawson T, Schlessinger J. Cell-contact-dependent signalling in axon growth and guidance: Eph receptor tyrosine kinases and receptor protein tyrosine phosphatase beta. *Curr Opin Neurobiol.* 1998;8:117-27.

[32] Hunter T. Signaling–2000 and beyond. *Cell* 2000;100:113–27.

[33] Jemal A, Siegel R, Xu J, et al. Cancer statistics, 2010. *CA Cancer J Clin.* 2010;60(5):277-300.

[34] Kalo MS, Pasquale EB: Multiple in vivo tyrosine phosphorylation sites in EphB receptors. *Biochemistry* 1999;38:14396-14408.

[35] Kalyankrishna S, Grandis JR. Epidermal growth factor receptor biology in head and neck cancer. *J Clin Oncol.* 2006;24(17):2666-72.

[36] Kashiwazaki H, Tonoki H, Tada M, Chiba I, Shindoh M, Totsuka Y, Iggo R, Moriuchi T. High frequency of p53 mutations in human oral epithelial dysplasia and primary squamous cell carcinoma detected by yeast functional assay. *Oncogene.* 1997;15:2667-2674.

[37] Kim S, Grandis JR, Rinaldo A, et al. Emerging perspectives in epidermal growth factor receptor targeting in head and neck cancer. *Head Neck.* 2008;30(5):667-74.

[38] Kim I, Ryu YS, Kwak HJ, Ahn SY, et al. EphB ligand, ephrinB2, suppresses the VEGF- and angiopoietin-1-induced Ras/mitogen-activated protein kinase pathway in venous endothelial cells. *Faseb J.* 2002;21:21.

[39] Kohama T, Olivera A, Edsall L, et al. Molecular cloning and functional characterization of murine sphingosine kinase. *J Biol Chem.* 1998; 273: 23722–23728.

[40] Krasnoperov V, Kumar SR, Ley E, et al. Novel EphB4 monoclonal antibodies modulate angiogenesis and inhibit tumor growth. *Am J Pathol.* 2010 Apr;176(4):2029-38.

[41] Kullander, K. and Klein, R., (2002). Mechanisms and functions of Eph and ephrin signaling. *Nat. Rev. Mol.Cell. Biol.* 3, 475-486.

[42] Kumar SR, Singh J, Xia G, et al. Receptor tyrosine kinase EphB4 is a survival factor in breast cancer. *Am J Pathol.* 2006;169(1):279-293.

[43] Kyzas PA, Cunha IW, Ioannidis JP. Prognostic significance of vascular endothelial growth factor immunohistochemical expression in head and neck squamous cell carcinoma: a meta-analysis. *Clin Cancer Res.* 2005;11:1434-40.

[44] Liu W, Ahmad SA, Jung YD, et al. Coexpression of ephrin-Bs and their receptors in colon carcinoma. *Cancer.* 2002;94(4):934-939.

[45] Lu Q, Sun EE, Klein RS, Flanagan JG. Ephrin-B reverse signaling is mediated by a novel PDZ-RGS protein and selectively inhibits G protein-coupled chemoattraction. *Cell.* 2001;105:69-79.
[46] Machiels JP, Henry S, Zanetta S, et al. Phase II study of sunitinib in recurrent or metastatic squamous cell carcinoma of the head and neck: GORTEC 2006-01. *J Clin Oncol.* 2010;28(1):21-8.
[47] Mao L, Lee JS, Fan YH, et al. Frequent microsatellite alterations at chromosomes 9p21 and 3p14 in oral premalignant lesions and their value in cancer assessment. *Nat Med.* 1996;2:682-5.
[48] Mandala SM, Thornton R, Tu Z, et al. Sphingoid base 1-phosphate phosphatase: a key regulator of sphingolipid metabolism and stress response. *Proc Natl Acad Sci.* 1998; 95: 150–155.
[49] Mashberg A, Boffetta P, Winkelman R, Garfinkel L. Tobacco smoking, alcohol drinking and cancer of the oral cavity and oropharynx among U.S. veterans. *Cancer.* 1993;72:1369-1375.
[50] Masood R, Kumar SR, Sinha UK, et al. EphB4 provides survival advantage to squamous cell carcinoma of the head and neck. *Int J Cancer.* 2006;119(6):1236-1248.
[51] Olivera A, Kohama T, Edsall L, et al. Sphingosine kinase expression increases intracellular sphingosine-1-phosphate and promotes cell growth and survival. *J Cell Biol.* 1999; 147: 545–558.
[52] Pasquale EB. The Eph family of receptors. *Curr Opin Cell Biol.* 1997;9(5):608-619.
[53] Pawson T. Protein modules and signalling networks. *Nature.* 1995;373:573-80.
[54] Paulovich AG, Toczyski DP, Hartwell LH. When checkpoints fail. *Cell.* 1997;88:315-321.
[55] Peng XH, Karna P, Cao Z, et al. Cross-talk between epidermal growth factor receptor and hypoxia-inducible factor-1alpha signal pathways increases resistance to apoptosis by up-regulating survivin gene expression. *J Biol Chem.* 2006 Sep 8;281(36):25903-14.
[56] Poeta ML, Manola J, Goldwasser MA, et al. TP53 mutations and survival in squamous-cell carcinoma of the head and neck. *N Engl J Med.* 2007 20;357(25):2552-61.
[57] Reiss M, Stash EB, Vellucci VF, Zhou ZL. Activation of the autocrine transforming growth factor alpha pathway in human squamous carcinoma cells. *Cancer Res.* 1991;51:6254-6262.
[58] Rodriguez T, Altieri A, Chatenoud L, et al. Risk factors for oral and pharyngeal cancer in young adults. *Oral Oncol.* 2004;40:207-213.
[59] Sankaranarayanan R, Masuyer E, Swaminathan R, Ferlay J, Whelan S. Head and neck cancer: a global perspective on epidemiology and prognosis. *Anticancer Res.* 1998;18(6B):4779-4786.
[60] Schlessinger J. Cell signaling by receptor tyrosine kinases. *Cell.* 2000;103:211-225.
[61] Shin DM, Lee JS, Choi LG. Prognostic significance of p53 expression in head and neck Squamous cell carcinoma. *Proc Am Soc Clin Onc* 1994;13:283-289.
[62] Sinha UK, Kundra A, Scalia P, et al. Expression of EphB4 in head and neck squamous cell carcinoma. *Ear Nose Throat J.* 2003;82(11):866, 869-870, 887.

[63] Sinha UK, Mazhar K, Chinn SB, et al. The association between elevated EphB4 expression, smoking status, and advanced-stage disease in patients with head and neck squamous cell carcinoma. *Arch Otolaryngol Head Neck Surg.* 2006;132(10):1053-1059.

[64] Sinha UK, Schorn VJ, Hochstim C, et al. Increased radiation sensitivity of head and neck squamous cell carcinoma with sphingosine kinase 1 inhibition. *Head Neck.* 2011;33:178-188.

[65] Smith BD, Smith GL, Carter D, et al. Prognostic significance of vascular endothelial growth factor protein levels in oral and oropharyngeal squamous cell carcinoma. *J Clin Oncol.* 2000;18:2046-52.

[66] Spiegel S, Milstien S. Functions of the multifaceted family of sphingosine kinases and some close relatives. *J Biol Chem.* 2007; 282: 2125–2129.

[67] Steinle JJ, Meininger CJ, Forough R, Wu G, Wu MH, Granger HJ. Eph B4 receptor signaling mediates endothelial cell migration and proliferation via the phosphatidylinositol3-kinase pathway. *J Biol Chem.* 2002;277:43830-43835.

[68] Strauss L, Volland D, Kunkel M, et al. Dual role of VEGF family members in the pathogenesis of head and neck cancer (HNSCC): possible link between angiogenesis and immune tolerance. *Med Sci Monit.* 2005;11:BR280-92.

[69] Vokes EE, Weichselbaum RR, Lippman SM, Hong WK. Head and neck cancer. *N Engl J Med.* 1993;328(3):184-194.

[70] Wang D, Ritchie JM, Smith EM, Zhang Z, Turek LP, Haugen TH. Alcohol dehydrogenase3 and risk of squamous cell carcinomas of the head and neck. *Cancer Epidemiol Biomarkers Prev.* 2005;14:626-632.

[71] Weinberg WC, Azzoli CG, Kadiwar N, Yuspa SH. p53 gene dosage modifies growth and malignant progression of keratinocytes expressing the v-rasHa oncogene. *Cancer Res.* 1994;54:5584-5592.

[72] Wimmer-Kleikamp, S.H. and Lackmann, M. (2005).Eph-modulated cell morphology, adhesion and motilityin carcinogenesis. *IUBMB Life* 57, 421-431.

[73] Wu, J. and Luo, H. (2005). Recent advances on T-cell regulation by receptor tyrosine kinases. *Curr. Opin. Hematol.* 12, 292-297.

[74] Wu Q, Suo Z, Kristensen GB, Baekelandt M, Nesland JM. The prognostic impact of EphB2/B4 expression on patients with advanced ovarian carcinoma. *Gynecol Oncol.* 2006;102(1):15-21.

[75] Wu X, Zhao H, Suk R, Christiani DC. Genetic susceptibility to tobacco-related cancer. *Oncogene.* 2004;23:6500-6523.26.

[76] www.clinicaltrials.gov

[77] Xia G, Kumar SR, Masood R, et al. EphB4 expression and biological significance in prostate cancer. *Cancer Res.* 2005;65(11):4623-4632.

[78] Xia G, Kumar SR, Stein JP, et al. EphB4 receptor tyrosine kinase is expressed in bladder cancer and provides signals for cell survival. *Oncogene.* 2006;25(5):769-780.

[79] Xu Z, Jin H, Qian Q. Humanized anti-EphB4 antibodies for the treatment of carcinomas and vasculogenesis-related diseases. *Expert Opin Ther Pat.* 2009 Jul;19(7):1035-7.

[80] Yamamoto T, Kamata N, Kawano H, Shimizu S, Kuroki T, Toyoshima K, Rikimaru K, Nomura N, Ishizaki R, Pastan I, et al. High incidence of amplification of the

epidermal growth factor receptor gene in human squamous carcinoma cell lines. *Cancer Res.* 1986; 46:414-416.

[81] Yarden Y. The EGFR family and its ligands in human cancer. Signaling mechanisms and therapeutic opportunities. *Eur J Cancer.* 2001;37 Suppl 4:S3-8.

[82] Yavrouian EJ, Sinha UK, Rice DH, et al. The significance of EphB4 and EphrinB2 expression and survival in head and neck squamous cell carcinoma. *Arch Otolaryngol Head Neck Surg.* 2008 Sep;134(9):985-91.

9

Involvement of Squamous Cell Carcinoma Antigen in Invasion and Metastasis of Squamous Cell Carcinoma of Uterine Cervix

Akihiro Murakami*, Keiko Yoshidomi and Norihiro Sugino
Yamaguchi University Graduate School of Medicine, Department of Obstetrics and Gynecology, Ube Japan

1. Introduction

A tumor-related protein, squamous cell carcinoma antigen (SCCA) was first discovered in uterine cervical squamous cell carcinoma [1], and subsequently has been used as a useful tumor marker for squamous cell carcinoma of various organs [2-4]. Cloning and characterization of *SCCA* cDNA has revealed that SCCA belongs to serine proteinase inhibitor (serpin) family [5]. Since SCCA is present not only in squamous cell carcinomas but also in normal squamous epithelium, the biological function of SCCA is of great interest. The present paper reviews the current understanding of SCCA, focusing on its biological function in uterine cervical squamous cell carcinoma.

2. Characteristics of SCCA

SCCA consists of more than 10 protein fractions with different isoelectric points, ranging from 5.9 to 6.6, which are roughly divided into two groups: the acidic SCCAs with pIs of less than 6.25 and the neutral SCCAs with pIs of 6.25 or higher [6]. The neutral SCCAs are generally present inside the cell, whereas the acidic SCCAs are often increased in squamous cell carcinomas and is easily secreted by the cell [6]. In 1991, our laboratory reported the cloning of *SCCA* cDNA, which consist of 1,170 nucleotides coding for 390 amino acids [5]. Schneider et al. also found two *SCCA* genes (*SCCA1* and *SCCA2*) and these two genes were tandemly arrayed at the human chromosome 18q21.3 locus [7, 8]. The predicted amino acid sequences of SCCA1 and SCCA2 are 92% identical and have identical predicted secondary structures, which suggests that *SCCA1* gene encodes the neutral SCCA, while *SCCA2* gene encodes the acidic SCCA [7]. SCCA1 inhibits the activities of serine proteinases, e.g. chymotrypsin and cysteine proteinases, e.g. cathepsin K, L, S and papain, whereas SCCA2 inhibits serine proteinases such as cathepsin G and chymase *in vitro* [9-12] (Table 1). For these reasons, SCCA1 and SCCA2 are thought to have different biological functions. It is thus of interest to better understand the biological behaviors of SCCAs in normal squamous epithelium and squamous cell carcinomas.

*Corresponding Author

group of proteinases	proteinases	inhibitors	
		SCCA1	SCCA2
Serine proteinase	chymotrypsin	+	-
	chymase	-	+
	cathepsin G	-	+
	plasmin	-	-
	plasminogen activator	-	-
	thrombin	-	-
	trypsin	-	-
Cysteine proteinase	cathepsin B	-	-
	cathepsin H	-	-
	cathepsin K	+	-
	cathepsin L	+	-
	cathepsin S	+	-
	papain	+	-

Table 1. Inhibitory effects of SCCAs on proteinases.

3. Evaluation of SCCA in clinical practice

Serum SCCA levels have been used as an indicator of a variety of squamous cell carcinomas, including skin cancers, head and neck cancers, esophageal cancers, lung cancers, bladder cancers, epidermoid cancers of the anal canal, and malignant transformation of mature cystic ovarian teratoma [13]. Serum SCCA levels are especially useful for monitoring treatment efficacy, disease progression and recurrence. In general, increased serum SCCA levels reflect disease progression and poor prognosis in squamous cell carcinomas [13]. In advanced cancers, pretreatment serum SCCA levels are associated with clinical stages, tumor sizes, and lymph node involvement. Furthermore, over 6 ng/ml of serum SCCA level shows a significant independent effect on survival and disease-free survival [14]. Even in the early stage of uterine squamous cell carcinomas, elevated serum SCCA levels predict pelvic lymph node involvement and are associated with a poor prognosis [15]. Recently, patients with elevated *SCCA2/SCCA1* mRNA ratios in uterine squamous cell carcinoma tissues were found to be at higher risk for recurrence in early stage uterine cervical cancers, suggesting SCCA2 is increased during cervical carcinogenesis [16]. In addition to malignant diseases, several benign and chronic inflammatory skin diseases, such as psoriasis, pemphigus, or eczema are often characterized by elevated SCCA levels [13]. SCCA will be a useful marker for monitoring the status of these diseases not only for malignant diseases but also for non-malignant diseases.

4. Role of SCCA in normal squamous epithelial cells

Human squamous epithelium is composed of four compartments; *stratum germinativus, stratum spinosum, stratum granulosum* and *stratum corneum*. Immunohistochemical staining shows that SCCA is present in the spinous and granular compartments, but not in the basal and parabasal cells [17] (Fig. 1). SCCA is not present in the epithelial region adjacent to the squamo-columnar junction of the uterine cervix. Interestingly, SCCA levels begin to increase at 18-20 weeks of pregnancy for the first time when the fetal epidermis begins to cornify during the development of human fetal skins [18]. *SCCA* genes has been found in most of the eutheria (placental mammals), but not in other vertebrates [19]. Furthermore, several eutherian species show heterogeneous patterns of *SCCA* nucleotides in Southern blot analyses [19]. This suggests that SCCA has had a role in the stratification and differentiation of integuments during evolutional change.

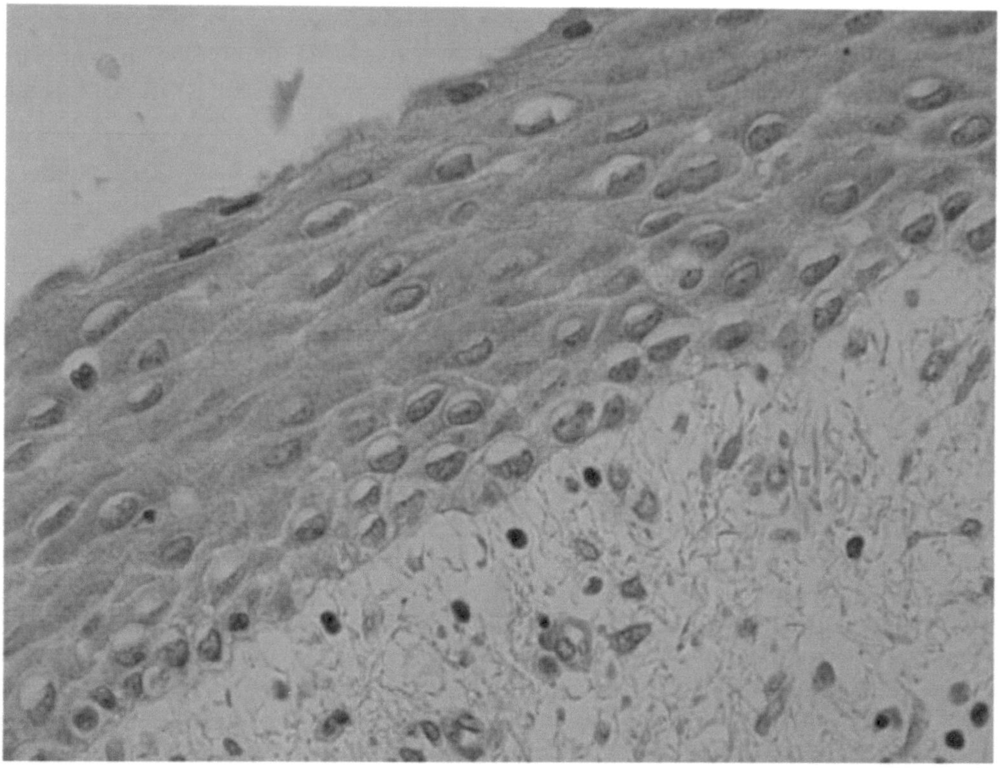

Fig. 1. Immunohistochemistry for SCCA expression in normal cervical squamous epithelium. SCCA is expressed in all epithelial layers except the basal layer (original magnification: X 100).

The stratification and cornification of normal squamous epithelial cells are influenced by extracellular calcium concentrations. Calcium concentrations are low in the parabasal layer but high in the granular layers. Keratinocytes begin to stratify and cornify in the presence of high concentrations of calcium [20]. High concentrations of calcium stimulate the production of neutral SCCA, whereas low concentration of calcium stimulate the production of acidic SCCA [21].

The final stage of differentiation of squamous epithelial cells is modulated by several cysteine proteinases, such as cathepsin L, calpain, and epidermal transglutaminase [20].

SCCA1 inhibits cathepsin L and some of the proteinases in the spinous and granular layers, suggesting that SCCA1 inhibits UV-induced apoptosis of squamous epithelial cells to maintain barrier functions in the squamous epithelium. On the other hand, SCCA2 may act outside of the cells to enhance the cell adhesion system in the parabasal layer [22, 23], suggesting that SCCA2 may play important roles to maintain the structure of the normal squamous epithelium, particularly structure of the thick stratum corneum in mammalian species.

5. Role of SCCA in squamous cell carcinoma of uterine cervix

Anti-tumor therapeutics inhibits the cancer cell proliferation and induce necrotic and apoptotic cell death. However, some cancer cells acquire the ability to resist anti-tumor therapeutics. Thus, proliferation, cell invasion and migration are the most crucial biological events in the progression of cancer.

Recently, much attention has been focused on the role of proteinases and their inhibitors in the malignant behavior of cancer cells. Proteinase inhibitors are thought to suppress the apoptotic process of cancer cells. Apoptosis involves complicated mechanisms with multistep pathways. Some serpins are involved in the apoptotic process. In squamous cell carcinoma tissues, the expression levels of SCCA2 are higher than those in normal squamous epithelial tissues, suggesting that SCCA2 plays a role in suppressing apoptotic cell death [24, 25]. Both SCCA1 and SCCA2 belong to the ov-serpin family, and some of the ov-serpins have been reported to inhibit apoptosis [5]. In fact, SCCA1 inhibits both serine proteinases and cysteine proteinases, and SCCA2 inhibits serine proteinases [9-12]. Although the target proteinases are different, both SCCA1 and SCCA2 inhibit apoptosis. SCCA1 suppresses apoptosis induced by activated natural killer cells, TNF-α, irradiation and anti-tumor agents, while SCCA2 suppresses apoptosis induced by irradiation and TNF-α [26-28]. Both SCCAs suppress the activity of caspase-3 and caspase-9 via down-regulation of p38 MAPK and/or MKK3/MKK6 [27]. These results suggest that SCCAs in tumor cells help to protect cancer cells from apoptotic cell death, both from therapeutic modalities and the immune systems. Proteinase inhibitors are also thought to suppress the invasion and metastasis of cancer cells by inhibiting proteinase activities that disrupt the cell-to-cell adhesion system. In the first step of cancer metastasis, loss of E-cadherin expression causes detachment of cancer cells from the primary tumor lesion. After the detachment from the primary tumor, cancer cells migrate, attach to vessels, and move to other organs through blood and lymph fluid flow. In fact, suppression of SCCA2 expression promoted cell invasion and cell migration with the decreased expression of E-cadherin [29, 30]. Blockage of E-cadherin action suppressed SCCA production in squamous cell carcinoma cell lines [31]. Our immunohistochemical study on cervical squamous cell carcinoma revealed that SCCA2 expression was significantly related with E-cadherin expression and that mixed pattern with loss and positive stained of SCCA2 and E-cadherin in primary lesions was strongly associated with high incidence of lymph node metastasis [32]. These facts strongly suggest that cancer cells with loss of SCCA2 expression, as well as loss of E-cadherin expression, metastasize to other organs including the lymph nodes. In contrast, increased expression of E-cadherin induces the increase of SCCA2 expression through a PI3K - Akt pathway in uterine squamous cell carcinoma cells [33]. These results suggest that the decrease in E-cadherin expression causes cancer cells to detach from the primary tumor, and acquire the activated E-cadherin - SCCA system, which leads to their aggregation, survival, and growth into metastatic tumors (Fig. 2).

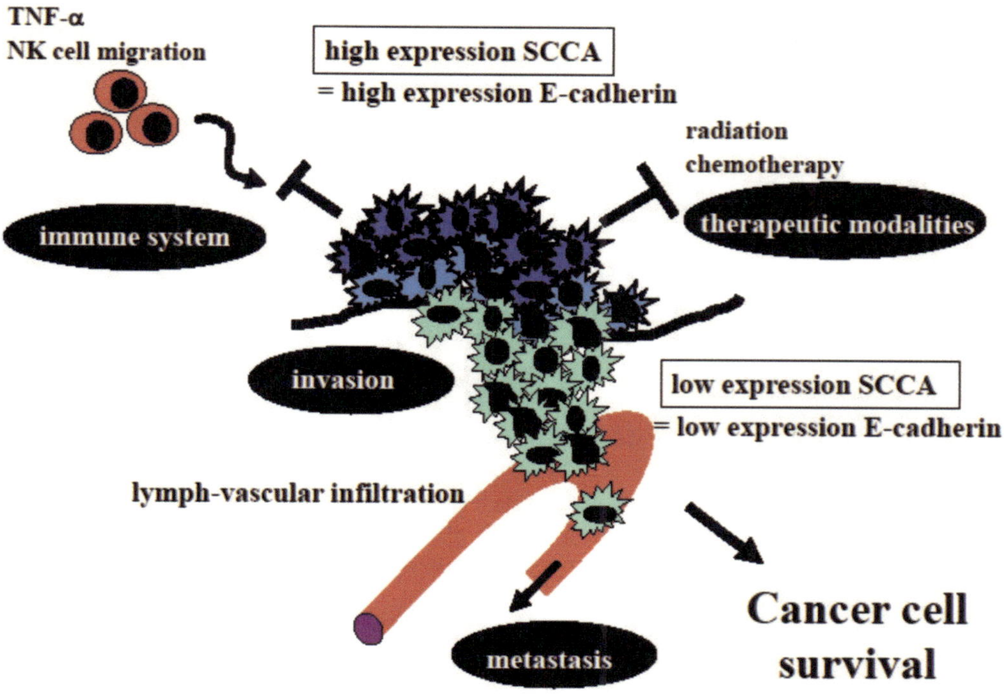

Fig. 2. Possible roles of SCCA in tumor cell survival and metastasis in uterine cervical squamous cell carcinoma. Cancer cells with abnormally high expression of SCCA are resistant to apoptosis induced by the immune system and therapeutic modalities. In contrast, cancer cells with abnormally low expression of SCCA show loss of E-cadherin expression, resulting in detachment from the primary tumor lesion. These cells migrate, attach to the vessels, and metastasize in other organs through blood and lymph fluid flow.

6. Conclusions

SCCAs have been regarded as a useful tumor marker for squamous cell carcinoma in clinical practice. Furthermore, they have some interesting biological functions. SCCAs are regarded as a useful tumor marker for squamous cell carcinoma in clinical practice. In normal squamous epithelium, SCCA may have roles in the stratification, cornification, barrier functions and structure of the epithelium. In squamous cell carcinomas, both SCCA1 and SCCA2 suppress apoptosis by inhibiting serine and cysteine proteinases concerned that function in the apoptotic pathway, resulting in the proliferation of cancer cells. Furthermore, suppression of SCCA2 promoted cancer cell invasion and migration with the decreased expression of E-cadherin, resulting in cancer cell metastases. Thus, SCCA appears to have roles not only in the normal squamous epithelium but also in the squamous cell carcinomas.

7. Conflict of interest

The authors declare no conflict of interest.

8. References

[1] Kato H and Torigoe T: Radioimmunoassay for tumour antigen of human cervical squamous cell carcinoma. Cancer 40: 1621-1628, 1977

[2] Kato H, Tamai K, Morioka H, Nagai M, Nagaya T, and Torigoe T: Prognostic significance of the tumour antigen TA-4 in squamous cell carcinoma of the uterine cervix. Am J Obstet Gynecol 145: 350-354, 1983

[3] Maruo T, Shibata K, Kimura A, Hoshina A, and Mochizuki M: Tumour-associated antigen, TA-4, in the monitoring of the effects of therapy for squamous cell carcinoma of the uterine cervix. Cancer 59: 302-308, 1985

[4] Brioschi PA, Bischof P, Delafosse C and Krauer F: Squamous cell carcinoma antigen (SCC-A) values related to clinical outcome of pre-invasive and invasive cervical carcinoma. Int J Cancer 47: 376-379, 1991

[5] Suminami Y, Kishi F, Sekiguchi K, and Kato H: Squamous cell carcinoma antigen is a new member of the serine protease inhibitors. Biochem Biophys Res Comm 181: 51-58, 1991

[6] Kato H, Nagaya T, and Torigoe T: Heterogeneity of a tumor antigen TA-4 of squamous cell carcinoma in regulation to its appearance in circulation. Gann 75: 433-435, 1984

[7] Schneider SS, Schick C, Fish KE, Miller E, Pena JC, Treter SD, Hui SM, and Silverman GA: A serine proteinase inhibitor locus at 18q21.3 contains a tandem duplication of the human squamous cell carcinoma antigen gene. Proc Natl Acad Sci USA 92: 3147-3151, 1995

[8] Kuwano A, Kondo I, Kishi F, Suminami Y, and Kato H: Assignment of the squamous cell carcinoma antigen locus (SCC) to 18q21 by in situ hybridization. Genomics 30: 626, 1995

[9] Nawata S, Tsunaga N, Numa F, Tanaka T, Nakamura K, and Kato H: Serine protease inhibitor activity of recombinant squamous cell carcinoma antigen towards chymotrypsin, as demonstrated by sodium dodecyl sulfate-polyacrylamide gel electrophoresis. Electrophoresis 16: 1027-1030, 1995

[10] Nawata S, Nakamura K, Tanaka T, Numa F, Suminami Y, Tsunaga N, Kakegawa H, Katsunuma N, and Kato H: Electrophoretic analysis of the"cross-class" interaction between novel inhibitory serpin, squamous cell carcinoma antigen-1 and cystein proteinases. Electrophoresis 18: 784-789, 1997

[11] Schick C, Kamachi Y, Bartuski A J, Çataltepe S, Schechter NM, Pemberton PA, and Silverman GA: Squamous cell carcinoma antigen 2 is a novel serpin that inhibits the chymotrypsin-like proteinases cathepsin G and mast cell chymase. J Biol Chem 17: 1849-1855, 1997

[12] Schick C, Pemberton PA, Shi GP, Kamachi Y, Çataltepe S, Bartuski AJ, Cornstein ER, Brömme D, Chapman HA, and Silverman GA: Cross-class inhibition of the cysteine proteinases cathepsin K, L, S by the serpin squamous cell carcinoma antigen 1: A kinetic analysis. Biochemistry 37: 5258-5266, 1998

[13] Kato H: Squamous cell carcinoma antigen, in: Sell S (ed), Serological Cancer markers. Human Press, Totowa, NJ, pp 437-451, 1992

[14] Ogino I, Nakayama H, Okamoto N, Kitamura T, and Inoue T: The role of pretreatment squamous cell carcinoma antigen level in locally advanced squamous cell carcinoma of the uterine cervix treated by radiotherapy. Int J Gynecol Cancer 16: 1094-1100, 2006

[15] van de Lande J, Davelaar EM, von Mendorff-Pouilly S, Water TJ, Berkhof J, van Baal WM, Kenemans P, and Verheijen RH: SCC-Ag, lymph node metastases and sentinel node procedure in early stage squamous cell cervical cancer. Gynecol Oncol 112: 119-125, 2009

[16] Hsu KF, Huang SC, Shiau AL, Cheng YM, Shen MR, Chen YF, Lin CY, Lee BH, and Chou CY: Increased expression level of squamous cell carcinoma antigen 2 and 1 ratio is associated with poor prognosis in early-stage uterine cervical cancer. Int J Gynecol Cancer 17: 174-181, 2007

[17] Suehiro Y, Kato H, Nagai M, Torigoe T: Flow cytometric analysis of tumor antigen TA-4 in cervical cytological specimens. Cancer 57: 1380-1384, 1986

[18] Takeshima N, Suminami Y, Takeda O, Abe H, and Kato H: Origin of CA125 and SCC antigen in human amniotic fluid. Asia Oceania J Obstet Gynecol 19: 199-204, 1993

[19] Michioka T, Takeshima N, Tsunaga N, Suminami Y, Nawata S, Kato H: Expression of squamous cell carcinoma antigen, a serine proteinase inhibitor, in the integment of vertebrates: possible role in stratification of epidermis. Acta Histochem Cytochem 27: 435-440, 1994

[20] Yuspa SH: The pathogenesis of squamous cell cancer: Lessons learned from studies of skin carcinogenesis-Thirty-third G.H.A. Clowes Memorial Award Lecture. Cancer Res 54: 1178-1189, 1994

[21] Tsunaga N: Effects of calcium on the production of squamous cell carcinoma antigen in normal human keratinocytes. Yamaguchi Igaku 43: 419-426, 1994 (abstract in English)

[22] Katagiri C, Nakanishi J, Kadoya K, and Hibino T: Serpin squamous cell carcinoma antigen inhibits UV-induced apoptosis via suppression of c-JUN NH_2-terminal kinase. J Cell Biol 172: 983-990, 2006

[23] Katagiri C, Negishi K, and Hibino T: c-JUN N-terminal kinase-1 (JNK1) but not JNK2 or JNK3 is involved in UV signal transduction in human epidermis. J Dermatol Sci 43: 171-179, 2006

[24] Nawata S, Murakami A, Hirabayashi K, Sakaguchi Y, Ogata H, Suminami Y, Numa F, Nakamura K, and Kato H: Identification of squamous cell carcinoma antigen-2 in tumor tissue by two-dimensional electrophoresis. Electrophoresis 20: 614-617, 1999

[25] Murakami A, Suminami Y, Sakaguchi Y, Nawata S, Numa F, Kishi F, and Kato H : Specific detection and quantitation of *SCC antigen 1* and *SCC antigen 2* mRNAs by fluorescence-based asymmetric semi-nested reverse transcription PCR. Tumour Biol 21: 224-234, 2000

[26] Suminami Y, Nagashima S, Vujanovic NL, Hirabayashi K, Kato H, and Whiteside TL: Inhibition of apoptosis in human tumour cells by the tumour-associated serpin, SCC antigen-1. Br J Cancer 82: 981-989, 2000

[27] Murakami A, Suminami Y, Hirakawa H, Nawata S, Numa F, and Kato H: Squamous cell carcinoma antigen suppresses radiation-induced cell death. Br J Cancer 84: 851-858, 2001

[28] McGettrick AF, Barnes RC and Worrall DM: SCCA2 inhibits TNF-mediated apoptosis in transfected HeLa cells. Eur J Biochem 268: 5868-5875, 2001

[29] Iwasaki M, Nishikawa A, Akutagawa N, Fujimoto T, Teramoto M, Sakaguchi Y, Kato H, Ito M, Yoshida K, Kudo R: E1AF/PEA3 reduces the invasiveness of SiHa cervical

cancer cells by activating serine proteinase inhibitor squamous cell carcinoma antigen. Exp Cell Res 299: 525-532, 2004

[30] Murakami A, Nakagawa T, Kaneko M, Nawata S, Takeda O, Kato H, Sugino N: Suppression of SCC antigen promotes cancer cell invasion and migration through the decrease in E-cadherin expression. Int J Oncol 29: 1231-1235, 2006

[31] Hirakawa H, Nawata S, Sueoka K, Murakami A, Takeda O, Numa F, Kato H, and Sugino N: Regulation of squamous cell carcinoma antigen production by E-cadherin mediated cell-cell adhesion, ion in squamous cell carcinoma cell line. Oncol Rep 11: 415-419, 2004

[32] Murakami A, Nakagawa T, Fukushima C, Torii M, Sueoka K, Nawata S, Takeda O, Ishikawa H, Sugino N: Relationship between decreased expression of squamous cell carcinoma antigen 2 and E-cadherin in primary cervical cancer lesions and lymph node metastasis. Oncol Rep 19: 99-104, 2008

[33] Nakagawa T, Murakami A, Torii M, Nawata S, Takeda O, and Sugino N: E-cadherin increases squamous cell carcinoma antigen expression through phosphatidylinositol-3 kinase-Akt pathway in squamous cell carcinoma cell lines. Oncol Rep 18: 175-179, 2007

Part 4

Role of Tumor Microenvironment in Head and Neck Squamous Cell Carcinoma

10

The Cellular Microenvironment of Head and Neck Squamous Cell Carcinoma

Maya Mathew and Sufi Mary Thomas*
Department of Otolaryngology, University of Pittsburgh and University of Pittsburgh Cancer Institute, Pittsburgh
USA

1. Introduction

Head and neck squamous cell carcinoma (HNSCC) tumors function much like organs with support from multiple cell lineages. Tobacco and alcohol abuse are strongly correlated with the disease. Environmental carcinogen exposure introduces genetic alterations not only in the epithelial cells but also in the surrounding stroma contributing to tumor initiation and progression [1]. Factors and cells that do not support tumor growth are commonly downregulated or mitigated in the tumor microenvironment. Several classes of stromal cells that exist in close proximity with HNSCC tumors have been identified. These include fibroblasts, immune cells and cells involved in vascular growth. Each of these cell types are involved in molecular cross-talk with the tumor resulting in tumor progression (Figure 1). Here we highlight each of the major cell types present in the HNSCC tumor microenvironment. Well characterized molecular markers have been used to identify the specific stromal cellular components (Table 1). There continues to be a tremendous need for improved understanding of the role of each of these cell types in tumor growth, dissemination and resistance to therapies. Tumor-associated stroma can support tumor cell proliferation, angiogenesis and invasion making them potential therapeutic targets. Since de novo acquisition of genetic mutations is not common in stromal cells they may be less prone to developing resistance to therapy via genomic instability. The synergistic relationship between stroma and tumor cells suggests that stroma targeted intervention may have a synergistic role in primary cancer therapy. However, fibrosis that follows surgery, chemotherapy and radiotherapy may trigger the release of stromal factors that support recurrence and metastasis. Thus stroma targeted therapies may emerge as important in adjuvant setting.

2. Tumor associated fibroblasts

Fibroblasts are important components of the mesenchymal stroma Though they appear morphologically similar, fibroblasts show large differences in their functions and patterns of gene expression depending on their anatomical site of origin. Under normal physiological conditions, fibroblasts help maintain the boundary between the epithelial cells and the

*Corresponding Author

underlying tissue by functioning as a physical barrier. Fibroblasts play a major role in regulating and maintaining extracellular homeostasis. Tissue injury triggers fibroblast activation [2]. Activated fibroblasts are responsible for wound contraction, fibrosis, scaring and regulation of inflammatory reactions. Upon activation, fibroblasts transdifferentiate into motile cells with abundant endoplasmic reticulum, Golgi and α-SMA stress fibers [3]. These α-SMA positive fibroblasts termed myofibroblasts synthesize extracellular matrix components, and several proteinases, growth factors and cytokines. Myofibroblasts have a morphology much like muscle cells with have highly contractile microfilaments. Tumors are frequently regarded as wounds that do not heal. HNSCC tumors are frequently associated with desmoplastic stromal myofibroblasts also known as tumor-associated fibroblasts (TAFs) or cancer associated fibroblasts.

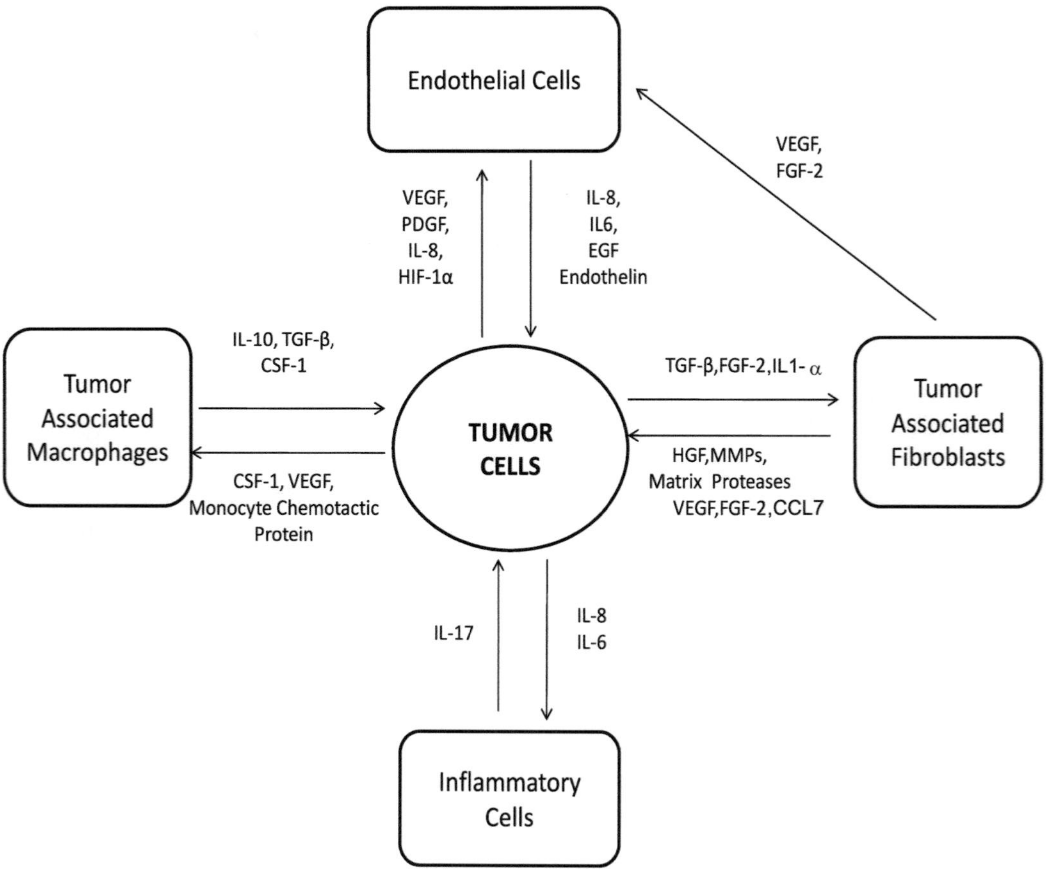

Fig. 1. Cross talk between HNSCC and stromal cellular components. Factors secreted by each cell type that influence target cells have been listed. Abbreviations include; VEGF-Vascular endothelial growth factor, PDGF-Platelet derived growth factor, IL-Interleukin, HIF-Hypoxia Inducible Factor, TGF-Transforming Growth Factor, CSF-Colony Stimulating Factor, EGF-Epithelial growth factor, HGF- Hepatocyte growth factor, MMP-Matrix metalloprotease, FGF- Fibroblast growth factor CCL7- Chemokine Ligand 7(C-C motif).

Cell Type	Molecular Marker
Tumor Associated Fibroblasts	α smooth muscle actin, Vimentin, Fibroblast activating protein
Tumor Associated Macrophages	CD-68, Macrophage inflammatory Protein-3α
Tumor Infiltrating Lymphocytes	
T cells	$CD\text{-}3^+$
NK cells	$CD16/56^+CD3^-$
T helper cells	$CD4^+$
Endothelial Cells	CD-31,CD34, VEGF-R1,VEGF-R2
Pericytes	α smooth muscle action
Mast Cell	Mast cell tryptase
Lymphatic Endothelial Cell	HIF-1alpha, VEGF-C

Table 1. Molecular markers commonly used to identify cellular components of the stroma

TAFs constitute a major cellular component of the tumor associated stroma and are characterized by increased proliferation and aberrant expression of extracellular matrix components. They have been reported to change the phenotype of normal keratinocytes to that resembling squamous cell carcinoma [4]. In other tumor types including prostate, TAFs are reported to play a role in tumor initiation [5-7]. In addition, they play a role in tumor progression as evidenced by a correlation with tumor stage, metastasis and poor prognosis [8]. Although epithelial tumors undergo epithelial-to-mesenchymal transition to acquire a fibroblast-like morphology, they express epithelial cytokeratin markers that are otherwise not expressed on fibroblasts. Epithelial cells with mesenchymal characteristics are not included in these discussions. Several markers have been used to identify TAFs including α-smooth muscle actin, vimentin and fibroblast activating protein [3, 9]. However, these markers show only partially overlapping expression and no single marker consistently labels TAFs. TAFs in the tumor microenvironment are primed to facilitate HNSCC tumor invasion [8]. They are important modulators of tumor growth, invasion and metastasis producing extracellular matrix and angiogenic factors [10-12]. TAFs may be derived not only from the fibroblasts in the locoregional vicinity of the tumor but also from circulating mesenchymal stem cells [13, 14]. TAFs are detected in both primary and metastatic HNSCC [15]. There are at least 4 possible explanations for the origin of the TAFs at metastatic sites; 1) they are derived from the stoma surrounding the metastatic site, 2) they co-metastasize along with the metastatic tumor cells from the primary tumor site or 3) they arrive at the metastatic site prior to the arrival of the tumor cells creating a metastatic niche permissible to the tumor growth or 4) they are derived from circulating mesenchymal stem cells. HNSCC stroma are either rich in TAFs dispersed throughout the tumor or have low levels of TAFs that are located at the periphery of HNSCC tumors or tumor islands [15]. TAFs are also commonly associated with the invasive margin of the tumor [10]. There is strong evidence to suggest that TAFs use protease and mechanical remodeling of the extracellular matrix to lay tracks along which HNSCC tumor cells invade [16]. They also influence the response of the tumors to conventional therapy [17]. Understanding the tumor microenvironment and the molecular mechanisms responsible for the highly invasive and metastatic nature of HNSCC tumors is vital in developing effective strategies to manage this disease.

TAFs differ in their phenotype, gene expression patterns and functionality from normal oral fibroblasts and normal-dermal fibroblasts derived from non-cancer patients [3, 4]. They are not contact inhibited and have a higher rate of proliferation than normal oral fibroblasts [3]. Somatic mutations such as in the *PTEN* and *TP53* tumor suppressor genes have been reported in TAFs derived from breast carcinoma [18]. There is extensive evidence to demonstrate that cross-talk between TAFs and HNSCC cells results in fibroblast activation and tumor promotion. Release of interleukin-1α from HNSCC cell lines was reported to induce chemokine receptor ligand CCL7 from TAFs. CCL7 binds to its receptors on HNSCC cells promoting cancer cell migration [19]. Other cytokines released by HNSCC cells under the influence of fibroblasts include interleukin-1β, -6, TNF-α and TGF-β [20, 21]. Several factors secreted by TAFs facilitate HNSCC invasion including MT1-matrix metalloprotease, [22]. Several aspects of the biology of TAFs suggest that targeting these cells may offer therapeutic benefits. Specific targeting of TAFs with CD8+ T-cells resulted in reduced growth and metastasis of colon and breast tumors [23]. Targeting galectin-1 expressed in TAFs reduced the secretion of monocyte chemotactic protein-1 mitigating HNSCC migration and metastasis [24]. Several studies have demonstrated that TAFs express the hepatocyte growth factor which promotes the expression of angiogenic factors in HNSCC cells via the oncogenic c-Met receptor and its downstream effectors PI3 kinase and MEK [12, 25, 26].

3. Tumor associated macrophages

Monocytes are recruited by cytokine and chemokine gradients into tissues where further differentiation to macrophages is regulated by environmental signals. In neoplasms tumor associated macrophages (TAMs) represent a major component of the infiltrating leukocytes. The presence of TAMs can be beneficial for the growth of the tumor and sometimes they can cause the death of the tumor cells. For example it has been shown that the amount of TAMs in tumors can be associated with increased neoangiogensis and worsened survival rates. TAMs also have potential for cytotoxicity towards tumor cells and some reports state an improvement in prognosis in relation to high number of TAMs in tumors. TAMs release various cytokines that cause further influx of monocytes in circulation into tumors. The cytokines released by the TAMs also play an important role in angiogenesis, lymphangiogenesis, invasion and metastasis. TAMs modulate the host immune response against the tumor cell mass by releasing cytokines, chemokines, and enzymes that influence the function of antigen presenting cells and host lymphocytes.

In normal homeostasis, macrophages play an important role in immune surveillance and wound healing engulfing debris and dying cells. In addition they provide factors necessary for tissue matrix remodeling [27]. Depending on signals in the local microenvironment, macrophages mature into 3 distinct functional phenotypes namely classically, type I and type II activated. Macrophages induced by microbial products are classified as classically activated. Type 1 macrophages are antigen presenting cells capable of producing factors including cytokines, TNFα, reactive oxygen that trigger microbial and tumor cell kill [28]. In contrast, type II macrophages are anti-inflammatory, scavenge cell debris and promote angiogenesis, tissue remodeling and repair [29]. Macrophages develop into type 1 or type 2 phenotypes reversibly in response to changes in the microenvironment [30]. Tumor associated macrophages (TAMs) are typically type II cells reported to promote growth of various tumors including breast, prostate and lung [31]. CD68 stained TAMs are present at higher levels in HNSCC and modulate angiogenesis during tumor progression [32, 33]. Primary HNSCC tumor with high TAM infiltration is a strong predictor of lymph node metastasis, extracellular capsular spread and advanced HNSCC stage [34]. Further, expression of macrophage inflammatory protein-3α was shown to promote oral SCC migration and invasion [35]. Thus, sufficient evidence exists to indicate that TAMs may be important therapeutic targets.

4. Tumor infiltrating lymphocytes

Pathologic examination of HNSCC demonstrates infiltration of cytotoxic T cell that are functionally inactive. Patients with stage 2 and stage 3 carcinoma of the glottis, tongue and hypo pharynx had significantly increased number of T lymphocytes compared to patients with stage 4 disease [36]. Further, increased T lymphocyte numbers at the margins of HNSCC tumors are associated with favorable prognosis. The T lymphocytes produce lymphokines and play an important role in the proliferation of cytotoxic effector cells, thereby play an important role in the local immune response in squamous cell carcinomas of head and neck.

T lymphocytes are the gatekeepers of autoimmune regulation. Failure of T lymphocytes to recognize and eradicate malignant cells contributes to tumor development [37, 38]. Tumors with a high infiltrate of lymphocytes are associated with improved prognosis [39-41]. HNSCC tumors are influenced by several classes of T lymphocytes including T helper cells, CD3, 4 or -8 positive T cells, natural killer cells, regulatory T cells and myeloid progenitor cells [42-45]. Depending up on the subtype of T cells infiltrating the tumor, the tumor experiences growth promotion or regression [46]. In Table 2 we list the tumor facilitating and tumor-promoting T cells. Myeloid-derived suppressor cells (MDSC) are reported to display antitumor effects or tumor promoting effects depending on the factors secreted in the tumor microenvironment [47]. In addition to modulating immune cells in its vicinity, HNSCC tumors actively recruit and trigger the production of tumor growth promoting interleukin-6 from CD34+ myeloid progenitor cells [48]. CD34+ progenitor cells differentiate into a variety of cell lineages including endothelial cells involved in angiogenesis [49]. Th17-T helper cells are characterized by the high levels of secreted pro-inflammatory cytokine interleukin-17. HNSCC tumor and draining lymph nodes are reported to be infiltrated with Th17 cells that are recruited by the tumor cells [45]. Interestingly, Th17 cells reduce HNSCC proliferation while increasing angiogenesis. Natural killer cells on the other hand, are capable of profound antitumor effects. A deficiency in invariant CD1d-restricted natural killer cells was reported to predict a poor clinical outcome in HNSCC patients [42]. Dendritic cells and T regulatory (Treg) cells also play a role in HNSCC tumor suppression [43, 50]. Under normal physiological conditions these cells are responsible for antigen presenting and for discriminating between self and non-self-antigens, respectively. HNSCC use multiple mechanisms to evade immune surveillance including downmodulation of immunologic molecules, prevention of immune cell activation, inactivation or by triggering functional deficiencies in immune cells [51-54]. Immune evasion occurs not only in the primary HNSCC tumor but also during the process of metastasis allowing dissemination to regional lymph nodes and distant sites [55]. Reconstitution of immune cells with anti-tumor capabilities may be a feasible adjuvant immunotherapeutic strategy for HNSCC. Not all immune cells with anti-tumor activities are suppressed in HNSCC. Although the mechanisms remain unknown, in human-papillomavirus associated oropharyngeal carcinoma, large numbers of CD3 positive tumor-infiltrating lymphocytes correlate with higher overall survival and a decreased incidence of metastasis [44].

TILs Facilitating Tumor	TILs Antagonistic To Tumor
CD 34 +ve myeloid progenitor Cells	Cytotoxic T Cells
Th 17 cells (increasing angiogenesis)	Helper T Cells
	Natural Killer Cells
	Myeloid derived Suppressor Cells(MDSC)
	Dendritic Cells
	T regulatory Cells

Table 2. Tumor infiltrating lymphocytes that influence HNSCC tumors

5. Endothelial cells

Endothelial cells when stimulated by the growth factors form blood vessels that facilitate tumor growth and dissemination [56, 57]. HNSCC cells directly bind to endothelial cells through adhesion molecules including intercellular cell adhesion molecule-1, CD44, lymphocyte function-associated antigen-3, integrin chains $\alpha6\beta1$ and sialyl Lewis (x) [58]. Direct binding of HNSCC to endothelial cells is a prerequisite for penetration of and metastasis through the vasculature. In addition, direct interaction between HNSCC and endothelial cells trigger Notch-1 signaling in endothelial cells promoting capillary tubule formation [59]. Angiogenesis and neo-vascularization are complex processes involving cross-talk between multiple cell lineages in the vicinity [60]. HNSCC tumors and stromal cells secrete cytokines and growth factors including vascular endothelial growth factor

(VEGF), platelet-derived growth factor and interleukin-8 inducing angiogenesis [61]. VEGF plays an important role in endothelial cell survival [62, 63]. On binding to its receptor VEGFR2, VEGF induces expression of Bcl-2 and autocrine signaling through chemokines CXCL1 and CXCL8 facilitating proliferation of endothelial cells and sprouting of microvessels [64]. Global gene expression profiling revealed that HNSCC tumors induce angiogenesis by either expressing high levels of VEGF/fibroblast growth factor (FGF-2) and low levels of interleukin-8/CXCL8 or low levels of VEGF/FGF2 and high levels of interleukin-8/CXCL8 [65]. Tumor hypoxia also plays an important role in the release of angiogenic growth factors. Under hypoxic conditions stabilization of the hypoxia inducible factor 1α (HIF-1α) in tumor cells allows transcription of genes involved in angiogenesis and other critical aspects of tumor maintenance [66, 67]. Semaphorin 4D strongly induced by HIF-1α, binds to plexin B1 on endothelial cells inducing migration [68]. In addition to the formation of new blood vessels, endothelial cells are also involved in a cross talk with squamous cell carcinoma cells resulting in a significant increase in tumor cell survival and migration [69]. Specifically, soluble factors secreted by endothelial cells including interleukin-8, interleukin-6, and epidermal growth factor induce phosphorylation of signal transducers and activators of transcription-3, extracellular-regulated kinase and Akt in HNSCC. Thus molecular targeting of endothelial cells may have tremendous therapeutic potential for HNSCC.

6. Lymphatic cells, pericytes, mast cells and other cells in the tumor microenvironment

In addition to blood vessels, HNSCC are typically infiltrated by lymphatic vessels a process known as lymphangiogenesis. Lymph vessels are typically distributed throughout the tumor as well as in the peritumoral regions [70-72]. Metastasis to regional lymph nodes commonly occurs in HNSCC and correlates with poor prognosis [73, 74]. Due to the paucity of lymphatic endothelial cell line models, most of the data generated pertaining to lymphangiogenesis are based on immunohistochemical analysis of xenograft or patient tissues. HNSCC tumors secrete VEGF-C, a member of the VEGF family, which plays an important role in tumor lymphangiogenesis [75]. Increased tumor lymphatic vessel density correlates with metastasis to lymph nodes in HNSCC [76, 77]. HNSCC tumors expressing high levels of HIF-1α and VEGF-C had high lymphatic vessel density and increased metastasis [78].

Pericytes are contractile stromal cells closely associated with vascular endothelial cells that stabilize the capillary walls [79-81]. In the absence of pericytes, blood vessels are unstable and undergo regression. [82]. Pericytes influence the proliferation, migration and maturation of endothelial cells [83]. In tumors, pericytes are loosely associated with endothelial cells resulting in increased capillary leakiness [84]. Very few studies have focused on pericytes in HNSCC. Majority of reports use markers such as α-smooth muscle actin to stain pericytes associated with endothelial cells via immunohistochemical analyses [85, 86].

Mast cells are white blood cells that directly associate with endothelial cells stimulating vascular tube formation [87]. As HNSCC progresses, there is an increase in mast cell numbers that correlated with angiogenesis suggesting a role in angiogenesis [88].

The oral cavity and associated areas of the head and neck region are exposed to several microorganisms. Metaproteomic analyses of human salivary microbiota revealed a large number of oral bacteria that are metabolically active and actively engaged in protein synthesis [89]. The role of the human oral microbiome in tumor pathogenesis remains largely unknown. It is well known that bacteria associated with periodontitis a condition caused by chronic inflammation of the gums, poses an independent risk factor for HNSCC [90]. Human papilloma virus (HPV) infection is a major risk factor for oropharyngeal squamous cell carcinoma [91, 92]. A recent study demonstrated that stromal cells expressing high levels of carbonic anhydrase IX (a sensitive marker for hypoxia) significantly correlated with reduced survival in HPV-negative HNSCC patients [93].

Tumor associated stroma are complex and influence tumor growth in a coordinated manner. Further studies on their contribution to tumor recurrence and new primaries are needed. The identification of promising targets for stroma-directed therapy will pave the way for enhanced anti-tumor effects and improved HNSCC patient survival.

7. Acknowledgements

This work was supported by a career development award from the University of Pittsburgh, Head and Neck Cancer SPORE P50 CA097190 and the Competitive Medical Research Fund (UPMC Health System) to SMT.

8. References

[1] Weber, F., et al., *Microenvironmental genomic alterations and clinicopathological behavior in head and neck squamous cell carcinoma.* JAMA, 2007. 297(2): p. 187-95.

[2] Werner, S., T. Krieg, and H. Smola, *Keratinocyte-fibroblast interactions in wound healing.* J Invest Dermatol, 2007. 127(5): p. 998-1008.

[3] Liu, Y., et al., *Separation, cultivation and biological characteristics of oral carcinoma-associated fibroblasts.* Oral Dis, 2006. 12(4): p. 375-80.

[4] Strnad, H., et al., *Head and neck squamous cancer stromal fibroblasts produce growth factors influencing phenotype of normal human keratinocytes.* Histochem Cell Biol, 2010. 133(2): p. 201-11.

[5] Cunha, G.R., et al., *Role of the stromal microenvironment in carcinogenesis of the prostate.* Int J Cancer, 2003. 107(1): p. 1-10.

[6] Bhowmick, N.A., E.G. Neilson, and H.L. Moses, *Stromal fibroblasts in cancer initiation and progression.* Nature, 2004. 432(7015): p. 332-7.

[7] Weber, F., et al., *Total-genome analysis of BRCA1/2-related invasive carcinomas of the breast identifies tumor stroma as potential landscaper for neoplastic initiation.* Am J Hum Genet, 2006. 78(6): p. 961-72.

[8] Park, C.C., M.J. Bissell, and M.H. Barcellos-Hoff, *The influence of the microenvironment on the malignant phenotype.* Mol Med Today, 2000. 6(8): p. 324-9.

[9] Mishra, P.J., et al., *Carcinoma-associated fibroblast-like differentiation of human mesenchymal stem cells.* Cancer Res, 2008. 68(11): p. 4331-9.

[10] Lewis, M.P., et al., *Tumour-derived TGF-beta1 modulates myofibroblast differentiation and promotes HGF/SF-dependent invasion of squamous carcinoma cells.* Br J Cancer, 2004. 90(4): p. 822-32.

[11] Dang, D., et al., *Matrix metalloproteinases and TGFbeta1 modulate oral tumor cell matrix.* Biochem Biophys Res Commun, 2004. 316(3): p. 937-42.

[12] Knowles, L.M., et al., *HGF and c-Met participate in paracrine tumorigenic pathways in head and neck squamous cell cancer.* Clin Cancer Res, 2009. 15(11): p. 3740-50.

[13] Spaeth, E.L., et al., *Mesenchymal stem cell transition to tumor-associated fibroblasts contributes to fibrovascular network expansion and tumor progression.* PLoS One, 2009. 4(4): p. e4992.
[14] De Boeck, A., et al., *Resident and bone marrow-derived mesenchymal stem cells in head and neck squamous cell carcinoma.* Oral Oncol, 2010. 46(5): p. 336-42.
[15] Vered, M., et al., *Cancer-associated fibroblasts and epithelial-mesenchymal transition in metastatic oral tongue squamous cell carcinoma.* Int J Cancer, 2010. 127(6): p. 1356-62.
[16] Gaggioli, C., et al., *Fibroblast-led collective invasion of carcinoma cells with differing roles for RhoGTPases in leading and following cells.* Nat Cell Biol, 2007. 9(12): p. 1392-400.
[17] Ostman, A. and M. Augsten, *Cancer-associated fibroblasts and tumor growth--bystanders turning into key players.* Curr Opin Genet Dev, 2009. 19(1): p. 67-73.
[18] Patocs, A., et al., *Breast-cancer stromal cells with TP53 mutations and nodal metastases.* N Engl J Med, 2007. 357(25): p. 2543-51.
[19] Jung, D.W., et al., *Tumor-stromal crosstalk in invasion of oral squamous cell carcinoma: a pivotal role of CCL7.* Int J Cancer, 2010. 127(2): p. 332-44.
[20] Koontongkaew, S., P. Amornphimoltham, and B. Yapong, *Tumor-stroma interactions influence cytokine expression and matrix metalloproteinase activities in paired primary and metastatic head and neck cancer cells.* Cell Biol Int, 2009. 33(2): p. 165-73.
[21] Rosenthal, E., et al., *Elevated expression of TGF-beta1 in head and neck cancer-associated fibroblasts.* Mol Carcinog, 2004. 40(2): p. 116-21.
[22] Zhang, W., et al., *Fibroblast-derived MT1-MMP promotes tumor progression in vitro and in vivo.* BMC Cancer, 2006. 6: p. 52.
[23] Loeffler, M., et al., *Targeting tumor-associated fibroblasts improves cancer chemotherapy by increasing intratumoral drug uptake.* J Clin Invest, 2006. 116(7): p. 1955-62.
[24] Wu, M.H., et al., *Targeting galectin-1 in carcinoma-associated fibroblasts inhibits oral squamous cell carcinoma metastasis by downregulating MCP-1/CCL2 expression.* Clin Cancer Res, 2011. 17(6): p. 1306-16.
[25] Dong, G., et al., *Hepatocyte growth factor/scatter factor-induced activation of MEK and PI3K signal pathways contributes to expression of proangiogenic cytokines interleukin-8 and vascular endothelial growth factor in head and neck squamous cell carcinoma.* Cancer Res, 2001. 61(15): p. 5911-8.
[26] Daly, A.J., L. McIlreavey, and C.R. Irwin, *Regulation of HGF and SDF-1 expression by oral fibroblasts--implications for invasion of oral cancer.* Oral Oncol, 2008. 44(7): p. 646-51.
[27] DiPietro, L.A., et al., *MIP-1alpha as a critical macrophage chemoattractant in murine wound repair.* J Clin Invest, 1998. 101(8): p. 1693-8.
[28] Gordon, S., *Alternative activation of macrophages.* Nat Rev Immunol, 2003. 3(1): p. 23-35.
[29] Mantovani, A., P. Allavena, and A. Sica, *Tumour-associated macrophages as a prototypic type II polarised phagocyte population: role in tumour progression.* Eur J Cancer, 2004. 40(11): p. 1660-7.
[30] Stout, R.D., et al., *Macrophages sequentially change their functional phenotype in response to changes in microenvironmental influences.* J Immunol, 2005. 175(1): p. 342-9.
[31] Sica, A., et al., *Macrophage polarization in tumour progression.* Semin Cancer Biol, 2008. 18(5): p. 349-55.
[32] Li, C., et al., *Infiltration of tumor-associated macrophages in human oral squamous cell carcinoma.* Oncol Rep, 2002. 9(6): p. 1219-23.
[33] El-Rouby, D.H., *Association of macrophages with angiogenesis in oral verrucous and squamous cell carcinomas.* J Oral Pathol Med, 2010. 39(7): p. 559-64.

[34] Marcus, B., et al., *Prognostic factors in oral cavity and oropharyngeal squamous cell carcinoma.* Cancer, 2004. 101(12): p. 2779-87.

[35] Chang, K.P., et al., *Overexpression of macrophage inflammatory protein-3alpha in oral cavity squamous cell carcinoma is associated with nodal metastasis.* Oral Oncol, 2011. 47(2): p. 108-13.

[36] Guo, M., et al., *Lymphocyte phenotypes at tumor margins in patients with head and neck cancer.* Head Neck Surg, 1987. 9(5): p. 265-71.

[37] Young, M.R., *Protective mechanisms of head and neck squamous cell carcinomas from immune assault.* Head Neck, 2006. 28(5): p. 462-70.

[38] Whiteside, T.L., *Immune suppression in cancer: effects on immune cells, mechanisms and future therapeutic intervention.* Semin Cancer Biol, 2006. 16(1): p. 3-15.

[39] Clark, W.H., Jr., et al., *Model predicting survival in stage I melanoma based on tumor progression.* J Natl Cancer Inst, 1989. 81(24): p. 1893-904.

[40] Clemente, C.G., et al., *Prognostic value of tumor infiltrating lymphocytes in the vertical growth phase of primary cutaneous melanoma.* Cancer, 1996. 77(7): p. 1303-10.

[41] Curiel, T.J., et al., *Specific recruitment of regulatory T cells in ovarian carcinoma fosters immune privilege and predicts reduced survival.* Nat Med, 2004. 10(9): p. 942-9.

[42] Molling, J.W., et al., *Low levels of circulating invariant natural killer T cells predict poor clinical outcome in patients with head and neck squamous cell carcinoma.* J Clin Oncol, 2007. 25(7): p. 862-8.

[43] Bergmann, C., et al., *T regulatory type 1 cells in squamous cell carcinoma of the head and neck: mechanisms of suppression and expansion in advanced disease.* Clin Cancer Res, 2008. 14(12): p. 3706-15.

[44] Rajjoub, S., et al., *Prognostic significance of tumor-infiltrating lymphocytes in oropharyngeal cancer.* Ear Nose Throat J, 2007. 86(8): p. 506-11.

[45] Kesselring, R., et al., *Human Th17 cells can be induced through head and neck cancer and have a functional impact on HNSCC development.* Br J Cancer, 2010. 103(8): p. 1245-54.

[46] Yu, P. and Y.X. Fu, *Tumor-infiltrating T lymphocytes: friends or foes?* Lab Invest, 2006. 86(3): p. 231-45.

[47] Pastula, A. and J. Marcinkiewicz, *Myeloid-derived suppressor cells: a double-edged sword?* Int J Exp Pathol, 2011. 92(2): p. 73-8.

[48] Nitsch, S.M., R. Pries, and B. Wollenberg, *Head and neck cancer triggers increased IL-6 production of CD34+ stem cells from human cord blood.* In Vivo, 2007. 21(3): p. 493-8.

[49] Grote, K., et al., *The angiogenic factor CCN1 promotes adhesion and migration of circulating CD34+ progenitor cells: potential role in angiogenesis and endothelial regeneration.* Blood, 2007. 110(3): p. 877-85.

[50] Reichert, T.E., et al., *Signaling abnormalities, apoptosis, and reduced proliferation of circulating and tumor-infiltrating lymphocytes in patients with oral carcinoma.* Clin Cancer Res, 2002. 8(10): p. 3137-45.

[51] Du, C. and Y. Wang, *The immunoregulatory mechanisms of carcinoma for its survival and development.* J Exp Clin Cancer Res, 2011. 30: p. 12.

[52] Jewett, A., C. Head, and N.A. Cacalano, *Emerging mechanisms of immunosuppression in oral cancers.* J Dent Res, 2006. 85(12): p. 1061-73.

[53] Uppaluri, R., G.P. Dunn, and J.S. Lewis, Jr., *Focus on TILs: prognostic significance of tumor infiltrating lymphocytes in head and neck cancers.* Cancer Immun, 2008. 8: p. 16.

[54] Ferris, R.L., T.L. Whiteside, and S. Ferrone, *Immune escape associated with functional defects in antigen-processing machinery in head and neck cancer.* Clin Cancer Res, 2006. 12(13): p. 3890-5.
[55] Kumagai, K., et al., *Evidence for the changes of antitumor immune response during lymph node metastasis in head and neck squamous cell carcinoma.* Oral Surg Oral Med Oral Pathol Oral Radiol Endod, 2010. 110(3): p. 341-50.
[56] Folkman, J., et al., *Isolation of a tumor factor responsible for angiogenesis.* J Exp Med, 1971. 133(2): p. 275-88.
[57] Folkman, J., *Tumor angiogenesis: therapeutic implications.* N Engl J Med, 1971. 285(21): p. 1182-6.
[58] Wenzel, C.T., R.L. Scher, and W.J. Richtsmeier, *Adhesion of head and neck squamous cell carcinoma to endothelial cells. The missing links.* Arch Otolaryngol Head Neck Surg, 1995. 121(11): p. 1279-86.
[59] Zeng, Q., et al., *Crosstalk between tumor and endothelial cells promotes tumor angiogenesis by MAPK activation of Notch signaling.* Cancer Cell, 2005. 8(1): p. 13-23.
[60] Hasina, R. and M.W. Lingen, *Angiogenesis in oral cancer.* J Dent Educ, 2001. 65(11): p. 1282-90.
[61] Choi, S. and J.N. Myers, *Molecular pathogenesis of oral squamous cell carcinoma: implications for therapy.* J Dent Res, 2008. 87(1): p. 14-32.
[62] Jain, R.K., et al., *Endothelial cell death, angiogenesis, and microvascular function after castration in an androgen-dependent tumor: role of vascular endothelial growth factor.* Proc Natl Acad Sci U S A, 1998. 95(18): p. 10820-5.
[63] Christopoulos, A., et al., *Biology of vascular endothelial growth factor and its receptors in head and neck cancer: Beyond angiogenesis.* Head Neck, 2010.
[64] Karl, E., et al., *Unidirectional crosstalk between Bcl-xL and Bcl-2 enhances the angiogenic phenotype of endothelial cells.* Cell Death Differ, 2007. 14(9): p. 1657-66.
[65] Hasina, R., et al., *Angiogenic heterogeneity in head and neck squamous cell carcinoma: biological and therapeutic implications.* Lab Invest, 2008. 88(4): p. 342-53.
[66] Brennan, P.A., N. Mackenzie, and M. Quintero, *Hypoxia-inducible factor 1alpha in oral cancer.* J Oral Pathol Med, 2005. 34(7): p. 385-9.
[67] Zhu, G.Q., et al., *Hypoxia inducible factor 1alpha and hypoxia inducible factor 2alpha play distinct and functionally overlapping roles in oral squamous cell carcinoma.* Clin Cancer Res, 2010. 16(19): p. 4732-41.
[68] Sun, Q., et al., *Hypoxia-inducible factor-1-mediated regulation of semaphorin 4D affects tumor growth and vascularity.* J Biol Chem, 2009. 284(46): p. 32066-74.
[69] Neiva, K.G., et al., *Cross talk initiated by endothelial cells enhances migration and inhibits anoikis of squamous cell carcinoma cells through STAT3/Akt/ERK signaling.* Neoplasia, 2009. 11(6): p. 583-93.
[70] Audet, N., et al., *Lymphatic vessel density, nodal metastases, and prognosis in patients with head and neck cancer.* Arch Otolaryngol Head Neck Surg, 2005. 131(12): p. 1065-70.
[71] O'Donnell, R.K., et al., *Immunohistochemical method identifies lymphovascular invasion in a majority of oral squamous cell carcinomas and discriminates between blood and lymphatic vessel invasion.* J Histochem Cytochem, 2008. 56(9): p. 803-10.
[72] Zhao, D., et al., *Intratumoral lymphangiogenesis in oral squamous cell carcinoma and its clinicopathological significance.* J Oral Pathol Med, 2008. 37(10): p. 616-25.

[73] Munoz-Guerra, M.F., et al., *Prognostic significance of intratumoral lymphangiogenesis in squamous cell carcinoma of the oral cavity.* Cancer, 2004. 100(3): p. 553-60.
[74] Franchi, A., et al., *Tumor lymphangiogenesis in head and neck squamous cell carcinoma: a morphometric study with clinical correlations.* Cancer, 2004. 101(5): p. 973-8.
[75] Kishimoto, K., et al., *Expression of vascular endothelial growth factor-C predicts regional lymph node metastasis in early oral squamous cell carcinoma.* Oral Oncol, 2003. 39(4): p. 391-6.
[76] Beasley, N.J., et al., *Intratumoral lymphangiogenesis and lymph node metastasis in head and neck cancer.* Cancer Res, 2002. 62(5): p. 1315-20.
[77] Sedivy, R., et al., *Expression of vascular endothelial growth factor-C correlates with the lymphatic microvessel density and the nodal status in oral squamous cell cancer.* J Oral Pathol Med, 2003. 32(8): p. 455-60.
[78] Liang, X., et al., *Hypoxia inducible factor-alpha expression correlates with vascular endothelial growth factor-C expression and lymphangiogenesis/angiogenesis in oral squamous cell carcinoma.* Anticancer Res, 2008. 28(3A): p. 1659-66.
[79] Allt, G. and J.G. Lawrenson, *Pericytes: cell biology and pathology.* Cells Tissues Organs, 2001. 169(1): p. 1-11.
[80] Hirschi, K.K. and P.A. D'Amore, *Pericytes in the microvasculature.* Cardiovasc Res, 1996. 32(4): p. 687-98.
[81] Shepro, D. and N.M. Morel, *Pericyte physiology.* FASEB J, 1993. 7(11): p. 1031-8.
[82] Papetti, M. and I.M. Herman, *Mechanisms of normal and tumor-derived angiogenesis.* Am J Physiol Cell Physiol, 2002. 282(5): p. C947-70.
[83] Egginton, S., et al., *The role of pericytes in controlling angiogenesis in vivo.* Adv Exp Med Biol, 2000. 476: p. 81-99.
[84] Morikawa, S., et al., *Abnormalities in pericytes on blood vessels and endothelial sprouts in tumors.* Am J Pathol, 2002. 160(3): p. 985-1000.
[85] Kimura, M., et al., *Soluble form of ephrinB2 inhibits xenograft growth of squamous cell carcinoma of the head and neck.* Int J Oncol, 2009. 34(2): p. 321-7.
[86] Bhattacharya, A., et al., *Tumor vascular maturation and improved drug delivery induced by methylselenocysteine leads to therapeutic synergy with anticancer drugs.* Clin Cancer Res, 2008. 14(12): p. 3926-32.
[87] Blair, R.J., et al., *Human mast cells stimulate vascular tube formation. Tryptase is a novel, potent angiogenic factor.* J Clin Invest, 1997. 99(11): p. 2691-700.
[88] Iamaroon, A., et al., *Increase of mast cells and tumor angiogenesis in oral squamous cell carcinoma.* J Oral Pathol Med, 2003. 32(4): p. 195-9.
[89] Rudney, J.D., et al., *A metaproteomic analysis of the human salivary microbiota by three-dimensional peptide fractionation and tandem mass spectrometry.* Mol Oral Microbiol, 2010. 25(1): p. 38-49.
[90] Tezal, M., et al., *Chronic periodontitis and the incidence of head and neck squamous cell carcinoma.* Cancer Epidemiol Biomarkers Prev, 2009. 18(9): p. 2406-12.
[91] Gillison, M.L., et al., *Distinct risk factor profiles for human papillomavirus type 16-positive and human papillomavirus type 16-negative head and neck cancers.* J Natl Cancer Inst, 2008. 100(6): p. 407-20.
[92] Ernster, J.A., et al., *Rising incidence of oropharyngeal cancer and the role of oncogenic human papilloma virus.* Laryngoscope, 2007. 117(12): p. 2115-28.
[93] Brockton, N., et al., *High stromal carbonic anhydrase IX expression is associated with decreased survival in P16-negative head-and-neck tumors.* Int J Radiat Oncol Biol Phys, 2011. 80(1): p. 249-57.

11

Role of Connective Tissue Growth Factor (CTGF/CCN2) in Oral Squamous Cell Carcinoma-Induced Bone Destruction

Tsuyoshi Shimo* and Akira Sasaki
Department of Oral and Maxillofacial Surgery,
Okayama University Graduate School of Medicine,
Dentistry and Pharmaceutical Sciences, Okayama
Japan

1. Introduction

Oral squamous cell carcinoma cells in the gingiva frequently invade the maxillary or mandibular bone. The clinical consequences of oral squamous cell carcinoma-induced bone destruction include a worse prognosis, a high morbidity rate, hypercalcemia, and nerve paralysis (Brown, et al., 2002; Hicks, et al., 1997; Shaw, et al., 2004). Patients with oral squamous cell carcinoma and associated bone invasion require bone resection, which has a major influence on their functional outcome. However, the mechanism of bone destruction by oral squamous cell carcinoma remains unresolved.

Localization of tumor cells within the bone leads to the production of tumor-associated factors synthesized either directly by the tumor cell itself or as a result of tumor/stromal interactions. These tumor-associated factors converge on the pre-osteoblast or stromal cell to cause an increase in the level of receptor activator of nuclear factor kappa β ligand (RANKL) and/or a decrease in that of osteoprotegerin (OPG), which ultimately results in the activation and survival of osteoclasts, with osteolytic lesions being the result (Roodman GD & Dougall WC, 2008). Bone destruction then leads to the release of growth factors derived from bone, including transforming growth factor-β (TGF-β), insulin-like growth factors (IGFs), fibroblast growth factors (FGFs), platelet-derived growth factor (PDGF), and bone morphogenetic proteins (BMPs; (Kayamori, et al., 2010; Roodman GD, 2004; Roodman GD & Dougall WC, 2008; Shibahara, et al., 2005). These factors increase the production of tumor-associated factors or promote tumor growth directly. Thus, tumor cell proliferation and production of tumor-associated factors through the signaling of these pathways are promoted, and the vicious cycle continues.

Connective tissue growth factor (CTGF/CCN2) is a member of the CCN family (Takigawa M, et al., 2003), which consists of 6 members: CCN1 (Cyr61), CCN2 (CTGF), CCN3 (NOV), CCN4 (WISP-1), CCN5 (WISP-2), and CCN6 (WISP-3; (Katsube K, et al., 2009; Kubota S & Takigawa M, 2007b; Perbal B, 2004), all of which possess an NH_2-terminal signal peptide

*Corresponding Author

indicative of their secreted-protein nature. CCN proteins share a common molecular structure consisting of an insulin-like growth factor (IGF)-binding protein-like module (IGFBP), von Willebrand factor type C repeat (VWC), thrombospondin type-1 repeat (TSP1), and C-terminal module (CT), except in the case of CCN5, which lacks the CT module. The N-terminal and C-terminal halves of the proteins are connected by a hinge region that is not conserved and is particularly sensitive to proteolysis (Dean, et al., 2007; Kireeva, et al., 1996). By means of these modules, the CCN2 protein interacts with a number of extracellular molecules. The IGFBP motif is responsible for binding IGF (Bork P, 1993), albeit studies with CCN2 have demonstrated that the interaction of CCN2 with IGF occurs with a much lower affinity than that of authentic IGFBPs (Yang DH, et al., 1998 Jul;). The VWC motif binds to integrin αvβ3 (Perbal B & Takigawa M, 2005) and has been implicated as a binding site for BMP-4 and TGF-β family members, this binding modulating their activity (Abreu JG, et al., 2002). The TSP-1 motif is involved in binding to integrin α6β1, αvβ3 (Perbal B & Takigawa M, 2005), LRP1 and LRP6 (Gao & Brigstock, 2003; Segarini PR, et al., 2001), and VEGF (Inoki I, et al., 2002). Finally, the CT motif binds integrin αvβ3 and cell-surface heparan sulfate proteoglycans (HSPGs; (Gao R & Brigstock DR, 2004). These different domains of CCN2 could be responsible for the differential signaling resulting in its various biological activities (Fig. 1).

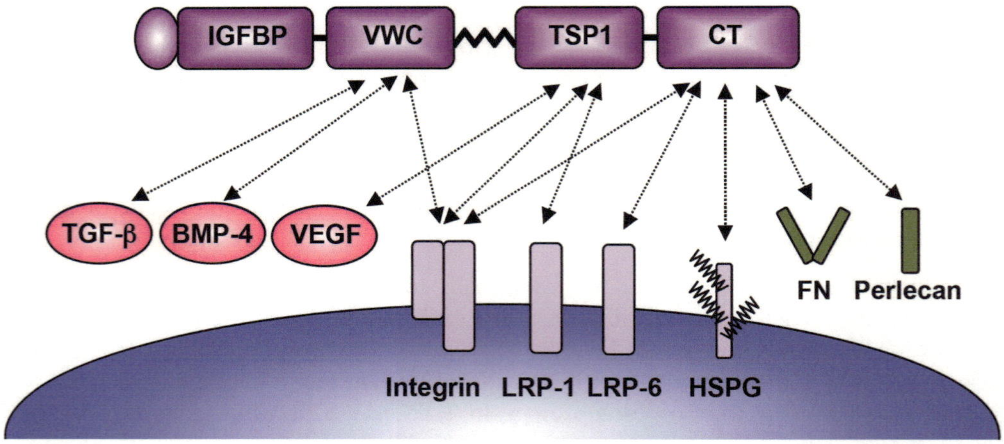

Fig. 1. CCN2-interacting proteins and receptors of CCN2. CCN2 protein interacts with a variety of cell-surface signal-transducing receptors and extracellular ligands, including various integrins, heparan sulfate proteoglycans (HSPG), and LRPs. Receptors and extracellular proteins that interact with 3 of the 4 conserved CCN2 domains are shown.

One of the most prominent functions of CCN2 is its role in cell adhesion. When immobilized on solid surfaces in cell cultures, CCN2 proteins can support the adhesion of most adherent-cell types through integrins and HSPGs and induce adhesive signaling. Adhesion of CCN2 to human skin fibroblasts occurs through α6β1-HSPGs and rapidly induces the formation of α 6β1-containing focal adhesion complexes, activation of focal adhesion kinase (FAK), paxillin, and Rac, as well as reorganization of the actin cytoskeleton and formation of filopodia and lamellipodia (C. C. Chen, et al., 2001). CCN2 can serve as an adaptor for other extracellular matrix proteins to promote cell adhesion, as exemplified by the binding of CCN2 to fibronectin and perlecan (Y. Chen, et al., 2004; Nishida, et al., 2003). In addition to supporting cell adhesion, one of the ubiquitous activities of CCN proteins is the regulation of cell migration.

CCN2 proteins stimulate the migration of many mesenchymal cell types (Babic, et al., 1999; Grzeszkiewicz, et al., 2001; Lin, et al., 2003; Shimo T, et al., 1998; Shimo T, et al., 1999).

CCN2 was originally discovered in, and purified from, the conditioned medium of cultured vein endothelial cells (Bradham, et al., 1991). In 1998, Shimo et al. reported that knockdown of *ccn2* expression results in the suppression of the proliferation and migration of normal vascular endothelial cells (Shimo T, et al., 1998). Subsequently, CCN2 was shown to induce angiogenesis in corneal implants (Babic, et al., 1999) and chick chorioallatonic membranes (Shimo T, et al., 1999). CCN2 also induces chemotaxis (inducing directional cell migration) and chemokinesis (random cell movement) in endothelial cells (Babic, et al., 1999; Babic, et al., 1998; Lin, et al., 2003; Shimo T, et al., 1999). Through direct binding to integrin $\alpha v\beta 3$, CCN2 can recapitulate angiogenic events *in vitro* by promoting endothelial cell adhesion, migration, proliferation, and tubule formation (Babic, et al., 1999; Leu, et al., 2002; Lin, et al., 2003; Shimo T, et al., 1999).

CCN2 knockout mice die just after birth due to respiratory failure (Ivkovic S, et al., 2003). This failure is attributed to hypoplasia of the thoracic skeleton and deformity of the oral cavity (palatal cleft and shortened mandible). CCN2 knockout mice also show skeletal dysmorphisms as a result of impaired chondrocyte proliferation and reduced extracellular matrix with altered composition within the hypertrophic chondrocytic zone in the growth plate. Histologically, angiogenesis and formation of tartrate-resistant acid phosphatase (TRAP)-positive osteoclast-like cells, as well as critical protease expression in the growth plate, are impaired and accompanied by defective replacement of cartilage by bone during endochondral ossification (Nakanishi T, et al., 2000; Nishida T, et al., 2000; Shimo T, et al., 2005). These results demonstrate that CCN2 is important for cell proliferation and matrix remodeling during chondrogenesis, and is a key regulator coupling extracellular matrix remodeling to angiogenesis at the growth plate. The biological activities of CCN2 also include the development of Meckel's cartilage (Shimo T, et al., 2004) and tooth germs (Shimo T, et al., 2002).

Next we will summarize research indicating the essential roles of CCN2 and related molecules in the bone destruction caused by cancer.

2. Cancers and CCN2

CCN2 proteins carry out their biological activity through binding and cell surface integrins (Lau LF & Lam SC, 1999), and elevated CCN2 expression has been observed in breast cancers (Xie D, et al., 2001), pancreatic cancers (Wenger C, et al., 1999), melanomas (Kubo M, et al., 1998), chondrosarcomas (Shakunaga T, et al., 2000), and squamous cell carcinomas (Shimo T, et al., 2008). Although CCN2 shows multiple roles in various cancer types, in breast tumor cells CCN2 over-expression has been linked to an increase in tumor size, lymph node metastasis (Chen PS, et al., 2007; Xie D, et al., 2001), and drug resistance through up-regulation of the survival pathway (Wang MY, et al., 2009). CCN2 is also regarded as a central mediator of tumor angiogenic factor in certain malignancies (Kondo S, et al., 2002; Shimo T, et al., 2001a; Shimo T, et al., 2001b). It should be noted that CCN2 is one of the contributors to bone metastasis, as it converts low-metastatic breast cancer cells to high-metastatic ones in collaboration with other factors (Kang Y, et al., 2003; Minn AJ, et al., 2005). Neutralizing antibodies against CCN2 significantly inhibit local tumor growth, angiogenesis, and osteolysis caused by metastatic human breast cancer cells (Shimo T, et al., 2006). CCN2 and PTHrP are strongly expressed in cancer cells that have invaded the bone matrix, and CCN2 expression is regulated by PTHrP through PKA, PKC, and ERK1/2 MAPK pathways (Shimo T, et al., 2006). Furthermore, the CCN2 gene is significantly over-expressed in overt metastatic tumor cells as compared with its expression in disseminated tumor cells in the bone marrow of breast cancer patients by CT-guided bone metastasis biopsy and bone marrow biopsy (Cawthorn, et al., 2009). Fig. 2A illustrates a representative radiographic pattern of invasive bone destruction observed in a patient with oral squamous cell carcinoma in the mandibular region. In such cases, as shown in Fig. 2B, tumor cells fill the bone marrow space and destroy both the trabecular and cortical bone of the mandible.

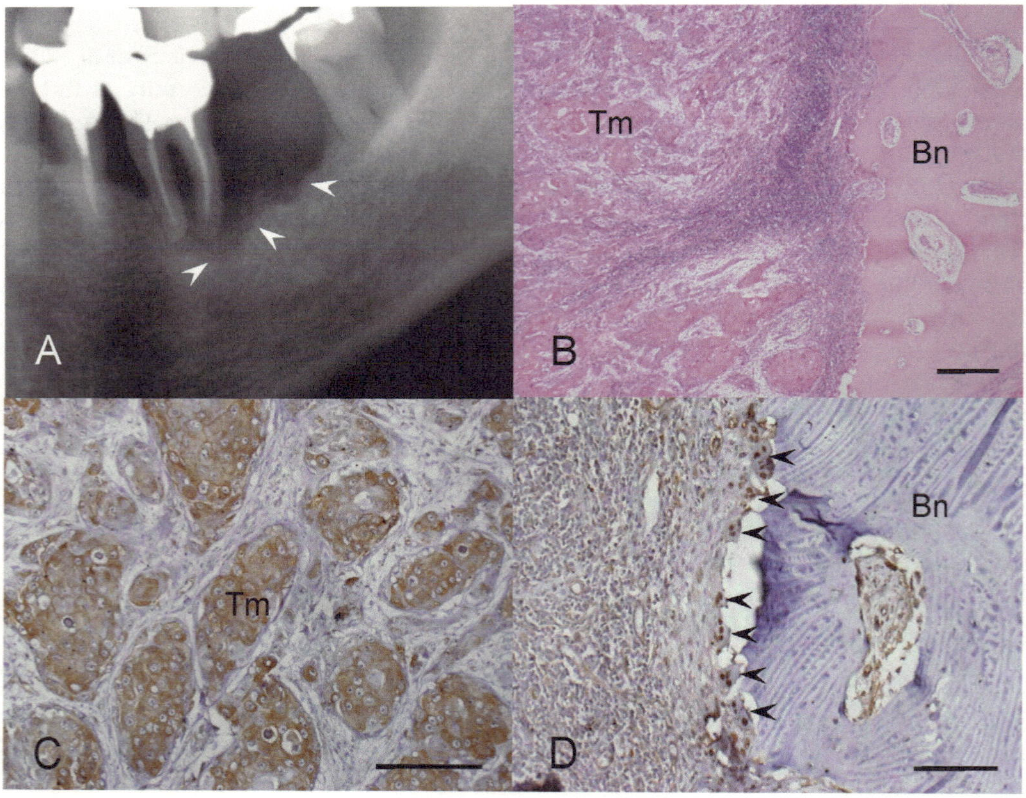

Fig. 2. Radiographic and immunohistochemical analysis of oral squamous cell carcinoma of the mandibular region. (A) Representative radiograph of an invasive oral squamous cell carcinoma in the mandibular region (arrowheads). (B) HE-stained sections of the resected mandible. Tumor tissue (Tm) has invaded into the marrow cavity and replaced the normal cellular elements. Significant loss of trabecular and cortical bone (Bn) has occurred. (C and D) Immunohistochemical staining of CCN2 in a section of invasive tumor (C) and of osteoclasts (D, arrowheads) of the resected mandible. Scale bar = 100 μm. Bn: Bone, Tm: Tumor. The data were modified from Shimo et al. (Shimo, et al., 2008) (B and D).

CCN2 is abundantly produced by the tumor cells that have invaded the bone matrix (Fig. 2C); and, interestingly, CCN2 is also present in the osteoclasts at the destroyed bone/tumor cell interface (Fig. 2D, arrowheads). Of note, up-regulation of CCN2 in oral squamous cell carcinoma of the mandible is associated with increased bone destruction (Shimo T, et al., 2008). These data suggest that CCN2 can be considered both a diagnostic marker and target for treatment of oral osteolytic mandibular squamous cell carcinoma.

3. Relation between CCN2 and tumor associated factors and signaling

3.1 Insulin-like growth factor (IGF) and CCN2

The insulin-like growth factor (IGF) is the most abundant factor stored in the bone matrix (Hauschka, et al., 1986). The IGF system comprises hormone-like growth factors (IGF-I and II), cell-surface receptors (IGF-IR, IGF-IIR and insulin receptor), circulating binding proteins (IGFBPs), and IGFBP proteases. Activation of IGF-I/IGFR signaling plays an important role in cancer cells, leading to an increase in cell proliferation, invasion/migration, to a decrease in apoptosis, and to resistance to antineoplastic agents, suggesting that IGF/IGFR plays an important role in mammary tumorigenesis (Brady, et al., 2007; Kimura, et al., 2010; Saxena, et al., 2008). A larger family of secreted cysteine-rich proteins, made so by inclusion of the Twisted gastrulation (TSG), IGFBP, and CCN families, is termed TIC (Flint, et al., 2008; Pell, et al., 2005). Interestingly, members of the CCN protein family bind IGF with low affinity (Hwa, et al., 1999). However, there are only a few published reports on the association between IGF system and CCN proteins.

3.2 Parathyroid hormone-related protein (PTHrP) and CCN2

Parathyroid hormone-related protein (PTHrP) has important developmental roles in the embryonic skeleton and other tissues. Detection or increased plasma concentrations of PTHrP have been found in 80% of hypercalcemia patients with solid tumor (Burtis WJ, et al., 1990). When it is produced in excess by cancer cells, it can cause hypercalcemia; and its local production by breast cancer cells has been implicated in the pathogenesis of bone metastasis in that disease. Localized production of PTHrP by cancer cells in such lesions was shown to promote the survival and proliferation of cancer cells and osteolysis in a mouse model (Guise TA, et al., 1996). PTHrP induces both the production of RANKL and down-regulation of OPG production by osteoblasts, thereby stimulating osteoclastogenesis (Horwood NJ, et al., 1998; Lee SK & Lorenzo JA, 1999). Oral squamous cell carcinoma cells provide a suitable microenvironment for osteoclast formation by producing PTHrP (Kayamori, et al., 2010). Knock-down of PTHrP in oral squamous cell carcinoma cell caused decreased osteoclast formation in vitro, and suppressed tumor bone invasion in vivo (Y. Takayama, et al., 2010). Sections of resected mandibles from patients with invasive oral squamous cell carcinoma showed strong expression of PTHrP in tumor cells and great number of osteoclasts at bone invasion sites (Y. Takayama, et al., 2010). Type I PTH/PTHrP receptor (PTH1R) expression is specifically observed in cancer cells producing PTHrP and CCN2 that have invaded the bone marrow, and PTHrP strongly up-regulates CCN2 in MDA-MB-231 cells *in vitro* (Shimo T, et al., 2006). CCN2 is also critically involved in osteolytic metastasis and is induced by PKA- and PKC-dependent activation of ERK 1/2 signaling by PTHrP (Shimo T, et al., 2006).

3.3 Transforming growth factor-β (TGF-β) and CCN2

TGF-β is by far the second abundant cytokine in bone, and must be considered as a central player in bone turnover (Bonewald LF & Mundy GR, 1990) and potentially able to couple bone resorption with bone formation (Karsdal MA, et al., 2001; Takeshita S, et al., 2000). Restricted to the bone environment, target cells of TGF-β include cancer cells as well as osteoblasts, osteoclasts, their precursors in the bone marrow, and stromal cells (Bonewald LF & Mundy GR, 1990; Karsdal MA, et al., 2001). TGF-β is a pleiotropic cytokine that plays a central role in maintaining epithelial homeostasis. In early carcinogenesis, TGF-β acts as a tumor suppressor by inhibiting cell proliferation (Massague J, et al., 2000; Sun L, 2004). However, several studies showed that primary tumor cells in the late stage can reprogram their response to TGF-β by dysregulation or mutational inactivation of various components of the TGF-β signaling pathway and through cross-interaction with other oncogenic pathways (Nagaraj & Datta, 2010). TGF-β transduces its signal through 2 highly conserved single transmembrane serine/threonine kinase receptors, termed type I (TβRI) and type II (TβRII). TβRII activates TβRI upon formation of a ligand–receptor complex by hyperphosphorylating serine/threonine residues in the GS region of TβRI. Activated TβRI in turn phosphorylates Smad2 and Smad3, which interact with Smad4. Their complex is translocated to the nucleus, where it regulates the transcription of target genes. This signalling cascade initiates broad cellular and noncellular processes including proliferation and differentiation, migration and motility, and deposition of extracellular matrix, as well as induces the production of cytokines contributing to tumorigenesis, metastasis, and angiogenesis (Ge, et al., 2006; Petersen, et al., 2010). Due to its central role in TGF-β signalling, TβRI is emerging as a novel target for the blockade of the tumor-promoting and metastasis activities of the TGF-β pathway (Shinto, et al., 2010). Consequently, the TGF-β signal becomes a bone metastasis-promoting one (Kang Y, et al., 2005; Kominsky SL, et al., 2007; Yin JJ, et al., 1999). TβRI-positive signals are closely associated with destructive invasion of the mandible by oral squamous cell carcinoma cells, and a TβRI-inhibitor greatly reduces oral squamous cell carcinoma cell-induced bone destruction and osteoclast formation both *in vivo* and *in vitro* (Goda, et al., 2010).

TGF-β is one of the most potent inducers of CCN2, promoting CCN2 expression in bone metastatic cancer cells (Kang Y, et al., 2003); and the induction occurs through a complex network of transcriptional interactions requiring Smads, protein kinase C, and ras/MEK/ERK, as well as an Ets-1/transcription enhancer factor-binding element in the CCN2 promoter (Chen Y, et al., 2002; Leask A, et al., 2002; Van Beek JP, et al., 2006). TGF-β released from the bone causes a further increase in the expression of the TGF-β-responsive osteoclast-inducing genes, *CCN2*, RANKL, and TNF-α in oral squamous cell carcinoma cells, thus establishing a composite positive-feedback cycle of metastasis (Kang Y, et al., 2003; Shimo T, et al., 2006).

3.4 RANKL and CCN2

The RANK and its ligand RANKL signaling pathway play pivotal role in osteoclast-mediated bone resorption in both normal bone remodeling and in pathological conditions, including bone metastasis (Boyle WJ, et al., 2003; Lacey DL, et al., 1998; Simonet WS, et al., 1997). RANK is a transmembrane signaling receptor of the tumor necrosis factor (TNF) receptor superfamily that is expressed on the surface of osteoclast precursors (Hsu H, et al., 1999; Nakagawa N, et al., 1998). Its cognate ligand, RANKL, is expressed almost exclusively within the bone marrow stromal cell compartment and is up-regulated by most hormones and factors that stimulate bone resorption (Boyle WJ, et al., 2003; Roodman GD & Dougall WC, 2008). The interaction between RANK and RANKL is necessary for osteoclast formation, function, and survival (Kong YY, et al., 1999; Lacey DL, et al., 1998). RANKL (50 ng/ml) stimulates osteoclastogenesis in mouse total bone marrow cells in the presence of 100 ng/ml CCN2 (Shimo T, et al., 2008). Stromal/osteoblastic cells are essential for *in vitro* osteoclastogenesis through cell-to-cell interactions (Kondo Y, et al., 2001). The expression of CCN2 is up-regulated in the cells of mouse macrophage cell line RAW264.7 after treatment with RANKL, and CCN2 synergistically promotes RANKL-induced osteoclast differentiation by interacting with dendritic cell-specific transmembrane protein (DC-STAMP) on the surface of osteoclast-like cells (Nishida, et al., 2011). Therefore, it has been hypothesized that CCN2 may facilitate cell-to-cell signaling by interacting with multiple molecules on the surface of these cells through integrin (Gao R & Brigstock DR, 2004; Hoshijima, et al., 2006), proteoglycans (Nishida, et al., 2003), and growth factors (Inoki I, et al., 2002).

3.5 Endothelin-1 (ET-1) and CCN2

Endothelin-1 (ET-1) is also a key mediator of osteoblastic bone metastasis, which is characteristic of breast and prostate cancers (Nelson JB, et al., 1995; Yin JJ, et al., 2003). Functional inhibition of ET-1 activity by blocking its receptor, ET_A, significantly decreases bone metastasis in an experimental bone metastasis model involving the osteoblastic breast cancer cell line ZR-75-1 (Guise, et al., 2003; Yin JJ, et al., 2003).

CCN2 is one of the secreted factors downstream of ET-1, as determined from microarray analysis of osteoblasts (Clines GA, et al., 2007). ET-1 activates the CCN2 promoter and induces CCN2 expression in cardiomyocyte cells (Recchia AG, et al., 2009). Furthermore, ET-1 induces CCN2 in an additive fashion with TGF-β through an element distinct from the TGF-β response element (Horstmeyer A, et al., 2005; Shi-Wen X, et al., 2008; Xu SW, et al., 2004).

3.6 Integrins and CCN2

Integrin have been shown to be critical in controlling how tumor cells interact with their microenvironment. The integrin $\alpha_v\beta_3$ is a receptor for osteopontin, fibronectin, and vitronectin, which are extracellular matrix proteins important in the bone matrix (Schneider, et al., 2011); and $\alpha_v\beta_3$ has been identified as one of the CCN2 receptors (C. C. Chen, et al., 2001). Bone metastatic cancer cells have a higher expression of $\alpha_v\beta_3$ than their primary tumor (Liapis, et al., 1996), promoting adherence to the bone matrix (S. Takayama, et al., 2005). The over-expression of $\alpha_v\beta_3$ in the tumor cells not only leads to increased tumor cell adhesion, migration, and invasion to bone, but also increases osteoclast recruitment at the tumor and bone interface (Pecheur, et al., 2002; Sloan, et al., 2006). Whereas, $\alpha_5\beta_1$, another signaling receptor mediating CCN2 action, plays a necessary role in the binding of prostate cancer tumor cells to the bone stroma (Van der

Velde-Zimmermann, et al., 1997), and in skeletal metastasis of breast cancer cells (Korah, et al., 2004).

Bone-invading destructive tumor cells enhance osteoclast function and recruitment. $\alpha_v\beta_3$ is the predominant integrin found on osteoclasts, and is responsible for mediating osteoclast-bone recognition (Crippes, et al., 1996; Liapis, et al., 1996; Ross, et al., 1993; Zambonin Zallone, et al., 1989) and subsequent attachment to the bone matrix (Chellaiah, 2006; Ross, et al., 1993). This signaling creates the characteristic resorptive ruffled membrane, as well as regulates OC spreading and the overall organization of the cytoskeleton (Faccio, et al., 2003; McHugh, et al., 2000).

3.7 Wnt signaling and CCN2

The Wnt signaling pathways are initiated by a combination of ligands and receptors formed from among 19 secreted Wnt ligands, 10 Frizzled receptors, with the involvement of the co-receptor LRP5/6, which is lipoprotein receptor-related protein 5/6. These ligand-receptor interactions then lead to the activation of multiple intermediate Wnt effectors including β-catenin, c-Jun-NH_2-kinase, and calcium-channel regulators. The accumulation of β-catenin in the cytoplasm and its translocation to the nucleus represent the hallmark of the activated canonical Wnt pathway. In the nucleus, β-catenin forms a complex with lymphocyte enhancer factor/T-cell factor family of transcription factors to activate many oncogenes, such as c-Myc, cyclin D1, metalloproteinases, c-Met, etc (Fuerer, et al., 2008; Rubin, et al., 2010).

The Wnt/β-catenin signaling pathway is an important target for eliminating cancer stem cell in head and neck squamous cell carcinomas (Song, et al., 2010). The importance of paracrine Wnt signaling in bone metastasis was first revealed in multiple myeloma (Tian, et al., 2003), a plasma cell leukemia that causes severe osteolytic bone disease. The results revealed that one of the tumor-secreted factors responsible for the enhanced osteolysis is the Wnt-inhibitor DKK-1 (Tian, et al., 2003). In prostate cancer cells, high DKK-1 expression is correlated with osteolytic disease, consistent with the findings in multiple myeloma; whereas low DKK-1 expression is associated with osteosclerotic bone metastases (Schwaninger, et al., 2007). Functional inhibition of Wnt singling by DKK-1 over-expression in prostate cancer cells favors the formation of osteolytic bone metastases (Hall, et al., 2005).

Si et al. (Si, et al., 2006) observed a significant up-regulation of CCN2 gene expression in mesenchymal stem cells that had been stimulated by Wnt3A. Osteoblasts and stromal cells of transgenic mice that over-express CCN2 display reduced Wnt-β-catenin signaling (Smerdel-Ramoya, et al., 2008). Over-expression of CCN2 in esophageal squamous carcinoma cells results in the accumulation and nuclear translocation of β-catenin leading to activation of TCF-LEF signaling and up-regulation of c-myc and cyclin D1 (Deng, et al., 2007).

4. Role of CCN2 in tumor/bone microenvironment

In the bone marrow microenvironment affected by a tumor, substantial bone marrow angiogenesis is present compared with that in healthy persons (Chavez-Macgregor, et al., 2005). CCN2, the best-characterized factor in its family is known to promote the proliferation

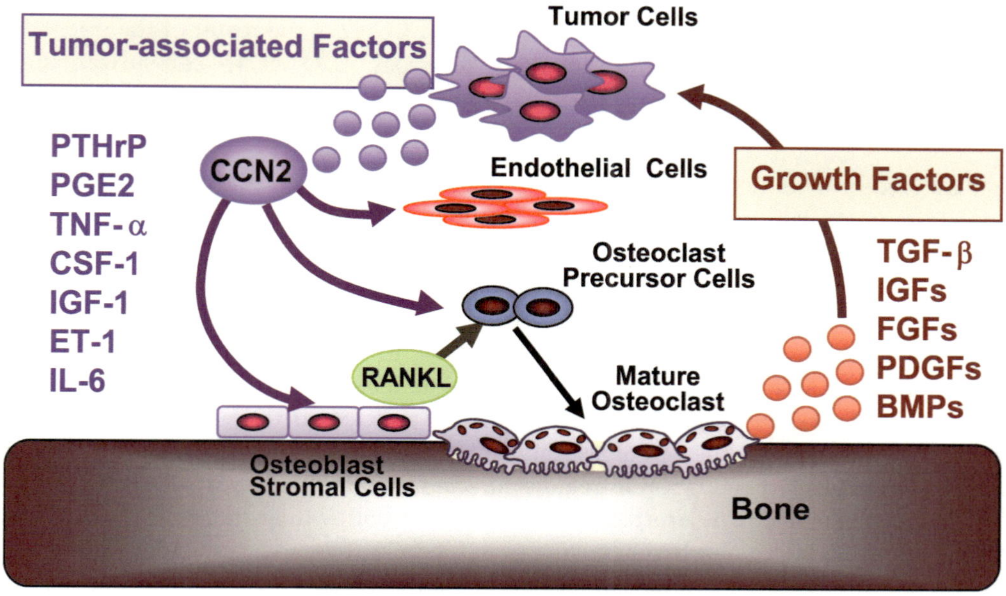

Fig. 3. Role of CCN2 in tumor-induced bone destruction. The cross-talk between tumor cells and osteoclasts is not direct, but involves molecular and cellular intermediates; e.g., tumor cells secrete parathyroid-hormone-related peptide (PTHrP), which is the primary stimulator of osteoblast production of RANKL (Roodman GD, 2004). PTHrP induces CCN2 in tumor cells (Shimo T, et al., 2008); on the other hand, PTHrP both up-regulates the production of RANKL and down-regulates OPG production by osteoblasts, thereby stimulating osteoclastogenesis (Horwood NJ, et al., 1998). Other factors produced and secreted by tumor cells (TNF-α, TGF-β, macrophage colony-stimulating factor (M-CSF), IL-6, and prostaglandin E2) also increase the expression of RANKL. The increased expression of RANKL in the tumor environment leads to increased formation, activation, and survival of osteoclasts, which cells cooperate with these tumor-induced growth factors (CCN2, TNF-α, TGF-β, and M-CSF), resulting in osteolytic lesions. Osteolysis then leads to the release of growth factors derived from bone, including transforming growth factor-β (TGF-β), insulin-like growth factors (IGFs), fibroblast growth factors (FGFs), platelet-derived growth factor (PDGF), and bone morphogenetic proteins (BMPs). These factors increase the production of PTHrP and CCN2 or promote tumor growth directly and cause neovascularization. Bone destruction increases local extracellular calcium (Ca^{2+}) concentrations, which have also been shown to promote tumor growth and the production of PTHrP (Roodman GD, 2004). Thus, tumor cell proliferation and production of tumor-associated factors through the signaling of positive-feedback pathways is promoted, thus giving rise to a "vicious cycle." The Scheme was modified from (Shimo T, et al., 2011).

and differentiation of not only vascular endothelial cells but also fibroblasts and osteoblasts (C. C. Chen, et al., 2001; Nishida T, et al., 2000; Shimo T, et al., 1998; Shimo T, et al., 1999). CCN2 protein is able to interact with multiple molecules in the bone microenvironment, which interaction results in the modulation of the extracellular molecular network therein. The angiogenic effect of CCN2 is the result of the interaction of it with adhesion molecules (Gao R & Brigstock DR, 2004), cell-surface signal transducing receptors (Wahab, et al., 2005), proteoglycans (Nishida, et al., 2003), and growth factors (Inoki I, et al., 2002).

Bone-derived growth factors, such as TGF-β, FGFs, PDGFs, BMPs, and IGF-1, are activated and released into the bone microenvironment. Elevated TGF-β does not appear to affect tumor growth, but rather leads to the production of PTHrP (Guise TA, 2000) and CCN2 (Kang Y, et al., 2003; Shimo T, et al., 2006) in cancer cells, thus establishing a continuously destructive cycle termed the "vicious cycle" through up-regulation of RANKL and accelerated bone resorption. Of note, CCN2 is known to interact with these growth factors (Abreu JG, et al., 2002; Inoki I, et al., 2002) or regulate the gene expression of some of them (Shimo T, et al., 2001b). As a result, CCN2 may be anticipated to modulate the effects of these growth factors on the osteoblast-induced RANKL and OPG expression, osteoclast formation or osteoclast activation in regions affected by bone metastasis (Fig. 3). The other critical function of CCN2 is exerted by its interaction with extracellular matrix molecules and cell-adhesion molecules. By interacting with integrins, functions and other proteins and proteoglycans, CCN2 may promote adhesion and migration of osteoclast precursor cells and stimulate osteoclast formation and activation (Shimo T, et al., 2008). CCN2 not only promotes the expression of DC-STAMP, which plays an important role in cell-cell fusion, but also interacts with this molecule to promote osteoclast differentiation (Nishida, et al., 2011). CCN2 may thus be an integrator/modulator of extracellular information and appears to allow the establishment and progression of tumor angiogenesis and bone destruction within the skeleton (Kubota S & Takigawa M, 2007a; Sasaki A, et al., 1998; Sasaki A, et al., 2003).

5. Conclusions

The initiation of osteoclastogenesis and angiogenesis is the most fundamental step leading to tumor-induced bone destruction. From a clinical point of view, osteoclast formation and angiogenesis would be the major targets of therapeutic drugs for tumor bone metastasis. The major modulator of these processes, referring to osteoclast formation and angiogenesis has been shown to be the CCN2 molecule, which is thus now regarded as a potential target of anti-osteoclastogenic and angiogenic therapy (Aikawa, et al., 2006; Shimo T, et al., 2006). These findings strongly suggest that CCN2 may be a suitable molecular target for therapy of advanced oral squamous cell carcinoma.

6. Acknowledgements

This work was partly supported by grants from the programs Grants-in-Aid for Young Scientists (A) (to T. S.), and Scientific Research (B) (to A. S.) from the Ministry of Education, Culture, Sports, Science, and Technology of Japan.

7. References

Abreu, J. G., Ketpura, N. I., Reversade, B. & De Robertis, E. M. (2002) Connective-tissue growth factor (CTGF) modulates cell signalling by BMP and TGF-beta. *Nat Cell Biol*, 4, 8, 599-604

Aikawa, T., Gunn, J., Spong, S. M., Klaus, S. J. & Korc, M. (2006) Connective tissue growth factor-specific antibody attenuates tumor growth, metastasis, and angiogenesis in an orthotopic mouse model of pancreatic cancer. *Mol Cancer Ther*, 5, 5, 1108-1116

Babic, A. M., Kireeva, M. L., Kolesnikova, T. V. & Lau, L. F. (1998) CYR61, a product of a growth factor-inducible immediate early gene, promotes angiogenesis and tumor growth. *Proc Natl Acad Sci U S A*, 95, 11, 6355-6360

Babic, A. M., Chen, C. C. & Lau, L. F. (1999) Fisp12/mouse connective tissue growth factor mediates endothelial cell adhesion and migration through integrin alphavbeta3, promotes endothelial cell survival, and induces angiogenesis in vivo. *Mol Cell Biol*, 19, 4, 2958-2966

Bonewald, L. F. & Mundy, G. R. (1990) Role of transforming growth factor-beta in bone remodeling. *Clin Orthop Relat Res*, 250, 261-276

Bork, P. (1993) The modular architecture of a new family of growth regulators related to connective tissue growth factor. *FEBS Lett*, 327, 2, 125-130

Boyle, W. J., Simonet, W. S. & Lacey, D. L. (2003) Osteoclast differentiation and activation. *Nature*, 423, 6937, 337-342

Bradham, D. M., Igarashi, A., Potter, R. L. & Grotendorst, G. R. (1991) Connective tissue growth factor: a cysteine-rich mitogen secreted by human vascular endothelial cells is related to the SRC-induced immediate early gene product CEF-10. *J Cell Biol*, 114, 6, 1285-1294

Brady, G., Crean, S. J., Naik, P. & Kapas, S. (2007) Upregulation of IGF-2 and IGF-1 receptor expression in oral cancer cell lines. *Int J Oncol*, 31, 4, 875-881

Brown, J. S., Lowe, D., Kalavrezos, N., D'Souza, J., Magennis, P. & Woolgar, J. (2002) Patterns of invasion and routes of tumor entry into the mandible by oral squamous cell carcinoma. *Head Neck*, 24, 4, 370-383

Burtis, W. J., Brady, T. G., Orloff, J. J., Ersbak, J. B., Warrell, R. P., Jr., Olson, B. R., Wu, T. L., Mitnick, M. E., Broadus, A. E. & Stewart, A. F. (1990) Immunochemical characterization of circulating parathyroid hormone-related protein in patients with humoral hypercalcemia of cancer. *N Engl J Med*, 322, 16, 1106-1112

Cawthorn, T. R., Amir, E., Broom, R., Freedman, O., Gianfelice, D., Barth, D., Wang, D., Holen, I., Done, S. J. & Clemons, M. (2009) Mechanisms and pathways of bone metastasis: challenges and pitfalls of performing molecular research on patient samples. *Clin Exp Metastasis*, 26, 8, 935-943

Chavez-Macgregor, M., Aviles-Salas, A., Green, D., Fuentes-Alburo, A., Gomez-Ruiz, C. & Aguayo, A. (2005) Angiogenesis in the bone marrow of patients with breast cancer. *Clin Cancer Res*, 11, 15, 5396-5400

Chellaiah, M. A. (2006) Regulation of podosomes by integrin alphavbeta3 and Rho GTPase-facilitated phosphoinositide signaling. *Eur J Cell Biol*, 85, 3-4, 311-317

Chen, C. C., Chen, N. & Lau, L. F. (2001) The angiogenic factors Cyr61 and connective tissue growth factor induce adhesive signaling in primary human skin fibroblasts. *J Biol Chem*, 276, 13, 10443-10452

Chen, P. S., Wang, M. Y., Wu, S. N., Su, J. L., Hong, C. C., Chuang, S. E., Chen, M. W., Hua, K. T., Wu, Y. L., Cha, S. T., Babu, M. S., Chen, C. N., Lee, P. H., Chang, K. J. & Kuo, M. L. (2007) CTGF enhances the motility of breast cancer cells via an integrin-alphavbeta3-ERK1/2-dependent S100A4-upregulated pathway. *J Cell Sci,* 120, Pt 12, 2053-2065

Chen, Y., Abraham, D. J., Shi-Wen, X., Pearson, J. D., Black, C. M., Lyons, K. M. & Leask, A. (2004) CCN2 (connective tissue growth factor) promotes fibroblast adhesion to fibronectin. *Mol Biol Cell,* 15, 12, 5635-5646

Chen, Y., Blom, I. E., Sa, S., Goldschmeding, R., Abraham, D. J. & Leask, A. (2002) CTGF expression in mesangial cells: involvement of SMADs, MAP kinase, and PKC. *Kidney Int,* 62, 4, 1149-1159

Clines, G. A., Mohammad, K. S., Bao, Y., Stephens, O. W., Suva, L. J., Shaughnessy, J. D. Jr., Fox, J. W., Chirgwin, J. M. & Guise, T. A. (2007) Dickkopf homolog 1 mediates endothelin-1-stimulated new bone formation. *Mol Endocrinol,* 21, 2, 486-498

Crippes, B. A., Engleman, V. W., Settle, S. L., Delarco, J., Ornberg, R. L., Helfrich, M. H., Horton, M. A. & Nickols, G. A. (1996) Antibody to beta3 integrin inhibits osteoclast-mediated bone resorption in the thyroparathyroidectomized rat. *Endocrinology,* 137, 3, 918-924

Dean, R. A., Butler, G. S., Hamma-Kourbali, Y., Delbe, J., Brigstock, D. R., Courty, J. & Overall, C. M. (2007) Identification of candidate angiogenic inhibitors processed by matrix metalloproteinase 2 (MMP-2) in cell-based proteomic screens: disruption of vascular endothelial growth factor (VEGF)/heparin affin regulatory peptide (pleiotrophin) and VEGF/Connective tissue growth factor angiogenic inhibitory complexes by MMP-2 proteolysis. *Mol Cell Biol,* 27, 24, 8454-8465

Deng, Y. Z., Chen, P. P., Wang, Y., Yin, D., Koeffler, H. P., Li, B., Tong, X. J. & Xie, D. (2007) Connective tissue growth factor is overexpressed in esophageal squamous cell carcinoma and promotes tumorigenicity through beta-catenin-T-cell factor/Lef signaling. *J Biol Chem,* 282, 50, 36571-36581

Faccio, R., Takeshita, S., Zallone, A., Ross, F. P. & Teitelbaum, S. L. (2003) c-Fms and the alphavbeta3 integrin collaborate during osteoclast differentiation. *J Clin Invest,* 111, 5, 749-758

Flint, D. J., Tonner, E., Beattie, J. & Allan, G. J. (2008) Role of insulin-like growth factor binding proteins in mammary gland development. *J Mammary Gland Biol Neoplasia,* 13, 4, 443-453

Fuerer, C., Nusse, R. & Ten Berge, D. (2008) Wnt signalling in development and disease. Max Delbruck Center for Molecular Medicine meeting on Wnt signaling in Development and Disease. *EMBO Rep,* 9, 2, 134-138

Gao, R. & Brigstock, D. R. (2003) Low density lipoprotein receptor-related protein (LRP) is a heparin-dependent adhesion receptor for connective tissue growth factor (CTGF) in rat activated hepatic stellate cells. *Hepatol Res,* 27, 3, 214-220

Gao, R. & Brigstock, D. R. (2004) Connective tissue growth factor (CCN2) induces adhesion of rat activated hepatic stellate cells by binding of its C-terminal domain to integrin alpha(v)beta(3) and heparan sulfate proteoglycan. *J Biol Chem,* 279, 10, 8848-8855

Ge, R., Rajeev, V., Ray, P., Lattime, E., Rittling, S., Medicherla, S., Protter, A., Murphy, A., Chakravarty, J., Dugar, S., Schreiner, G., Barnard, N. & Reiss, M. (2006) Inhibition of growth and metastasis of mouse mammary carcinoma by selective inhibitor of transforming growth factor-beta type I receptor kinase in vivo. *Clin Cancer Res,* 12, 14 Pt 1, 4315-4330

Goda, T., Shimo, T., Yoshihama, Y., Hassan, N. M., Ibaragi, S., Kurio, N., Okui, T., Honami, T., Kishimoto, K. & Sasaki, A. (2010) Bone destruction by invading oral squamous carcinoma cells mediated by the transforming growth factor-beta signalling pathway. *Anticancer Res,* 30, 7, 2615-2623

Grzeszkiewicz, T. M., Kirschling, D. J., Chen, N. & Lau, L. F. (2001) CYR61 stimulates human skin fibroblast migration through Integrin alpha vbeta 5 and enhances mitogenesis through integrin alpha vbeta 3, independent of its carboxyl-terminal domain. *J Biol Chem,* 276, 24, 21943-21950

Guise, T. A., Yin, J. J. & Mohammad, K. S. (2003) Role of endothelin-1 in osteoblastic bone metastases. *Cancer,* 97, 3 Suppl, 779-784

Guise, T. A., Yin, J. J., Taylor, S. D., Kumagai, Y., Dallas, M., Boyce, B. F., Yoneda, T. & Mundy, G. R. (1996) Evidence for a causal role of parathyroid hormone-related protein in the pathogenesis of human breast cancer-mediated osteolysis. *J Clin Invest,* 98, 7, 1544-1549

Guise, T. A. (2000) Molecular mechanisms of osteolytic bone metastases. *Cancer,* 88, 12 Suppl, 2892-2898

Hall, C. L., Bafico, A., Dai, J., Aaronson, S. A. & Keller, E. T. (2005) Prostate cancer cells promote osteoblastic bone metastases through Wnts. *Cancer Res,* 65, 17, 7554-7560

Hauschka, P. V., Mavrakos, A. E., Iafrati, M. D., Doleman, S. E. & Klagsbrun, M. (1986) Growth factors in bone matrix. Isolation of multiple types by affinity chromatography on heparin-Sepharose. *J Biol Chem,* 261, 27, 12665-12674

Hicks, W. L., Jr., Loree, T. R., Garcia, R. I., Maamoun, S., Marshall, D., Orner, J. B., Bakamjian, V. Y. & Shedd, D. P. (1997) Squamous cell carcinoma of the floor of mouth: a 20-year review. *Head Neck,* 19, 5, 400-405

Horstmeyer, A., Licht, C., Scherr, G., Eckes, B. & Krieg, T. (2005) Signalling and regulation of collagen I synthesis by ET-1 and TGF-beta1. *FEBS J,* 272, 24, 6297-6309

Horwood, N. J, Elliott, J., Martin, T. J. & Gillespie, M. T. (1998) Osteotropic agents regulate the expression of osteoclast differentiation factor and osteoprotegerin in osteoblastic stromal cells. *Endocrinology,* 139, 11, 4743-4746

Hoshijima, M., Hattori, T., Inoue, M., Araki, D., Hanagata, H., Miyauchi, A. & Takigawa, M. (2006) CT domain of CCN2/CTGF directly interacts with fibronectin and enhances cell adhesion of chondrocytes through integrin alpha5beta1. *FEBS Lett,* 580, 5, 1376-1382

Hsu, H., Lacey, D. L., Dunstan, C. R., Solovyev, I., Colombero, A., Timms, E., Tan, H. L., Elliott, G., Kelley, M. J., Sarosi, I., Wang, L., Xia, X. Z., Elliott, R., Chiu, L., Black, T., Scully, S., Capparelli, C., Morony, S., Shimamoto, G., Bass, M. B. & Boyle, W. J. (1999) Tumor necrosis factor receptor family member RANK mediates osteoclast differentiation and activation induced by osteoprotegerin ligand. *Proc Natl Acad Sci U S A,* 96, 7, 3540-3545

Hwa, V., Oh, Y. & Rosenfeld, R. G. (1999) The insulin-like growth factor-binding protein (IGFBP) superfamily. *Endocr Rev,* 20, 6, 761-787

Inoki, I., Shiomi, T., Hashimoto, G., Enomoto, H., Nakamura, H., Makino, K., Ikeda, E., Takata, S., Kobayashi, K. & Okada, Y. (2002) Connective tissue growth factor binds vascular endothelial growth factor (VEGF) and inhibits VEGF-induced angiogenesis. *FASEB J,* 16, 2, 219-221

Ivkovic, S., Yoon, B. S., Popoff, S. N., Safadi, F. F., Libuda, D. E., Stephenson, R. C., Daluiski, A. & Lyons, K. M. (2003) Connective tissue growth factor coordinates chondrogenesis and angiogenesis during skeletal development. *Development,* 130, 12, 2779-2791

Kang, Y., Siegel, P. M., Shu, W., Drobnjak, M., Kakonen, S. M., Cordón-Cardo, C., Guise, T. A. & Massagué, J. (2003) A multigenic program mediating breast cancer metastasis to bone. *Cancer Cell,* 3, 6, 537-549

Karsdal, M. A., Fjording, M. S, Foged, N. T, Delaissé, J. M & Lochter, A. (2001) Transforming growth factor-beta-induced osteoblast elongation regulates osteoclastic bone resorption through a p38 mitogen-activated protein kinase- and matrix metalloproteinase-dependent pathway. *J Biol Chem,* 276, 42, 39350-39358

Katsube, K., Sakamoto, K., Tamamura, Y. & Yamaguchi, A. (2009) Role of CCN, a vertebrate specific gene family, in development. *Dev Growth Differ,* 51, 1, 55-67

Kayamori, K., Sakamoto, K., Nakashima, T., Takayanagi, H., Morita, K., Omura, K., Nguyen, S. T., Miki, Y., Iimura, T., Himeno, A., Akashi, T., Yamada-Okabe, H., Ogata, E. & Yamaguchi, A. (2010) Roles of interleukin-6 and parathyroid hormone-related peptide in osteoclast formation associated with oral cancers: significance of interleukin-6 synthesized by stromal cells in response to cancer cells. *Am J Pathol,* 176, 2, 968-980

Kimura, T., Kuwata, T., Ashimine, S., Yamazaki, M., Yamauchi, C., Nagai, K., Ikehara, A., Feng, Y., Dimitrov, D. S., Saito, S. & Ochiai, A. (2010) Targeting of bone-derived insulin-like growth factor-II by a human neutralizing antibody suppresses the growth of prostate cancer cells in a human bone environment. *Clin Cancer Res,* 16, 1, 121-129

Kireeva, M. L., Mo, F. E., Yang, G. P. & Lau, L. F. (1996) Cyr61, a product of a growth factor-inducible immediate-early gene, promotes cell proliferation, migration, and adhesion. *Mol Cell Biol,* 16, 4, 1326-1334

Kondo, S., Kubota, S., Shimo, T., Nishida, T., Yosimichi, G., Eguchi, T., Sugahara, T. & Takigawa, M. (2002) Connective tissue growth factor increased by hypoxia may initiate angiogenesis in collaboration with matrix metalloproteinases. *Carcinogenesis,* 23, 5, 769-776

Kondo, Y., Irie, K., Ikegame, M., Ejiri, S., Hanada, K. & Ozawa, H. (2001) Role of stromal cells in osteoclast differentiation in bone marrow. *J Bone Miner Metab,* 19, 6, 352-358

Kong, Y. Y., Yoshida, H., Sarosi, I., Tan, H. L., Timms, E., Capparelli, C., Morony, S., Oliveira-dos-Santos, A. J., Van, G., Itie, A., Khoo, W., Wakeham, A., Dunstan, C. R., Lacey, D. L., Mak, T. W., Boyle, W. J. & Penninger, J. M. (1999) OPGL is a key regulator of osteoclastogenesis, lymphocyte development and lymph-node organogenesis. *Nature,* 397, 6717, 315-323

Korah, R., Boots, M. & Wieder, R. (2004) Integrin alpha5beta1 promotes survival of growth-arrested breast cancer cells: an in vitro paradigm for breast cancer dormancy in bone marrow. *Cancer Res,* 64, 13, 4514-4522

Kubo, M., Kikuchi, K., Nashiro, K., Kakinuma, T., Hayashi, N., Nanko, H. & Tamaki, K. (1998) Expression of fibrogenic cytokines in desmoplastic malignant melanoma. *Br J Dermatol,* 139, 2, 192-197

Kubota, S. & Takigawa, M. (2007a) CCN family proteins and angiogenesis: from embryo to adulthood. *Angiogenesis,* 10, 1, 1-11

Kubota, S. & Takigawa, M. (2007b) Role of CCN2/CTGF/Hcs24 in bone growth. *Int Rev Cytol,* 257, 1-41

Lacey, D. L., Timms, E., Tan, H. L., Kelley, M. J., Dunstan, C. R., Burgess, T., Elliott, R., Colombero, A., Elliott, G., Scully, S., Hsu, H., Sullivan, J., Hawkins, N., Davy, E., Capparelli, C., Eli, A., Qian, Y. X., Kaufman, S., Sarosi, I., Shalhoub, V., Senaldi, G., Guo, J., Delaney, J. & Boyle, W. J. (1998) Osteoprotegerin ligand is a cytokine that regulates osteoclast differentiation and activation. *Cell,* 93, 2, 165-176

Lau, L. F. & Lam, S. C. (1999) The CCN family of angiogenic regulators: the integrin connection. *Exp Cell Res,* 248, 1, 44-57

Leask, A., Abraham, D. J., Finlay, D. R., Holmes, A., Pennington, D., Shi-Wen, X., Chen, Y., Venstrom, K., Dou, X., Ponticos, M., Black, C., Bernabeu, C., Jackman, J. K., Findell, P. R. & Connolly, M. K. (2002) Dysregulation of transforming growth factor beta signaling in scleroderma: overexpression of endoglin in cutaneous scleroderma fibroblasts. *Arthritis Rheum,* 46, 7, 1857-1865

Lee, S. K. & Lorenzo, J. A. (1999) Parathyroid hormone stimulates TRANCE and inhibits osteoprotegerin messenger ribonucleic acid expression in murine bone marrow cultures: correlation with osteoclast-like cell formation. *Endocrinology,* 140, 8, 3552-3561

Leu, S. J., Lam, S. C. & Lau, L. F. (2002) Pro-angiogenic activities of CYR61 (CCN1) mediated through integrins alphavbeta3 and alpha6beta1 in human umbilical vein endothelial cells. *J Biol Chem,* 277, 48, 46248-46255

Liapis, H., Flath, A. & Kitazawa, S. (1996) Integrin alpha V beta 3 expression by bone-residing breast cancer metastases. *Diagn Mol Pathol,* 5, 2, 127-135

Lin, C. G., Leu, S. J., Chen, N., Tebeau, C. M., Lin, S. X., Yeung, C. Y. & Lau, L. F. (2003) CCN3 (NOV) is a novel angiogenic regulator of the CCN protein family. *J Biol Chem,* 278, 26, 24200-24208

Massague, J., Blain, S. W. & Lo, R. S. (2000) TGFbeta signaling in growth control, cancer, and heritable disorders. *Cell,* 103, 2, 295-309

McHugh, K. P., Hodivala-Dilke, K., Zheng, M. H., Namba, N., Lam, J., Novack, D., Feng, X., Ross, F. P., Hynes, R. O. & Teitelbaum, S. L. (2000) Mice lacking beta3 integrins are osteosclerotic because of dysfunctional osteoclasts. *J Clin Invest,* 105, 4, 433-440

Minn, A. J., Kang, Y., Serganova, I., Gupta, G. P., Giri, D. D., Doubrovin, M., Ponomarev, V., Gerald, W. L., Blasberg, R. & Massagué, J. (2005) Distinct organ-specific metastatic potential of individual breast cancer cells and primary tumors. *J Clin Invest,* 115, 1, 44-55

Nagaraj, N. S. & Datta, P. K. (2010) Targeting the transforming growth factor-beta signaling pathway in human cancer. *Expert Opin Investig Drugs,* 19, 1, 77-91

Nakagawa, N., Kinosaki, M., Yamaguchi, K., Shima, N., Yasuda, H., Yano, K., Morinaga, T. & Higashio, K. (1998) RANK is the essential signaling receptor for osteoclast differentiation factor in osteoclastogenesis. *Biochem Biophys Res Commun,* 253, 2, 395-400

Nakanishi, T., Nishida, T., Shimo, T., Kobayashi, K., Kubo, T., Tamatani, T., Tezuka, K. & Takigawa, M. (2000) Effects of CTGF/Hcs24, a product of a hypertrophic chondrocyte-specific gene, on the proliferation and differentiation of chondrocytes in culture. *Endocrinology,* 141, 1, 264-273

Nelson, J. B., Hedican, S. P., George, D. J., Reddi, A. H., Piantadosi, S., Eisenberger, M. A. & Simons, J. W. (1995) Identification of endothelin-1 in the pathophysiology of metastatic adenocarcinoma of the prostate. *Nat Med,* 1, 9, 944-949

Nishida, T., Kubota, S., Fukunaga, T., Kondo, S., Yosimichi, G., Nakanishi, T., Takano-Yamamoto, T. & Takigawa, M. (2003) CTGF/Hcs24, hypertrophic chondrocyte-specific gene product, interacts with perlecan in regulating the proliferation and differentiation of chondrocytes. *J Cell Physiol,* 196, 2, 265-275

Nishida, T., Emura, K., Kubota, S., Lyons, K. M. & Takigawa, M. (2011) CCN family 2/connective tissue growth factor (CCN2/CTGF) promotes osteoclastogenesis via induction of and interaction with dendritic cell-specific transmembrane protein (DC-STAMP). *J Bone Miner Res,* 26, 2, 351-363

Nishida, T., Nakanishi, T., Asano, M., Shimo, T. & Takigawa, M. (2000) Effects of CTGF/Hcs24, a hypertrophic chondrocyte-specific gene product, on the proliferation and differentiation of osteoblastic cells in vitro. *J Cell Physiol,* 184, 2, 197-206

Pecheur, I., Peyruchaud, O., Serre, C. M., Guglielmi, J., Voland, C., Bourre, F., Margue, C., Cohen-Solal, M., Buffet, A., Kieffer, N. & Clezardin, P. (2002) Integrin alpha(v)beta3 expression confers on tumor cells a greater propensity to metastasize to bone. *FASEB J,* 16, 10, 1266-1268

Pell, J. M., Salih, D. A., Cobb, L. J., Tripathi, G. & Drozd, A. (2005) The role of insulin-like growth factor binding proteins in development. *Rev Endocr Metab Disord,* 6, 3, 189-198

Perbal, B. (2004) CCN proteins: multifunctional signalling regulators. *Lancet,* 363, 9402, 62-64

Perbal, B. & Takigawa, M. (2005) CCN Proteins a New Family of Cell Growthad Differentiation Regulators. *Imperial College Press, London,*

Petersen, M., Pardali, E., van der Horst, G., Cheung, H., van den Hoogen, C., van der Pluijm, G. & Ten Dijke, P. (2010) Smad2 and Smad3 have opposing roles in breast cancer bone metastasis by differentially affecting tumor angiogenesis. *Oncogene,* 29, 9, 1351-1361

Recchia, A. G., Filice, E., Pellegrino, D., Dobrina, A., Cerra, M. C. & Maggiolini, M. (2009) Endothelin-1 induces connective tissue growth factor expression in cardiomyocytes. *J Mol Cell Cardiol,* 46, 3, 352-359

Roodman, G. D. (2004) Mechanisms of bone metastasis. *N Engl J Med,* 350, 16, 1655-1664

Roodman, G. D. & Dougall, W. C. (2008) RANK ligand as a therapeutic target for bone metastases and multiple myeloma. *Cancer Treat Rev,* 34, 1, 92-101

Ross, F. P., Chappel, J., Alvarez, J. I., Sander, D., Butler, W. T., Farach-Carson, M. C., Mintz, K. A., Robey, P. G., Teitelbaum, S. L. & Cheresh, D. A. (1993) Interactions between the bone matrix proteins osteopontin and bone sialoprotein and the osteoclast integrin alpha v beta 3 potentiate bone resorption. *J Biol Chem,* 268, 13, 9901-9907

Rubin, E. M., Guo, Y., Tu, K., Xie, J., Zi, X. & Hoang, B. H. (2010) Wnt inhibitory factor 1 decreases tumorigenesis and metastasis in osteosarcoma. *Mol Cancer Ther,* 9, 3, 731-741

Sasaki, A., Alcalde, R. E., Nishiyama, A., Lim, D. D., Mese, H., Akedo, H. & Matsumura, T. (1998) Angiogenesis inhibitor TNP-470 inhibits human breast cancer osteolytic bone metastasis in nude mice through the reduction of bone resorption. *Cancer Res,* 58, 3, 462-467

Sasaki, A., Yoshioka, N. & Shimo, T. (2003) Angiogenetic factor. *THE BONE,* 17, 2, 51-55 (In Japanese)

Saxena, N. K., Taliaferro-Smith, L., Knight, B. B., Merlin, D., Anania, F. A., O'Regan, R. M. & Sharma, D. (2008) Bidirectional crosstalk between leptin and insulin-like growth factor-I signaling promotes invasion and migration of breast cancer cells via transactivation of epidermal growth factor receptor. *Cancer Res,* 68, 23, 9712-9722

Schneider, J. G., Amend, S. R. & Weilbaecher, K. N. (2011) Integrins and bone metastasis: integrating tumor cell and stromal cell interactions. *Bone,* 48, 1, 54-65

Schwaninger, R., Rentsch, C. A., Wetterwald, A., van der Horst, G., van Bezooijen, R. L., van der Pluijm, G., Lowik, C. W., Ackermann, K., Pyerin, W., Hamdy, F. C., Thalmann, G. N. & Cecchini, M. G. (2007) Lack of noggin expression by cancer cells is a determinant of the osteoblast response in bone metastases. *Am J Pathol,* 170, 1, 160-175

Segarini, P. R., Nesbitt, J. E., Li, D., Hays, L. G., Yates, J. R. 3rd. & Carmichael, D. F. (2001) The low density lipoprotein receptor-related protein/alpha2-macroglobulin receptor is a receptor for connective tissue growth factor. *J Biol Chem,* 276, 44, 40659-40667

Shakunaga, T., Ozaki, T., Ohara, N., Asaumi, K., Doi, T., Nishida, K., Kawai, A., Nakanishi, T., Takigawa, M. & Inoue, H. (2000) Expression of connective tissue growth factor in cartilaginous tumors. *Cancer,* 89, 7, 1466-1473

Shaw, R. J., Brown, J. S., Woolgar, J. A., Lowe, D., Rogers, S. N. & Vaughan, E. D. (2004) The influence of the pattern of mandibular invasion on recurrence and survival in oral squamous cell carcinoma. *Head Neck,* 26, 10, 861-869

Shi-Wen, X., Leask, A. & Abraham, D. (2008) Regulation and function of connective tissue growth factor/CCN2 in tissue repair, scarring and fibrosis. *Cytokine Growth Factor Rev,* 19, 2, 133-144

Shibahara, T., Nomura, T., Cui, N. H. & Noma, H. (2005) A study of osteoclast-related cytokines in mandibular invasion by squamous cell carcinoma. *Int J Oral Maxillofac Surg,* 34, 7, 789-793

Shimo, T., Nakanishi, T., Kimura, Y., Nishida, T., Ishizeki, K., Matsumura, T. & Takigawa, M. (1998) Inhibition of endogenous expression of connective tissue growth factor by its antisense oligonucleotide and antisense RNA suppresses proliferation and migration of vascular endothelial cells. *J Biochem,* 124, 1, 130-140

Shimo, T., Nakanishi, T., Nishida, T., Asano, M., Kanyama, M., Kuboki, T., Tamatani, T., Tezuka, K., Takemura, M., Matsumura, T. & Takigawa, M. (1999) Connective tissue growth factor induces the proliferation, migration, and tube formation of vascular endothelial cells in vitro, and angiogenesis in vivo. *J Biochem,* 126, 1, 137-145

Shimo, T., Kubota, S., Kondo, S., Nakanishi, T., Sasaki, A., Mese, H., Matsumura, T. & Takigawa, M. (2001a) Connective tissue growth factor as a major angiogenic agent that is induced by hypoxia in a human breast cancer cell line. *Cancer Lett,* 174, 1, 57-64

Shimo, T., Nakanishi, T., Nishida, T., Asano, M., Sasaki, A., Kanyama, M., Kuboki, T., Matsumura, T. & Takigawa, M. (2001b) Involvement of CTGF, a hypertrophic chondrocyte-specific gene product, in tumor angiogenesis. *Oncology,* 61, 4, 315-322

Shimo, T., Wu, C., Billings, P. C., Piddington, R., Rosenbloom, J., Pacifici, M. & Koyama, E. (2002) Expression, gene regulation, and roles of Fisp12/CTGF in developing tooth germs. *Dev Dyn,* 224, 3, 267-278

Shimo, T., Kanyama, M., Wu, C., Sugito, H., Billings, P. C., Abrams, W. R., Rosenbloom, J., Iwamoto, M., Pacifici, M. & Koyama, E. (2004) Expression and roles of connective tissue growth factor in Meckel's cartilage development. *Dev Dyn,* 231, 1, 136-147

Shimo, T., Koyama, E., Sugito, H., Wu, C., Shimo, S. & Pacifici, M. (2005) Retinoid signaling regulates CTGF expression in hypertrophic chondrocytes with differential involvement of MAP kinases. *J Bone Miner Res,* 20, 5, 867-877

Shimo, T., Kubota, S., Yoshioka, N., Ibaragi, S., Isowa, S., Eguchi, T., Sasaki, A. & Takigawa, M. (2006) Pathogenic role of connective tissue growth factor (CTGF/CCN2) in osteolytic metastasis of breast cancer. *J Bone Miner Res,* 21, 7, 1045-1059

Shimo, T., Kubota, S., Goda, T., Yoshihama, Y., Kurio, N., Nishida, T., Ng, P. S., Endo, K., Takigawa, M. & Sasaki. A. (2008) Clinical significance and pathogenic function of connective tissue growth factor (CTGF/CCN2) in osteolytic mandibular squamous cell carcinoma. *Anticancer Res,* 28, 4C, 2343-2348

Shimo, T. & Sasaki, A. (2011) Mechanism of cancer-induced bone destruction: An association of connective tissue growth factor (CTGF/CCN2) in the bone metastasis. *Japanese Dental Science Review,* 47, 1, 13-22

Shinto, O., Yashiro, M., Kawajiri, H., Shimizu, K., Shimizu, T., Miwa, A. & Hirakawa, K. (2010) Inhibitory effect of a TGFbeta receptor type-I inhibitor, Ki26894, on invasiveness of scirrhous gastric cancer cells. *Br J Cancer,* 102, 844-51,

Si, W., Kang, Q., Luu, H. H., Park, J. K., Luo, Q., Song, W. X., Jiang, W., Luo, X., Li, X., Yin, H., Montag, A. G., Haydon, R. C. & He, T. C. (2006) CCN1/Cyr61 is regulated by the canonical Wnt signal and plays an important role in Wnt3A-induced osteoblast differentiation of mesenchymal stem cells. *Mol Cell Biol,* 26, 8, 2955-2964

Sloan, E. K., Pouliot, N., Stanley, K. L., Chia, J., Moseley, J. M., Hards, D. K. & Anderson, R. L. (2006) Tumor-specific expression of alphavbeta3 integrin promotes spontaneous metastasis of breast cancer to bone. *Breast Cancer Res,* 8, 2, R20

Smerdel-Ramoya, A., Zanotti, S., Stadmeyer, L., Durant, D. & Canalis, E. (2008) Skeletal overexpression of connective tissue growth factor impairs bone formation and causes osteopenia. *Endocrinology,* 149, 9, 4374-4381

Song, J., Chang, I., Chen, Z., Kang, M. & Wang, C. Y. (2010) Characterization of side populations in HNSCC: highly invasive, chemoresistant and abnormal Wnt signaling. *PLoS One,* 5, 7, e11456

Sun, L. (2004) Tumor-suppressive and promoting function of transforming growth factor beta. *Front Biosci,* 9, 1925-1935

Takayama, S., Ishii, S., Ikeda, T., Masamura, S., Doi, M. & Kitajima, M. (2005) The relationship between bone metastasis from human breast cancer and integrin alpha(v)beta3 expression. *Anticancer Res,* 25, 1A, 79-83

Takayama, Y., Mori, T., Nomura, T., Shibahara, T. & Sakamoto, M. (2010) Parathyroid-related protein plays a critical role in bone invasion by oral squamous cell carcinoma. *Int J Oncol,* 36, 6, 1387-1394

Takeshita, S., Kaji, K. & Kudo, A. (2000) Identification and characterization of the new osteoclast progenitor with macrophage phenotypes being able to differentiate into mature osteoclasts. *J Bone Miner Res,* 15, 8, 1477-1488

Takigawa, M., Nakanishi, T., Kubota, S. & Nishida, T. (2003) Role of CTGF/HCS24/ecogenin in skeletal growth control. *J Cell Physiol,* 194, 3, 256-266

Tian, E., Zhan, F., Walker, R., Rasmussen, E., Ma, Y., Barlogie, B. & Shaughnessy, J. D., Jr. (2003) The role of the Wnt-signaling antagonist DKK1 in the development of osteolytic lesions in multiple myeloma. *N Engl J Med,* 349, 26, 2483-2494

Van Beek, J. P., Kennedy, L., Rockel, J. S., Bernier, S. M. & Leask, A. (2006) The induction of CCN2 by TGFbeta1 involves Ets-1. *Arthritis Res Ther,* 8, 2, R36

Van der Velde-Zimmermann, D., Verdaasdonk, M. A., Rademakers, L. H., De Weger, R. A., Van den Tweel, J. G. & Joling, P. (1997) Fibronectin distribution in human bone marrow stroma: matrix assembly and tumor cell adhesion via alpha5 beta1 integrin. *Exp Cell Res,* 230, 1, 111-120

Wahab, N. A., Weston, B. S. & Mason, R. M. (2005) Connective tissue growth factor CCN2 interacts with and activates the tyrosine kinase receptor TrkA. *J Am Soc Nephrol,* 16, 2, 340-351

Wang, M. Y., Chen, P. S., Prakash, E., Hsu, H. C., Huang, H. Y., Lin, M. T., Chang, K. J. & Kuo, M. L. (2009) Connective tissue growth factor confers drug resistance in breast cancer through concomitant up-regulation of Bcl-xL and cIAP1. *Cancer Res,* 69, 8, 3482-3491

Wenger, C., Ellenrieder, V., Alber, B., Lacher, U., Menke, A., Hameister, H., Wilda, M., Iwamura, T., Beger, H. G., Adler, G. & Gress, T. M. (1999) Expression and differential regulation of connective tissue growth factor in pancreatic cancer cells. *Oncogene,* 18, 4, 1073-1080

Xie, D., Nakachi, K., Wang, H., Elashoff, R. & Koeffler, H. P. (2001) Elevated levels of connective tissue growth factor, WISP-1, and CYR61 in primary breast cancers associated with more advanced features. *Cancer Res,* 61, 24, 8917-8923

Xu, S. W., Howat, S. L., Renzoni, E. A., Holmes, A., Pearson, J. D., Dashwood, M. R., Bou-Gharios, G., Denton, C. P., du Bois, R. M., Black, C. M., Leask, A. & Abraham, D. J. (2004) Endothelin-1 induces expression of matrix-associated genes in lung fibroblasts through MEK/ERK. *J Biol Chem,* 279, 22, 23098-23103

Yang, D. H., Kim, H. S., Wilson, E. M., Rosenfeld, R. G. & Oh, Y. (1998 Jul;) Identification of glycosylated 38-kDa connective tissue growth factor (IGFBP-related protein 2) and proteolytic fragments in human biological fluids, and up-regulation of IGFBP-rP2 expression by TGF-beta in Hs578T human breast cancer cells. *J Clin Endocrinol Metab,* 83, 7, 2593-2596

Yin, J. J., Mohammad, K. S., Käkönen, S. M., Harris, S., Wu-Wong, J. R., Wessale, J. L., Padley, R. J., Garrett, I. R., Chirgwin, J. M. & Guise, T. A. (2003) A causal role for endothelin-1 in the pathogenesis of osteoblastic bone metastases. *Proc Natl Acad Sci U S A,* 100, 19, 10954-10959

Zambonin Zallone, A., Teti, A., Gaboli, M. & Marchisio, P. C. (1989) Beta 3 subunit of vitronectin receptor is present in osteoclast adhesion structures and not in other monocyte-macrophage derived cells. *Connect Tissue Res,* 20, 1-4, 143-149

12

Role of Inflammation in Oral Squamous Cell Carcinoma

Kıvanç Bektaş-Kayhan
Istanbul University, Faculty of Dentistry, Department of Oral Surgery and Medicine
Turkey

1. Introduction

The most common malignant oral disease is oral squamous cell carcinoma (OSCC), and most of the time this term is used synonymously with oral cancer (1). Oral cancer is a serious and growing problem in many parts of the world. When grouped together with pharyngeal cancers, it is the sixth most common cancer globally (2). There is a wide geographic variation in the incidence of this cancer. This usually depends on the culture, life style factors and level of country development (1). In the South and Southeast Asia, parts of Western (e.g. France) and Eastern Europe, parts of Latin America and the Caribbean and in the Pacific regions, oral cancer rates are higher than the other parts of the world (3). The major risk factors of the disease are cigarette smoking (4), alcohol abuse (5), and viral infections such as HPV (6). These risk factors are primarily based on life style but do not adequately explain the increasing incidence of this cancer among the young population (7) and non- smoking females (8). In addition, genetic susceptibility may play an important role (9, 10, 11). Epidemiological studies have shown that chronic inflammation is associated with various types of cancer (12). It is estimated that 15–20% of all deaths from cancer worldwide are linked to infections and inflammatory responses (13). In the last two decades most chronic diseases, including cancer, have been associated with dysregulated inflammatory response. The identification of transcript factors such as NF-κB, AP-1 and STAT3 and their gene products such as tumor necrosis factor (TNF), interleukin-1 (IL-1), interleukin-6 (IL-6), chemokines, cyclooxygenase-2 (COX-2), 5 lipooxygenase, matrix metalloproteases (MMP) and vascular endothelial growth factor (VEGF), adhesion molecules and others has provided the molecular basis for the role of inflammation in cancer. These inflammatory pathways are activated by tobacco, stress, dietary agents, obesity, alcohol, infectious agents, irradiation, and environmental stimuli, which, combined, account for as much as 95% of all cancers (14).

2. Inflammation and cancer

2.1 A short overview of inflammation

Inflammation is a crucial, complex host defense against biologic, chemical, physical, and endogenous irritants. The contribution of inflammation to physiological and pathological processes such as wound healing and infection needs to be understood for a better understanding of the role of inflammation in cancer formation. When tissues are injured, a multifactorial network of chemical signals initiates and maintains a host response designed to heal the afflicted tissue. The response includes activation and directed migration of leukocytes (neutrophils, monocytes and eosinophils) from the venous system to sites of damage. Neutrophils are thought to coordinate recruitment of these inflammatory cells to sites of tissue injury and to the provisional extracellular matrix (ECM). This is a four-step mechanism: first come selectins that include adhesion molecules (L- P-, and E-selectin) that facilitate rolling along the vascular endothelium; signals are then generated that activate and upregulate leukocyte integrins mediated by cytokines and leukocyte-activating molecules; neutrophils on the surface of the vascular endothelium are immobilized by means of tight adhesion through α4β1 and α4β7 integrins binding to endothelial vascular cell-adhesion molecule-1 (VCAM-1) and MadCAM-1, respectively; this brings about transmigration through the endothelium to sites of injury and is presumably facilitated by extracellular proteases, such as matrix metalloproteinases (MMPs) (15).

Cellular components

Platelet activation and aggregation, in addition to accelerating coagulation, provide a bolus of secreted proteins and α-granule contents to the immediate area, all of which help initiate and accelerate the inflammatory response by the host. Examples of such secreted proteins include arachidonic acid metabolites, heparin, serotonin, thrombin, coagulation factors (factor V), adhesive proteins (fibrinogen and von Willebrand factor), plasma proteins (immunoglobulin-γ and albumin), cell growth factors (platelet-derived growth factor (PDGF), platelet-derived angiogenesis factor, transforming growth factor-α (TGF-α), TGF-β and basic fibroblast growth factor (bFGF)), enzymes (heparinase and factor XIII) and protease inhibitors (plasminogen activator inhibitor-1, α2-macroglobulin and α2-antiplasmin). Following platelet-induced hemostasis and release of TGF-β1 and PDGF, formation of granulation tissue is facilitated by chemotaxis of neutrophils, monocytes, fibroblasts and myofibroblasts, as well as synthesis of new extracellular matrix (ECM) and neoangiogenesis.

Neutrophils produce cytokines/chemokines required for effector cell recruitment, activation and response (16). These phagocytic cells initiate wound healing by serving as a source of early-response pro-inflammatory cytokines such as tumor necrosis factor-α (TNF-α) (17), and interleukin (IL)-1α and IL-1β (18). These cytokines mediate leukocyte adherence to the vascular endothelium, restricting leukocytes to areas of repair, and initiate repair by inducing expression of matrix metalloproteinases (MMPs) and keratinocyte growth factor (KGF/FGF-7) by fibroblasts (19).

Mononuclear phagocytes migrate from the venous system to the site of tissue injury, in response to tissue injury. Chemotactic factors, including PF-4, TGF-β, PDGF, chemokines (monocyte chemoattractant protein-1, -2 and -3 (MCP-1/CCL2, MCP-2/CCL8 and MCP-3/CCL7), macrophage inflammatory protein-1α and -1β (MIP-1α/CCL3 and MIP-1β/CCL4), and the cytokines IL-1β and TNF-α, guide them to the site. Deployment of monocytes/macrophages to the site of injury causes the number of neutrophils to decline as they are phagocyted by macrophages. Once present, however, they differentiate into mature macrophages or immature dendritic cells. After activation, macrophages are the main source of growth factors and cytokines (TGF-β1, PDGF, bFGF, TGF-α, insulin-like growth factor (IGF)-I and -II, TNF-α and IL-1) that modulate tissue repair. Cells in their local microenvironment (e.g., endothelial, epithelial, mesenchymal or neuroendocrine cells) are profoundly affected by macrophage products (20, 21). Following their activation, mast cells are full of stored and newly synthesized inflammatory mediators. This cell type synthesizes and stores histamine, cytokines and proteases complexed to highly sulphated proteoglycans within granules, as well as producing, lipid mediators and cytokines upon stimulation. Once activated by complement or by the binding of antigens to immunoglobulin E (IgE) bound to high-affinity IgE receptors (FcεRI), mast cells degranulate, releasing mediators including heparin, heparinase, histamine, MMPs and serine proteases, and various polypeptide growth factors, including bFGF and vascular endothelial growth factor. These function both in the early initiation phase of inflammation (e.g. vascular reaction and exudation), and in the late phase where leukocyte accumulation and wound healing takes place (15).

Chemotactic cytokines

Chemokines represent the largest family of cytokines (~41 human members), forming a complex network for the chemotactic activation of all leukocytes. Chemokine receptors, members of the seven-transmembrane-spanning G-protein-coupled receptors, vary by cell type and degree of cell activation (22). There is considerable redundancy in chemokine-receptor interaction, as many ligands bind to different receptors.

The composition of chemokines produced at sites of tissue wounding not only recruits downstream effector cells, but also dictates the natural evolution of immune reactivity. For example, MCP-1/CCL2, a potent chemotactic protein for monocytes and lymphocytes, simultaneously induces expression of lymphocyte-derived IL-4 in response to antigen challenge while decreasing expression of IL-12 (23). The net effect of this alteration facilitates a switch from a TH1-type to a TH2-type inflammatory response (15).

Tissue repair

In response to wounding, fibroblasts migrate into the wound bed and initially secrete collagen type III, which is later replaced by collagen type I. Synthesis and deposition of these collagens by fibroblasts is stimulated by factors including TGF-β1, -β2 and -β3, PDGF, IL-1α, -1β and -4, and mast cell tryptase. Once sufficient collagen has been generated, its synthesis stops; thus, during wound repair, production as well as degradation of collagens is under precise spatial and temporal control.

The final phase of the healing process is re-epithelialization and migration of epithelial cells across this amalgam. This is a process that requires both dissolution of the fibrin clot and degradation of the underlying dermal collagen. Epithelial cells at the leading edge of the wound express the uPA receptor, which is important for focal activation of uPA and the collagenolytic enzymes of the MMP family. In the absence of the fibrinolytic enzyme plasmin, derived from plasminogen after activation by uPA and tissue-PA, re-epithelialization is dramatically delayed (24).

The profile of cytokine/chemokines persisting at an inflammatory site is important in the development of chronic disease. The pro-inflammatory cytokine TNF-α (tumor necrosis factor-α) controls inflammatory cell populations and also mediates many of the other aspects of the inflammatory process. In addition, TGF-β1 is important, because it influences the processes of inflammation and repair in both a positive and negative manner. The key idea is that normal inflammation – i.e., inflammation associated with wound healing – is usually self-limiting; however, dysregulation of any of the converging factors can lead to abnormalities and ultimately, pathogenesis. This seems to be the case during neoplastic progression (15).

3. OSCC and inflammation

Pathologists have known for more than 100 years that almost all tumors are accompanied by inflammatory cells. At present, there is almost unanimous agreement about the causes. The functional association dates back to Virchow, who in 1863 hypothesized that cancer arises in sites of inflammation (12). Today it is accepted that chronic inflammation resulting from low grade, persistent chemical, bacterial, viral agents predisposes the formation of the preneoplastic foci and promotes tumor development (25).

Infectious agents such as *Helicobacter pylori,* with its strong association to gastric cancer, or the relationship of non-infectious chronic inflammation like chronic pancreatitis to pancreatic cancer (12, 15) are examples of infection and inflammation leading to tumor growth. Chronic inflammation caused by infections and chronic irritations are being deeply researched in order to locate the exact mechanism that triggers the cancer.

3.1 Infections of oral cavity and OSCC

OSCC is a multifactorial disease where no single clearly recognizable causative factor has been identified. Inflammation or infection-related carcinogenesis of the oral cavity is currently under investigation. Considering the oral cavity which comprises a variety of different surfaces with a huge diversity of microorganisms, including more than 750 distinct taxa of bacteria, it is not surprising that one or more of these microbes would take part in the carcinogenesis of their habitat (26). Table 1 summarizes the infectious agents and related carcinogenic mechanisms in OSCC development.

The first species of bacteria that has been classified as a definitive cause of cancer in humans is *Helicobacter pylori,* which is associated with gastric adenocarcinoma (27). After this discovery many other possibilities were investigated. Gall bladder carcinoma was associated with *Salmonella typhi,* cervical carcinoma with *Chlamydia trachomatis,* lung cancer with *Chlamydia pneumonia* and intestinal cancer with *Streptococcus bovis* (28). No such direct link was established in OSCC. As mentioned before, the oral cavity is home to a rich microflora which changes composition and quantity from person to person and throughout the lifetime of an individual as a response to a variety of factors (26). In the studies with OSCC, it is essential to identify the organisms in the tumor specimens. Specific bacteria detected in the tumor specimen were *Exiguobacterium oxidotolerans, Prevotella melaninogenica, Staphylococcus aureus* and *Veillonella parvula* (29). In another study using saliva samples, out of 40 samples three bacteria were found to be elevated in OSCC, namely *Capnocytophaga gingivalis, Prevotella meninogenica* and *Streptococcus mitis* (30).

It has been suggested that specific oral bacteria play a part in carcinogenesis, either through induction of chronic inflammation or by interference, either directly or indirectly, with eukaryotic cell cycle and signaling pathways, or by metabolism of potentially carcinogenic substances like acetaldehyde causing mutagenesis (28).

There are also a number of yeasts sharing the same environment with the bacteria. The most common yeast found in the human oral mucosa and generally regarded as commensals is a species of *Candida* (26). When host defense mechanisms are compromised or when changes occur in the local oral microenvironment *Candida spp.* act as 'opportunistic pathogens' leading to a wide range of oral mucosal infections (31). Besides being opportunistic, it has been shown that leukoplakia with candidal infection (formerly known as candidal leukoplakia) has a higher rate of malignant transformation than non-infected leukoplakia, and the estimated rate is up to 10% (32). Moreover, it has been observed that oral carriage of the most common type of candida, *Candida Albicans*, is higher in patients presenting with leukoplakia or OSCC than in patients without oral pathology (33). *C. albicans* may have a direct or indirect role in oral carcinogenesis. *Candida* might induce OSCC by directly producing carcinogenic compounds (e.g. nitrosamines) (26). The tubular hyphal structure of *C. albicans* is an important factor as it allows access of precursors from saliva and the release of nitrosamine product to keratinocytes, potentially initiating OSCC (34). In a recent study in a mouse model of oral carcinogenesis Dwivedi et al. (35), found that infection with *C. albicans* alone was not capable of inducing dysplasia or OSCC, but it was suggested that *Candida* creates an environment favorable to cell proliferation that may lead to clonal expansion of genetically altered cells. Alcohol consumption is a well-known risk factor in OSCC development. Although ethanol itself is not carcinogenic, its metabolites comprise highly toxic compounds such as acetaldehyde, hydoxyethyl radicals, ethoxy radicals, and hydroxyl radicals (31). The metabolism of alcohol starts in the oral cavity with the conversion of ethanol with enzymes catalyzed by alcohol dehydrogenase (ADH) from the epithelium and also from the oral microorganisms. Acetaldehyde in the mouth can also be derived from tobacco smoke, which contains a number of toxic aldehydes and other substances. Therefore tobacco and alcohol use has a synergistic effect on the risk of developing OSCC (5, 26, 31). From the molecular perspective, mucosal bacterial infections may influence carcinogenesis by inducing chronic inflammation in the adjacent connective tissue leading to upregulation of cytokines and growth factors. Similarly, *C. albicans* has been found to induce IL-8 secretion of endothelial cells by stimulating the cells to produce TNF-α (31, 36).The transcript factor NF-κB, a key coordinator of innate immunity and inflammation, is also an important tumor promoter (14, 15). Candidal infection may activate particular toll-like receptors (TLRs), which are known to be activated after tissue damage and microbial infection. They can also communicate with the tumor promoter NF-κB. NF-κB is involved in carcinogenesis, especially where cancer-related inflammation is evident. The association between *C. albicans*, TLR and NF-κB, and the production of cytokines and enzymes in the prostoglandin synthesis pathway, such as COX-2, is another potential mechanism that shows how *C. albicans* might influence the development of OSCC (31). Hooper *et al.* (26) suggested that 'Whether or not there is a causal relation between microbes and cancer, there is also a possibility that changes commensal microflora occur in conjunction with cancer development, which could have been used as a diagnostic indicator'. Meurman (37) proposed that it would be fascinating to control oral cancer by controlling oral microbes. The idea is truly fascinating and may not be as far-fetched as thought.

Apart from bacteria and yeasts there is also evidence that viruses take part in oral carcinogenesis. The role of the human papilloma viruses (HPV) and herpes simplex viruses (HSV) has been investigated in a number of studies (38, 39, 40). More than 100 types of HPV are identified, but only 12 types of HPV isolated from the oral cavity were associated with malignant lesions, including HPV-2,-3,-6, -11,-13,-16,-18,-31,-33,-35,-52 and -57 (41). Studies indicated that HPV-16 and -18 were the most common types detected in individuals with OSCC (42). HPV-16 DNA, in particular, was detected predominantly in oropharyngeal SCCs located in the lingual and palatine tonsillar regions (39). Although the role of HPV in OSCC is smaller than in oropharyngeal cancers, it is important to distinguish HPV (+) OSCC since they are regarded as different entities (43, 44). HPV (+) OSCC are clinically found at young ages and generally in subjects without tobacco or chronic alcohol consumption. The histologically well differentiated and faster growing cancers which respond to chemo-radiotherapy have a clinical outcome—in term of overall survival—better than HPV (-) OSCC patients (44).

Recent studies revealed a synergistic effect between alcohol and HPV, but surprisingly tobacco use did not affect their relation (45). The mechanism of oral carcinogenesis by HPV is related with the E6 and E7 genes. Its genome is made up of early genes (E) with a primary function of episomal replication and late genes (L), which encode viral capsid proteins (41). There are 7 early genes identified and two of these, E6 and E7, have the capacity to immortalize the keratinocytes through inactivation of tumor growth suppression genes p53 and Retinoblastoma (Rb) respectively (39, 41). Generally, there is no clinic lesion or sign of inflammation in HPV (+) OSCC patients, but there is a relation proposed by Tezal et al. (40) that chronic inflammation in periodontal pockets may give an opportunity to initiate HPV infection and its persistency. In this study the base of tongue in squamous cell carcinoma patients were found to be 70% positive for HPV-16 and HPV (+) tumors, and had significantly higher rates of alveolar bone loss, which is indicative of chronic periodontitis.

Infections in the oral cavity are likely to play a role in oral carcinogenesis. Since there are numerous factors that cannot yet be distinguished, further studies with larger sample sizes are warranted.

Risk factor	Potential carcinogenic mechanism	Reference
Oral biofilm (Dental plaque)	Induction of cellular proliferation, inhibition of apoptosis, interference with cellular signalling mechanisms	46
	Mutagenic interaction with saliva	47
Periodontal disease	Microbial action on oncogenic inflammatory reactions and proto-oncogenes	48
	Providing oppurtunity to initiate HPV infection and serve resevoir for latent virus	40
Viridans streptococci	Interference with cellular signalling mechanism	49
	Converting ethanol to acetaldehyde	50
Candida albicans	Dysplastic changes in oral leukoplakia	26
	Converting ethanol to acetaldehyde	51
Human papilloma virus	Epithelial cell immortalization	52
Herpes simplex virus	Activation of proto-oncogenes inactivation of p53 tumor supressor gene	52

Modified from ref 37.

Table 1. Infectious agents and attributed carcinogenic mechanisms in oral carcinogenesis

3.2 Non-Infectious chronic inflammation and OSCC

Chronic inflammatory diseases such as ulcerative colitis, atrophic gastritis and Barret's esophagus (53) have been causally associated with cancer development. Within the oral cavity, the best example of chronic inflammation are periodontal disease (as mentioned before) and oral lichen planus (OLP), which is regarded as having a malignant potential in a wide range of 0-12,5% (48, 53, 54). OLP was proposed as a unique disease model for studying non-infectious chronic inflammation and its relation to cancer in a recent publication. In the tissue microenvironment of OLP it is expected to find cytokines/chemokines directly associated with oral carcinogenesis, and suggested that OLP-related OSCC is very likely to develop from another pathway than non-OLP OSCC (53). Chronic traumas in the oral cavity were also associated with oral carcinogenesis in some recent studies and case reports (55, 56, 57). Recently, we conducted a study on the etiological factors of tongue carcinoma. Patient and control groups each consisted of 30 male and 17 female subjects with mean ages 53,17 (± 12,565) and 52,55 (± 11,542) respectively. Smoking and alcohol abuse proportions were significantly higher in the patient group as expected ($p=0.0001$, $p<0.0001$ respectively). Chronic traumas were observed in 44,7% of the patients and 17% of the control group ($p=0.004$). On regression analysis chronic traumas, such as alcohol abuse or a family history of cancer and smoking ($p=0.0001$) (58) appeared as significant etiologic factors.

We believe that field cancerization is evident in oral and orofarengeal mucosa (in the existence of epigenetic factors) with multiple steps of molecular changes starting from the first sign of dysplasia. In our opinion, the nuance is that, the site of chronic trauma reaches the point of cancer before any other competitive sites of oral mucosa. This finding might be supported by studies that associate inflammation with OSCC.

4. Role of chemokines in cancer

Chemokines are low molecular weight proteins (approximately 8-17kDa) and were originally defined as potent attractants for leukocytes in all inflammatory settings—as well as being regarded as mediators of acute and chronic inflammation (59, 60). More than 45 non-allelic chemokine genes and more than 20 chemokine receptors, which interact combinatorial, have been identified in human genome (59). Chemokines are classified on the basis of the presence of variations on their cysteine group. The first group, the CC subfamily, is composed of 28 members, whereas the CXC subfamily comprises 17 members. The other two smaller subfamilies are the CX3C and XC families, and each is presented with one member. The CXC chemokines are further classified into ELR+ and ELR- subgroups based on presence or absence of their 'glu-leu-arg' motif. ELR+ CXC chemokines are angiogenic, whereas ELR- members (except CXCL12) function as angiostatic to inhibit the formation of blood vessels (60). These are shown in Table 2 with their subgroups, receptors and tumoral impacts.

Chemokines carry a great significance in many biological events, both in physiological such as embryogenesis, lymphoid organ development, in pathology as wound healing angiogenesis, Th1/Th2 development, leukocyte homeostasis and inflammatory diseases (25). Chemokines attract leukocytes to the site of inflammation. Chemokines affect both the pro- and anti-tumor effect in the tumor microenvironment by regulating immune cell infiltration (12).

Systematic name	Chemokine reseptor	P/M/A
CXC chemokine		
ELR+ chemokines		
CXCL1	CXCR2>CXCR1	P
CXCL2	CXCR2	P
CXCL3	CXCR2	P
CXCL4	Unknown	A
CXCL5	CXCR2	P
CXCL6	CXCR1,CXCR2	P
CXCL7	CXCR2	P
CXCL8	CXCR1,CXCR2	P
ELR- chemokines		
CXCL9	CXCR3	A
CXCR10	CXCR3	A
CXCR11	CXCR3	A
CXCR12	CXCR4,CXCR7	M,P
CXCR13	CXCR5	
CXCR14	Unknown	P
CXCR16	CXCR6	
CC chemokine		
CCL1	CCR3	P
CCL2	CCR2	P
CCL3	CCR1,5	P
CCL3L1	CCR1,5	
CCL4	CCR5	P
CCL5	CCR1,3,5	P
CCL6	Unknown	
CCL7	CCR1,2,3	P
CCL8	CCR3,5	P
CCL9/10	CCR1	
CCL11	CCR3	P
CCL12	CCR3	
CCL13	CCR2,3	
CCL14	CCR1,5	
CCL15	CCR1,3	P
CCL16	CCR1,2	P
CCL17	CCR4	
CCL18	Unknown	P
CCL19	CCR7	P
CCL20	CCR6	P
CCL21	CCR7	P,lymph node metastasis
CCL22	CCR4	
CCL23	CCR1	P/M
CCL24	CCR3	
CCL25	CCR9	
CCL26	CCR3	
CCL27	CCR10	
CCL28	CCR3,10	
C chemokine		
XCL1	XCL1	
CX_3CL1 chemokine		
CX_3CL1	CX_3CL1	P/M

P-tumor progression; M-metastasis; A-Angiostatic (Modified from ref 25)

Table 2. Chemokine superfamily and their receptors

Leukocytes infiltrate the tumor in response to chemokines secreted by the tumor itself. This immune cell recruitment may promote anti-tumor activities such as elimination of tumor cells by macrophages and recruitment of innate and adaptive immune cells (25). As the tumor progresses, the attraction of immune cells by chemokines being secreted from the tumor tissue itself results in an accumulation of leukocytes in order to increase tumor growth and angiogenic mediators for tumor vasculature. Mostly, receptors of these particular chemokines are up-regulated in tumor cells which allow them to take advantage of the persistent chemokines in their microenvironment. Tumors act as immune cells which have the ability to secrete chemokines for progression. The best example is macrophages present in the tumor lesions which secrete chemokines involved in tumor cell proliferation and survival as well as angiogenesis and metastasis (12, 13). In studies based on solid tumors such as breast and prostate cancers, cancer cells were found to express higher levels of chemokine receptors CXCR4, CCR7, CCR9 and CCR10 (61, 62). This might explain the metastatic tropism of each type of cancer, depending on the receptor present on cancer cells and chemokines produced at the site of metastasis. The ligand of CXCR4, CXCL12, is best expressed in the lung, liver and lymph nodes, which are frequently involved in tumor metastasis. Moreover, CCL21, the ligand of CCR7, is produced by lymph nodes, and CCL27, the ligand of CCR10, is secreted by skin (63). The step of tumor progression includes growth of the primary tumor, angiogenesis and metastasis. The chemokines and their receptors described in these steps are as follows: CXCR4/CXCL12 is the most efficient chemokine/chemokine receptor pair in enhancing cell growth (60), CXCR2 ligands, CXCL1, CXCL2 and CXCL8 in promoting angiogenesis (64), CXCR4/CXCL12 (in bone metastasis), CCL19-CCL21/CCR7 (in lymph node metastasis) and CCL27/CCR10 (in skin metastasis) pairs in metastasis (63). Recently, chemokines and their receptors have been identified as molecular targets of cancer therapy. CXCR4 is the most targeted receptor in these studies since it was the first chemokine receptor found to be related with metastasis. CXCR4 antagonists significantly reduced the size of primary tumors in mouse models of melanoma, osteosarcoma, breast and prostate tumors (65). Another promising target is the angiogenic chemokine receptor, CXCR2, and antagonists for this receptor are under consideration for melanoma therapy. Some others, such as CCR5 antagonist, have been approved by the FDA for the treatment of HIV-infected patients. Clinical trials involving a CCR9 antagonist are also in progression for Crohn's disease (60).

4.1 Chemokines and OSCC

Ammar et al. (66) conducted one of the first studies in oral squamous cell carcinoma and chemokine expression and revealed the association of CXCR4 expression in primary site and lymph node metastasis, mode of invasion, tumor recurrence and prognosis of the patients. Parallel with this finding Ishikawa et al. (67) found a highly significant correlation ($p=0.0035$) between CXCR4 expression and lymph node metastasis of OSCC. Another study on chemokine expression and OSCC was reported in 2004, investigating the role of tumor-associated macrophages in oral cavity and oropharyngeal squamous cell carcinoma. CCL2 was found to be up-regulated significantly in tumors compared with normal mucosa (68). Later on Ferreira et al. (69) reported the role of CCL2 in lymph node metastasis of OSCC. Lymph node metastasis was also associated with other chemokine expressions. For example, CCR7 was found to be significantly associated with five clinical factors, including lymph node metastasis. Other factors were large tumors, progressive stages, local recurrences and cancer death (70).

The association of CCR7 expression and lymph node metastasis was confirmed by another study in 2009 that demonstrated CCL21 stimulation increased the ability of CCR7-positive cells, which in turn showed stronger adhesion to lymph nodes (71). Another axis related with lymph nodes was CCL3/CCR1. Silva et al. (72) reported that CCL3/CCR1 expression was significantly higher in OSCC patients than controls and they suggested that CCL3/CCR1 axis may have a role in the spread of tumoral cells to the lymph nodes.

CCL5/CCR5 axis is also studied in OSCC and found related with enhanced migration of oral cancer cells through the increase of matrix metalloproteinase (MMP)-9 production (73).

Beyond the expression profiles there is another important factor related with predisposition and progression of cancer. Single nucleotid polymorphisms (SNPs), in genes for susceptibility factors, may influence gene expression, protein function and disease predisposition in certain individuals (74). Recently, many studies revealed certain functional polymorphisms influencing expression of genes related with inflammation, and have been correlated with an increased risk for developing oral malignancies (75, 76, 77). Vairaktaris et al. (74) studied polymorphisms of a group of interleukins and tumor necrosis factors -α and -β 162 OSCC patients. Among studied cytokines, IL-6 and TNF-α polymorphisms were found to be related with OSCC occurrence. Gupta et al. (78) confirmed the results of the previously mentioned study in tobacco-related OSCC in Asian Indians. They studied SNPs in TNF-α and TNF receptor genes and TNF- α -308 G/A was found related with susceptibility to OSCC. In a Southern Thailand study on polymorphism of proinflammatory cytokines genes, susceptibility to OSCC appeared to be influenced by variants in inflammatory and immunomodulatory genes (79). Another study, again from the Greek group, was published in 2009, showing that PAI-1, MMP-9, TIMP-2 and ACE polymorphisms, which effect their expression, contributed significantly in OSCC prediction (80). Currently there are not many studies on OSCC and polymorphism of chemokines. In one study for SDF-1 (CXCL12) and CCR5 polymorphisms in head-neck cancers, only SDF-1 genotypes among studied polymorphisms were found to be significantly different from the control group distribution and this was correlated with susceptibility of SCC of the head and neck—but salivary gland tumors were excluded (81). In the other study on CCR5 and its receptor CCL5 polymorphism conducted in Taiwan, 253 OSCC patients were enrolled and SNPs in CCL5-28 and -403 genes revealed increased risk for OSCC, whereas the combined effect of CLL5-28 CG and -403 TT genes were found to increase the risk of OSCC but reduce the clinicopathological development of OSCC patients (82).

There is also a recently published study about chemokine polymorphism and OSCC of our group from Istanbul University (83). We studied the CCL2/CCR2 axis since CCL2 has been identified as a major chemokine inducing the recruitment of macrophages in human tumors, including those of the bladder, cervix, ovary, lung and breast (84, 85, 86, 87, 88). CCL2 expression was detected at the protein level in tumor cells, both in primary tumors and in the metastatic sites (89). Studies indicated that lower levels of CCL2 did form tumors but with substantial delay in onset and growth rate (90). It is shown that the polymorphism A-2518G in the regulatory region of the CCL2 gene influences CCL2 expression in response to inflammatory stimuli (91). The level of expression may vary due to polymorphism in CCL2 and its receptor CCR2 (89). In Istanbul University we therefore studied CCL2 and its receptor CCR2 polymorphisms in OSCC, and to the best of our knowledge it was the first time in the literature. In this study, we hypothesized that genetic polymorphisms in chemokines and their receptors (CCL2 A-2518G and CCR2-V64I) are involved in leukocyte trafficking and may thus influence the risk of OSCC.

We found a statistically significant difference between the control and OSCC groups for CCL2 *A2518G* genotypes (p=0.012). The frequencies of CCL2 2518 GG genotype and G allele in the OSCC group were higher than those of the control group (p=0.043 and p=0.006, respectively). Individuals carrying the G allele (GG+AG genotypes) had a 1.89-fold increased risk for OSCC (p=0.011; χ^2=6.45; OR=1.89; 95%CI= 1.15-3.09).

The CCR2 V64I genotype frequencies for controls and cases were not significantly different (p=0.08). CCR2 V64I wt/wt genotype frequency in the control group was higher than that of patient group (p=0.027; χ^2=4.88) and individuals carrying the 64I allele and wt/64I genotype had an increased risk for OSCC individuals (p=0.027, χ^2=4.88; p=0.048; χ^2=3.91 respectively).

While CCL2 G allele, CCL2 GG genotype, CCR2 64I allele, gender, smoking and alcohol consumption were associated with OSCC in univariate analysis, only CCL2 G allele, CCR2 64I allele, gender and alcohol consumption were associated with this disease in multivariate logistic regression analysis.

Association of tumor progression and the possibility of CCL-2 *A2518G* and *CCR2* V64I polymorphism playing a role in OSCC as a prognostic marker has been studied. No statistically significant differences were found between genotypes.

The genotype distributions of both CCL2 A-2518G and its receptors CCR2-V64I vary in many cancer studies (92, 93, 94). Our findings indicated a relation between CCL2 A- 2518 GG genotype and G allele and OSCC (p=0.043 and p=0.006 respectively). It seems that individuals carrying the G allele had increased risk for development of OSCC (p=0.011). To our best knowledge, six papers have reported an association of CCL2 2518 A/G polymorphism with various cancer types including breast (93), bladder (95, 96), nasopharynx (94), endometrial (97) and non-small cell lung cancer (98). Among these studies CCL2 2518G GG genotype was found to be a risk factor in endometrial cancer (6.7-fold increased risk) (97) and in bladder cancer (3-fold increased risk) (95). In a breast cancer study CCL2 2518 GG genotype and G allele frequency were also found to be significantly different (p=0.020 and 0.026 respectively) in patients with metastatic tumors (93). These studies indicated that GG genotype and mutant G allele stand on the tumor side as reported in our study. These results are also consistent with the report suggesting the association of G allele with higher levels of CCL2 expression (89). However, in a nasopharynx cancer study (94), CCL2 2518G AA and AG genotypes, which were suggested to have an association with relatively lower expression of CCL2, were found to be more prone to distant metastasis than those with GG genotype. GG genotype and G allele were also found significantly decreased in non-small cell lung cancer (98) and bladder cancer (96) patients.

The CCR2 V64I wt/wt genotype frequency in the control group was higher than the patient group (p=0.027; χ^2=4.88), and individuals carrying the 64I allele and wt/64I genotype had increased risk to develop OSCC.

Although results presented in the current study have suggested that CCR2-V64I polymorphism leading to increased risk for OSCC is similar to bladder (95) and endometrial cancer (97) types in Turkish population, the other results related to hepatocellular carcinoma (99) and non-small cell lung cancers (98) remain controversial.

These conflicting results may be explained in many different ways. First, as these studies were mostly conducted in different countries; ethnic differences may play a part. Several CCL2 A-2518G and CCR2-V64I polymorphism studies were conducted around the world, and the distribution of control group data in these studies reveals genetic variations in distinct geographic areas. These results strengthen the idea that ethnic variations affect gene polymorphisms. Secondly, all mentioned studies were unique in cancer types and none was repeated either in the same or different nation. Thirdly, the sample sizes in the studies are relatively small when compared with the number of patients in their own nation—including our study.

The current study is the first report showing the influences of CCL2 and its receptor CCR2 gene variants on OSCC. Our results suggest that the genetic variants in the CCL2 and CCR2 genes may be associated with susceptibility of OSCC in the Turkish population. We can speculate that CCL2 polymorphism might increase the biological activity of the CCR2 receptor and the development of OSCC risk within this group.

5. Conclusion

Inflammation is a recently defined contributor of oral carcinogenesis. In this multi-step process, inflammation might have a role in initiation as well as progression. Important components of this association are cytokines and chemokines produced by activated innate immune cells, which stimulate tumor growth and progression. Moreover, genetic susceptibility and gene/environment interactions are becoming more important in the attempt to eliminate the burden of cancer. The evidence found so far is sending out signals that OSCC may cease to exist in the future, and the referral will only be for a group of diseases that manifests symptoms of a similar sort. Further studies with larger sample groups in premalignant diseases of oral mucosa as well as OSCC are required to confirm these findings.

6. Summary

Oral cancer accounts more than 2% of all body cancers worldwide and more than 95% of them were found to be squamous cell carcinoma. Despite its relative rareness, high mortality rates (survival is not more than 50% in 5 years), which have not improved over the past 3 decades, have drawn the attention of the investigators. The well- known risk factors of oral squamous cell carcinoma (OSCC) like smoking, alcohol abuse and HPV infection, which are mainly based on life -style factors, seem inadequate to explain the increasing incidence especially among young population. In addition, genetic susceptibility may play an important role but the underlying mechanism of the disease still remains obscure.

Many theories about pathogenesis of the disease have been produced as a result of the clinical observations. One of the best known is about inflammation. Clinicians have experienced that tumor mass is almost always accompanied by an inflammatory zone and pathologists have always observed inflammatory cells in and around the tumors. This is not a new finding and in fact so old, which dates back to famous hypothesis by Virchow in 19th Century and even ancient back to Celsius in the year 50 BC. So what is new? The new issues are the molecular developments which elucidate many unanswered questions about cancer. The relation between inflammation and cancer was one of them.

In clinical researches about the relationship between inflammation and cancer, oral squamous cell carcinoma has an important advantage which is being easily detected by naked eye. Our previous clinical studies about etiology of tongue squamous cell carcinomas revealed that chronic traumas and irritations which lead to chronic inflammation were associated with tongue SCC formation. This encouraged us to move another step into the molecular field to understand the mechanism.

It is suggested that the relationship between cancer and inflammation occurs through two pathways: an extrinsic pathway driven by inflammatory signals such as infections and an intrinsic pathway driven by genetic alterations that cause both inflammation and neoplasia. Main mediators at the intersection of these pathways include transcription factors and primary proinflammatory cytokines.

Chemokines are a family of cytokines which are important mediators of leukocyte trafficking. They involve in defense of microbial infection, angiogenesis and metastasis. Several important polymorphisms of chemokine and chemokine receptors which deregulate chemokine system have been found and it is suggested that they may interfere with inflammatory and other diseases.

This chapter will include a brief review of molecular mechanisms of inflammation that seem responsible for etiology, pathogenesis and prognosis of oral squamous cell carcinoma and the new findings of our study group on chemokine.

7. References

[1] Zini A, Czerninski R, Sgan-Cohen HD. Oral cancer over four decades: epidemiology, trends, histology, and survival by anatomic sites. J Oral Pathol Med 2010; 39: 299-305.
[2] Parkin DM, Bray F, Ferlay J, Pisani P. Global cancer statistics, 2002. CA Cancer J Clin 2005; 55: 74-108.
[3] Warnakulasuriya S. Global epidemiology of oral and oropharyngeal cancer. Oral Oncol 2009; 45: 309-16.
[4] Warnakulasuriya S, Sutherland G, Scully C. Tobacco, oral cancer, and treatment of dependence. Oral Oncol 2005; 41: 244-60.
[5] Ogden GR and Wight AJ: Aetiology of oral cancer: Alcohol. BR J Oral Maxillofac Surg 1998; 36: 247-51.
[6] Syrjänen S. Human papillomavirus (HPV) in head neck cancer. J Clin Virol 2005; 32 (Suppl): 59-66.
[7] Llewellyn CD, Linklater K, Bell J, Johnson NW, Warnakulasuriya KAAS. Squamous cell carcinoma of the oral cavity in patients aged 45 years and under: a descriptive analysis of 116 cases diagnosed in the South East of England from 1990 to 1997. Oral Oncol 2003; 39: 106-14.
[8] Bleyer A. Cancer of the oral cavity and pharynx in young females: increasing incidence, role of human papilloma virus, and lack of survival improvement. Semin Oncol 2009; 36: 451-9.
[9] Bau DT, Tsai MH, Huang CY et al. Relationship between polymorphisms of nucleotide excision repair genes and oral cancer risk in Taiwan: evidence for modification of smoking habit. Chin J Physiol. 2007; 50: 294–300.

[10] Hatagima A, Costa EC, Marques CF, Koifman RJ, Boffetta P, Koifman S. Glutathione S-transferase polymorphisms and oral cancer: a case-control study in Rio de Janeiro, Brazil. Oral Oncol 2008; 44: 200–7.

[11] Kietthubthew S, Sriplung H, Au WW, Ishida T. Polymorphism in DNA repair genes and oral squamous cell carcinoma in Thailand. Int J Hyg Environ Health 2006; 209: 21-9.

[12] Balkwill, F and Mantovani A. Inflammation and cancer: back to Virchow? Lancet 2001; 357: 539–45.

[13] Mantovani A, Allavena P, Sica A, Balkwill F. Cancer-related inflammation. Nature 2008; 24: 436-44.

[14] Aggarwal BB, Gehlot P. Inflammation and cancer: how friendly is the relationship for cancer patients? Current Opinion in Pharmacology 2009; 9: 351-69.

[15] Coussens LM, Werb Z. Inflammation and cancer. Nature 2002; 420:860-7.

[16] Brigati C, Noonan DM, Albini A, Benelli R. Tumors and inflammatory infiltrates: friends or foes? Clin Exp Metastasis 2002; 19: 247–58.

[17] Feiken E, Romer J, Eriksen J, Lund LR. Neutrophils express tumor necrosis factor-alpha during mouse skin wound healing. J Invest Dermatol 1995; 105: 120–3.

[18] Hubner G, et al. Differential regulation of pro-inflammatory cytokines during wound healing in normal and glucocorticoid-treated mice. Cytokine 1996; 8:548–56.

[19] Chedid M, Rubin JS, Csaky KG, Aaronson SA. Regulation of keratinocyte growth factor gene expression by interleukin 1. J Biol Chem 1994; 269:10753–7.

[20] Eming SA, Krieg T, Davidson JM. Inflammation in wound repair: Molecular and cellular mechanisms. J Oral Invest Dermatol 2007; 127: 514-25.

[21] Osusky R, Malik P, Ryan SJ. Retinal pigment epithelium cells promote the maturation of monocytes to macrophages in vitro. Ophthalmic Res 1997; 29: 31–6.

[22] Rossi D, Zlotnik A. The biology of chemokines and their receptors. Annu Rev Immunol 2000; 18: 217–42.

[23] Chensue SW, Ruth JH, Warmington K, Lincoln P, Kunkel SL. In vivo regulation of macrophage IL-12 production during type 1 and type 2 cytokine-mediated granuloma formation. J Immunol 1995; 155:3546–51.

[24] Romer J, et al. Impaired wound healing in mice with a disrupted plasminogen gene. Nature Med 1996; 2: 287–92.

[25] Raman D, Baugher PJ, Thu YM, Richmond A. Role of chemokines in tumor growth. Cancer Letters 2007; 256: 137-65.

[26] Hooper SJ, Wilson MJ, Crean SJ. Exploring the link between microorganisms and oral cancer: A systematic review of the literature. Head Neck 2009; 31: 1228-39.

[27] Correa P, Houghton J. Carcinogenesis of *Helicobacter pylori*. Gastroenterology 2007; 133: 659-72.

[28] Chocolatewala N, Chaturverdi P, Desale R. The role of bacteria in oral cancer. Indian Journal of Medical and Paediatric Oncology 2010; 31: 126-31.

[29] Hooper SJ, Crean SJ. Fardy MJ et al. A molecular analysis of the bacteria present within oral squamous cell carcinomas. J Med Microbiol 2007; 56: 1651-9.

[30] Mager DL, Haffajee AD, Devlin PM, Norris CM, Posner MR, Goodson JM. The salivary microbiota as a diagnostic indicator of oral cancer: A descriptive, non-randomized study of cancer-free and oral squamous cell carcinoma subjects. J Translational Med 2005; 3:27.

[31] Bakri MM, Hussaini HM, Holmes AR, Cannon RD, Rich AM. Revisiting the association between candidal infection and carcinoma, particularly oral squamous cell carcinoma. J Oral Microbiol 2010; 2: 5780.
[32] Bartie KL, Williams DW, Wilson MJ, Potts AJ, Lewis MA. Differential invasion of *Candida albicans* isolates in an *in vitro* model of oral candidosis. Oral Microbiol Immunol 2004; 19: 293-6.
[33] McCullough M, Jaber M, Barret AW, Bain L, Speight PM, Porter SR. Oral yeast carriage correlates with presence of oral epithelial dysplasia. Oral Oncol 2002; 38: 391-3.
[34] Krogh P, Hald B, Holmstrup P. Possible mycological etiology of oral mucosal cancer: catalytic potential of infecting *Candida albicans* and other yeast in production of N-nitrosobenzyl-methylamine. Carcinogenesis 1987; 8: 1543-8.
[35] Dwivedi PP, Mallya S, Dongari-Bagtzoglou A. A novel immunocompetent murine model for *Candida albicans*-promoted oral epithelial dysplasia. Med Mycol 2009; 47: 157-67.
[36] Orozco AS, Zhou X, Filler SG. Mechanisms of the proinflammatory response of endothelial cells to *Candida albicans* infection. Infect Immun 2000; 68: 1134-41.
[37] Meuman JH. Infections and dietary risk factors of oral cancer. Oral Oncol 2010; 46: 411-3.
[38] Shillitoe EJ. The role of viruses in squamous cell carcinoma of the oropharyngeal mucosa. Oral Oncol 2009; 45: 351-5.
[39] Gillison ML, D'Souza G, Westra W, Sugar E, Weihong Xiao, Begum S, Viscidi R. Distinct risk factor profiles for Human Papillomavirus type 16-positive and Human Papillomavirus type 16-negative head and neck cancers. J Natl Cancer Inst 2008; 100: 407-20.
[40] Tezal M, Nasca MS, Stoler DL, Melendy T, Hyland A, Smaldino PJ, Rigual NR, Loree TR. Chronic periodontitis-Human Papillomavirus synergy in base of tongue cancers. Arch Otolaryngol Head Neck Surg. 2009; 135: 391-6.
[41] Pinheiro RS, Franca TRT, Ferreira DC, Ribeiro CMB, Leao JC, Castro GF. Human Papillomavirus in the oral cavity of children. J Oral Pathol Med 2011; 40: 121-6.
[42] Miller CS, Johnstone B. Human Papillomavirus as a risk factor for oral squamous cell carcinoma: a meta-analysis, 1982-1997. Oral Surg Oral Med Oral Radiol Endod 2001; 91: 622-35.
[43] Machado J, Reis PP, Zhang T et al. Low prevalence of Human Papillomavirus in oral city carcinomas. Head Neck Oncol 2010; 2:6.
[44] Pannone G, Santoro A, Papagerakis A, Muzio LL, De Rosa G, Bufo P. The role of Human Papillomavirus in the pathogenesis of head and neck squamous cell carcinoma: an overview. Infectious Agents and Cancer 2011; 6:4.
[45] Smith EM, Ritchie JM, Summersgill KF, Hoffman HT, Wang DH, Haugen TH, Turek LP. Human Papillomavirus in oral exfoliated cells and risk of head and neck cancer. J Natl Cancer Inst 2004; 96: 449-55.
[46] Lax AJ, Thomas W. How bacteria could cause cancer: one step at a time. Trends Microbiol 2002; 10: 293-9.
[47] Bloching M, Reich W, Schubert J, Grummt T, Sandner A. The influence of oral hygiene on salivary quality in the Ames test, as a marker for genotoxic effects. Oral Oncol 2007; 43: 933-9.

[48] Tezal M, Sullivan MA, Hyland A et al. Chronic periodontitis and the incidence of head and neck squamous cell carcinoma. Cancer Epidemiol Biomarkers Prev 2009; 18: 2406-12.

[49] Narikiyo M, Tanabe C, Yamada Y et al. Frequent and preferential infection of *Treponema denticola, Streptococcus mitis, and streptococcus anginosus* in esophageal cancers. Cancer Sci 2004; 95: 569-74.

[50] Homann N, Tillonen J, Meurman JH et al. Increased salivary acetaldehyde levels in heavy drinkers and smokers: a microbiological approach to oral cavity cancer. Carcinogenesis 2000; 21: 663-8.

[51] Nieminen MT, Uittamo J, Salaspuro M, Rautemaa R. Acetaldehyde production from ethanol and glucose by non-Candida albicans yeasts in vitro. Oral Oncol 2009; 45: e245-8.

[52] Park NH, Li SL, Xie JF, Cherrick HM. In vitro and animal studies of the role of viruses in oral carcinogenesis. Eur J Cancer B Oral Oncol 1992; 28B: 145-52.

[53] Liu Y, Messadi DV, Wu H, Hu S. Oral lichen planus is a unique disease model for studying chronic inflammation and oral cancer. Medical Hypotheses 2010; 75: 492-4.

[54] Gandolfo S, Richiardi L, Carrozo M et al. Oral Oncol 2004; 40: 77-83.

[55] Piemonte ED, Lazos JP, Brunotto M. Relationship between chronic trauma of the oral mucosa, oral potentially malignant disorders and oral cancer. J Oral Pathol Med 2010; 39:513-7.

[56] Compilato D, Cirillo N, Termine N et al. Long-standing oral ulcers: proposal for a new 'S-C-D classification system' J Oral Pathol Med 2009; 38: 241-53.

[57] Gallego L, Junquera L, Llorente S. Oral carcinoma associated with implant-supported overdenture trauma: a case report. Dental Traumatol 2009; 25: e3-e4.

[58] Bektaş-Kayhan K, Ünür M, Hafiz G, Karadeniz A, Altun M, Meral R. Carsinoma of the tongue: A case-control study on etiologic factors and dental trauma. Oral Oncol 2007; (supp 2):154-155.

[59] Rollins BJ. Inflammatory chemokines in cancer growth and progression. Eur J Cancer 2006; 42: 760-7.

[60] Lazennec G, Richmond A. Chemokines and chemokine reseptors: new insights into cancer-related inflammation Trends Mol Med 2010; 16: 133-44.

[61] Ali S, Lazennec G. Chemokines: novel targets for breast cancer metastasis. Cancer Metastasis Rev 2007; 26: 401–20.

[62] Vindrieux D, Escobar P, Lazennec G. Emerging roles of chemokines in prostate cancer. Endocr Relat Cancer 2009; 16: 663–73.

[63] Ben-Baruch A. Organ selectivity in metastasis: regulation by chemokines and their receptors. Clin Exp Metastasis 2008; 25: 345–56.

[64] Mehrad B, Keane MP, Strieter RM. Chemokines as mediators of angiogenesis. Thromb Haemost 2007; 97: 755–62.

[65] Allavena P, Germano G, Marchesi F, Mantovani A. Chemokines in cancer related inflammation. Exp Cell Res 2011; 317: 664-73.

[66] Ammar A, Uchida D, Begum NM et al. The clinicopathological significance of the expression of CXCR4 protein in oral squamous cell carcinoma. Int J Oncol 2004; 25: 65-71.

[67] Ishikawa T, Nakashiro K, Hara S et al. H.CXCR4 expression is associated with lymph-node metastasis of oral squamous cell carcinoma. Int J Oncol 2006; 28: 61-6.
[68] Marcus B, Arenberg D, Lee J et al. Prognostic factors in oral cavity and oropharyngeal squamous cell carcinoma. Cancer 2004; 12: 2779-87.
[69] Ferreira FO, Ribeiro FL, Batista AC, Leles CR, de Cássia Gonçalves Alencar R, Silva TA. Association of CCL2 with lymph node metastasis and macrophage infiltration in oral cavity and lip squamous cell carcinoma. Tumour Biol 2008; 29: 114-21.
[70] Tsuzuki H, Takahashi N, Kojima A, Narita N, Sunaga H, Takabayashi T, Fujieda S. Oral and oropharyngeal squamous cell carcinomas expressing CCR7 have poor prognoses. Auris Nasus Larynx 2006; 33: 37-42.
[71] Shang ZJ, Liu K, Shao Z. Expression of chemokine receptor CCR7 is associated with cervical lymph node metastasis of oral squamous cell carcinoma. Oral Oncol. 2009; 45: 480-5.
[72] Chuang JY, Yang WH, Chen HT et al. CCL5/CCR5 axis promotes the motility of human oral cancer cells. J Cell Physiol 2009; 220: 418-26.
[73] Silva TA, Ribeiro FLL, Oliveira-Neto HH et al. Dual role of CCL3/CCR1 in oral squamous cell carcinoma: Implications in tumor metastasis and local host defense. Oncol Rep 2007; 18: 1107-13.
[74] Vairaktaris E, Yapijakis C, Serefoglou Z et al. Gene expression polymorphisms of interleukins-1 beta, -4, -6, -8, -10, and tumor necrosis factors-alpha, -beta: regression analysis of their effect upon oral squamous cell carcinoma. J Cancer Res Clin Oncol 2008; 134: 821-32.
[75] Tsai MH, Chen WC, Tsai CH, Hang LW, Tsai FJ. Interleukin-4 gene, but not the interleukin-1 beta gene polymorphism, is associated with oral cancer. J Clin Lab Anal 2005; 19: 93-8.
[76] Wong YK, Chang KW, Cheng CY, Liu CJ. Association of CTLA-4 gene polymorphism with oral squamous cell carcinoma. J Oral Pathol Med 2006; 35: 51-4.
[77] Vairaktaris E, Yiannopoulos A, Vylliotis A et al. Strong association of interleukin-6 -174 G>C promoter polymorphism with increased risk of oral cancer. J Biol Markers 2006; 21: 246-50.
[78] Gupta R, Sharma SC, Das SN. Association of TNF-α and TNFR1 promoters and 3′ UTR region of TNFR2 gene polymorphisms with genetic susceptibility to tobacco-related oral carcinoma in Asian Indians. Oral Oncol 2008; 44: 455-63.
[79] Kietthubthew S, Wickliffe J, Sriplung H, Ishida T, Chonmaitree T, Au WW. Association of polymorphisms in proinflammatory cytokine genes with the development of oral cancer in Southern Thailand. Int J Hyg Environ Health 2010; 213: 146-52.
[80] Vairaktaris E, Serefoglou Z, Avgoustidis D et al. Gene polymorphisms related to angiogenesis, inflammation and thrombosis that influence risk for oral cancer. Oral Oncol 2009; 45: 247-53.
[81] Khademi B, Razmkhah M, Efrani N, Gharagozloo M, Ghaderi A. SDF-1 and CCR5 genes polymorphism in patients with head and neck cancer. Pathol Oncol Res 2008; 14: 45-50.
[82] Weng CJ, Chien MH, Kin CW et al. Effect of CC chemokine ligand 5 and CC chemokine receptor 5 genes polymorphisms on the risk and clinicopathological development of oral cancer. Oral Oncol 2010; 46: 767-72.

[83] Bektas-Kayhan K, Unur M, Boy-Metin Z, Cakmakoglu B. MCP-1 and CCR2 gene variants in oral squamous cell Oral Diseases (2011) doi:10.1111/j.1601-0825.2011.01843.x

[84] Amann B, Perabo FG, Wirger A, Hugenschmidt H, Schultze- Seemann W. Urinary levels of monocyte chemoattractant protein-1 correlate with tumour stage and grade in patients with bladder cancer. Br J Urol 1998; 82: 118– 21.

[85] Riethdorf L, Riethdorf S, Gutzlaff K, Prall F, Loning T. Differential expression of the monocyte chemoattractant protein-1 gene in human papillomavirus-16-infected squamous intraepithelial lesions and squamous cell carcinomas of the cervix uteri. Am J Pathol 1996; 149: 1469–76.

[86] Negus RP, Stamp GW, Relf MG et al. The detection and localization of monocyte chemoattractant protein-1 (MCP-1) in human ovarian cancer. J Clin Invest 1995; 95: 2391– 6.

[87] Arenberg DA, Keane MP, DiGiovine B et al. Macrophage infiltration in human non-small-cell lung cancer: the role of CC chemokines. Cancer Immunol Immunother 2000; 49: 63– 70.

[88] Ueno T, Toi M, Saji H et al. Significance of macrophage chemoattractant protein-1 in macrophage recruitment, angiogenesis, and survival in human breast cancer. Clin Cancer Res 2000; 6: 3282– 9.

[89] Soria G and Ben-Baruch A. The inflammatory chemokins CCL2 and CCL5 in breast cancer. Cancer Letters 2008; 267: 271-85.

[90] Conti I, Rollins BJ. CCL2 (monocyte chemoattractant protein-1) and cancer. Semin Cancer Biol 2004; 14: 149-54.

[91] Rovin BH, Lu L, Saxena R. A novel polymorphism in the *MCP-1* gene regulatory region that influences MCP-1 expression. Biochem Biophys Res Commun 1999; 259: 344- 8.

[92] Yeh CB, Tsai HT, Chen YC et al. Genetic polymorphism of CCR2-64I increased the susceptibility of hepatocellular carcinoma. J Surg Oncol 2010; 102: 264-70.

[93] Ghilardi G, Biondi ML, Torre A, Battaglioli L, Scorza R. Breast cancer progression and host polymorphism in the chemokine system: Role of macrophage chemoattractant protein-1 (MCP-1) -2518 G allele. Clin Chem 2005; 51: 452-5.

[94] Tse K, Tsang N, Chen K et al. MCP-1 promoter polymorphism at -2518 is associated with metastasis of nasopharyngeal carcinoma after treatment. Clin Cancer Res 2007; 13: 6320-6.

[95] Narter KF, Agachan B, Sozen S, Cincin ZB, Isbir T. CCR2-64I is a risk factor for development of bladder cancer. Genet Mol Res 2010; 9: 685-92.

[96] Vázquez-Lavista LG, Lima G, Gabilondo F and Llorente L Genetic association of monocyte chemoattractant protein 1 (MCP-1)-2518 polymorphism in Mexican patients with transitional cell carcinoma of the bladder. Urology 2009; 74: 414-8.

[97] Attar R, Agachan B, Kuran SB et al. Association of *CCL2* and *CCR2* gene variants with endometrial cancer in Turkish women. In Vivo 2010; 24: 243-8.

[98] Yang L, Shi GL, Song CX, XU SF. Relationship between genetic polymorphism of MCP-1 and non-small-cell lung cancer in Han nationality of North China. Genetics and Molecular Res 2010; 9: 765-71.

[99] Nahon P, Sutton A, Rufat P et al. Chemokine system polymorphism, survival and hepatocellular carcinoma occurrence in patients with hepatitis C virus-related cirrhosis. World J Gastroenterol 2008; 14: 713-9.

Part 5

Cancer Stem Cells in Squamous Cell Carcinoma

13

Molecular Mechanisms Involving Therapeutic Resistance in Head and Neck Squamous Cell Carcinoma (HNSCC) – Roles of Hypoxic Microenvironment and Cancer Stem Cell

Xiaoming Li, Qingjia Sun and Yupeng Shen
Bethune International Peace Hospital
China

1. Introduction

Locally advanced diseases accounting for most HNSCC have a poor prognosis. The main reason for this is that corresponding symptoms of HNSCC are not always obvious or ignored by patients at early stage, which is mostly reflected by the fact that more than 2/3 HNSCC patients present with stage III/IV disease (AL-Sarraf, 1987; Argiris, 2008). Patients characterized with advanced HNSCC are subjected to worse prognosis than those with confined disease, exhibiting 5-year survival of 10-40%, cure rate of 30% and median survival time of 6-10 months (Argiris, 2008; Vokes et al, 1993; Cohen et al, 2004). Our recent study in a large series (X. Li et al, 2009) demonstrated that overall survival rates of patients with distant metastases in clinic were 56.8% at 1 year, 9.1% at 3 years, and 6.8% at 5 years, respectively. In addition, traditional treatment related morbidities could negatively influence quality life of patients, which involves loss of speech, permamant tracheostomy or gastrostomy dependence, dysphagia and other systematic side effects. Therefore, it is necessary to seek novel strategies to cure advanced HNSCC aiming at organ preservation, prevention of metastases as well as second malignancies and improvement in quality of life.

2. Necessities for adjuvant therapies in HNSCC

Surgical ablation plays a major role in the management of locoregional diseases of HNSCC. At early stage of HNSCC, current novel surgical alternatives, such as laser surgery, can achieve curable effects for 5-year survival rate of 80% even without prominent functional detriments. However, many tumors in the advanced stage are inoperable either due to the invasion of some major structures by tumor or due to the unfavorable general conditions of patients. Moreover, even with very skillful surgeons, some tumors remain after surgical resection, leading to postoperative recurrence if additional complimentary treatment is not carried out. In tumors with regional lymph node metastasis, extracapsular nodal spread always implicates poor prognosis even after a comprehensive neck dissection. For these conditions, adjuvant therapies such as radiotherapy, chemotherapy and chemoratiation are due to undertake to increase the chance of cure or to prolong duration of survival of advanced cases.

2.1 Traditional adjuvant therapies improve outcome of advanced HNSCC

The participation of radiotherapy improved effects of surgery alone. In 2008, *Cancer* journal (Lavaf et al, 2008) reported a large-scale analysis with regard to effects of combined surgery and radiotherapy on survival of patients with lymph node-positive HNSCC patients. In 8795 patients meeting the inclusion criteria, 54.9% of 3-year overall survival and 43.2% of 5-year overall survival for adjuvant therapy could be gotten compared with 44.4% and 33.4% for surgery alone. More recently, a new analysis with large series (Shrime, 2010) reported that postoperative radiotherapy improved 5-year overall survival rate in patients with $T_{1-2}N_1$ oral squamous carcinoma (41.4% for surgery alone vs. 54.2% for surgery plus radiotherapy). Although statistically significant, slight improvement in survival has to indicate the limitation of single radiotherapy addition, which appeals the need of chemotherapy in the management of advanced HNSCC. In 2009, the journal of *The Lancet Oncology* published a 10-year follow-up report of a trial for chemoradiotherapy for locally advanced head and neck cancer conducted by The UK Head and Neck (UKHAN) cancer group (Tobias et al, 2009). In this follow-up analysis, patients who did not undergo previous surgery benefited from scheduled simultaneous addition of chemicals to radiotherapy, exhibiting 4-7 years in the median overall survival. However, the median overall survival of patients undergoing surgery was still higher without substantial benefit from chemotherapy alone. Furthermore, sequent toxicity reactions, such as mucositis and xerostomia, are due to occur. All these findings suggest that the effects of traditional chemicals in treating the HNSCC are limited due to their unspecific hallmarks.

2.2 Limitations of traditional adjuvant chemoradiation therapies

As is known, HNSCC depend on many intrinsic or extrinsic factors to protect against traditional chemotherapeutic agents, such as cisplatin and 5- fluorouracil. As evidenced by clinical observations, HNSCC possesses a decreased sensitivity and increased resistance to chemo- and radiotherapy, giving rise to a poor tumor control efficacy of these treatment modalities. This situation is mostly reflected by the fact that many HNSCCs (including primary and recurrent carcinomas) have less or no response to the adopted treatment regimens in the course of chemotherapy and/or radiotherapy. For this reason, some tumors regenerate or relapse following a short- or long-term paracmasis during which time the tumor bulk contracts or even disappears visually in response to therapy. Therefore, chemo- and radiotherapeutic resistance and post-treatment relapse has been always a puzzling problem that needs to be solved urgently.

3. Role of hypoxia in therapeutic resistance in HNSCC

The mechanisms underlying resistance to chemo- and/or radiotherapy by HNSCC are very complicated. Among various factors that are associated with therapeutic resistance in HNSCC, hypoxic microenvironment resulting from hypoxia in local cancer lesions is thought to be important one. It has been demonstrated that, most solid tumors have a lower pressure of oxygen (PO_2) compared with normal tissues from which they originate. Hypoxia occurs due to rapid proliferation of cells and/or insufficient supplies of blood. The latter attributes to poor drugs delivery, leading to a common cause of chemoresistance. In addition, activated intrinsic pathways within tumor cells contribute to comprehensive radio- and chemo-resistance under hypoxic condition. In this section, we will focus on these intrinsic responses underlying resistance under hypoxia.

3.1 The general responses to hypoxia in tumor cells

General responses of tumor cells under hypoxia include translation inhibition, paradoxical translation and genetic instability. ATP defect caused by hypoxia invokes global translation inhibition for maintaining energy homeostasis. However, paradoxically, tumor cells activate some factors which are always unexpressed under normal conditions for adaptation to hypoxic stress. These proteins act as mediators of PH and metabolism, as well as function to propagate therapeutic resistance. In the long run, hypoxia-induced reactive oxygen species (ROS) and/or defective DNA repair induce mutagenesis of tumor cells to confer selection of heterogeneous population with hypoxia tolerance (see Fig. 1).

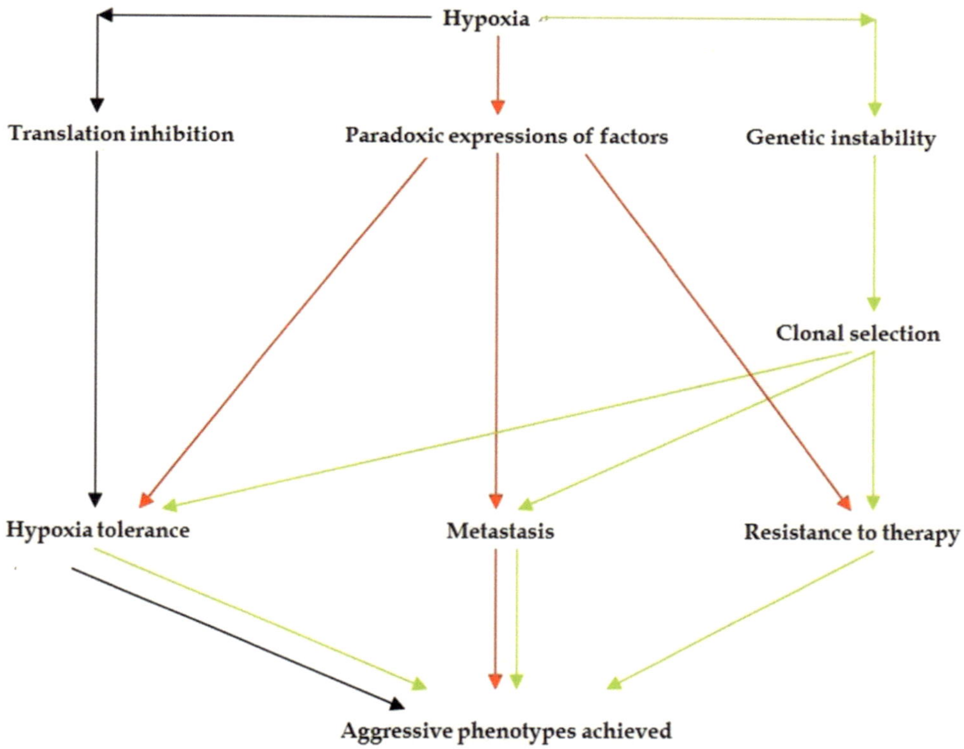

Fig. 1. General responses to hypoxia of tumor. Hypoxic tumor cells inhibit translation via mTOR pathways as well as UPR for energy homeostasis. Meanwhile paradoxically, they express some factors, such as HIF-1α and GRP78, to degrade nonfunctioning protein, regulate PH and counter apoptosis. These factors also act as resistance to therapy and metastasis. Hypoxia induced mutagenesis select clonal subset characterized with aggressive phenotypes, which confer more malignant biological behaviors including therapeutic resistance.

3.2 Hypoxia-related translation inhibition

3.2.1 The mammalian target of rapamycin (mTOR) pathways

Protein synthesis is processed as a result of energy-consumption. To date, emerging data have evidenced that inhibition of translation is an important category of cellular hypoxic tolerance, and the process occurs during the initial step of translation. The initiation of translation involves two components, the eukaryotic initiation factor 4F (eIF4F) as well as 43S preinitiation complex. The former consists of the cap binding protein eIF4E, a scaffolding protein eIF4G and an ATP-dependent helicase eIF4A (RNA helicase activity), among which eIF4E and eIF4G mostly participate in the regulation of initiation of translation. Under nutrient and/or oxygen repletion, mTOR phosphorylates eukaryotic initiation factor 4E binding protein 1 (4EBP1) that has a high affinity with eIF4E to low the affinity. Together with eIF4G, released eIF4E contributes to assembly of eIF4F complex that binds to the 5′m^{7}GpppN cap structure of mRNA to facilitate the recruitment of 43S preinitiation complex that includes the 40S ribosomal subunit and the ternary complex (eIF2-GTP and the methionine-loaded initiator tRNA) for the start of translation initiation. The ribosomal constituents of preinitiation complex scan though the 5′ untranslated region (5'UTR) until the AUG initiation codon is recognized. Sequently, the 60S ribosomal subunit joins to form 80S ribosome for the elongation of translation. Lots of recent reports have implicated that hypoxia can disturb the process above via hypoxic activation of the tuberous sclerosis protein 1 (TSC1)–TSC2 complex-mediated downregulation of mTOR. Thereby, corresponding expressions of translation initiation-related proteins, such as phosphorylated 4EBP1 and eIF4F, other mTOR-mediated targets and S6 protein kinases (S6K 1 and 2), all of which also function in translation, would be inactivated accordingly. In addition, hypoxia also interferes with formation of preinitiation complex to inhibit translation via PERK-mediated cascade of unfolded protein responses.

3.2.2 Unfolded protein responses (UPR)

UPR is an evolutionary conserved protective response to microenvironment stress. Because of abnormal vascular structure and aggressive cellular growth, hypoxia and glucose starvation always occur in tumor microenvironment, resulting in defective usage of energy in response to accumulation of many unfolded protein in endocytoplasmic reticulum (ER). Tumor cells must adapt to this stress though inhibiting mRNA and protein synthesis as well as degrading excessive useless protein, which is executed though activation of UPR. Glucose-regulated protein 78 (GRP78/BiP) is the core regulator in ER-stress and overexpressed in most tumor as a predictor of poor prognosis. Routinely, GRP78 binds to ER-stress sensors, IRE1α (inositol-requiring 1 alpha), PERK (double-strand RNA-activated protein kinase-like ER kinase), and ATF6 (activating transcription factor 6), to inactivate their downstream targets. Once ER-stress occurs, the role of GRP78 is shifted towards that of a chaperone. After dissociation, GRP78 handles unfolded protein to facilitate degradation and binds to Ca^{2+} to inhibit apoptosis. Importantly, the dissociation activates these integral ER membrane sensors PERK, IRE-1 and ATF6. Activated PERK phosphorylates eukaryotic initiation factor 2 subunit α (eIF2α), leading to either inhibition of global protein translational attenuation or paradoxical expression of the transcription factor 4 (ATF4) that immediately blocks eIF2α phosphorylation and sequently encodes genes upregulating stress-adaptive factors, such as GRP78 and hypoxia inducible factors (HIFs). UPR also includes IRE-1 and ATF6 arms. Activated IRE-1 serves as an endoribonuclease to remove a 26 nucleotide intron from X-box binding protein 1 (XBP1) pre-mRNA. The resulting XBP1 protein by spliced XBP1 mRNA can activate lots of ER chaperones and enzymes to remove mis/unfolded protein and help ER-localized protein maturation as well as ER-associated degradation. Similar with XBP1, ATF6 needs cleavage for its activation. Briefly, upon UPR activation, ATF6 is transmitted from ER to Golgi apparatus where ATF6 completes its splicing process. Subsequently, cleaved ATF6 also activates target genes functioning in protein degradation and upregulation of molecular chaperones. As a matter of fact, their functions and target genes overlap one another. Overall, these sensors play a critical role in inhibition of mRNA and protein synthesis and upregulation of stress-adaptive factors. As a final step, unfolded protein is transported to cytoplasm and degraded via ubiquitin-proteasome pathway (UPP) or autophagy. To our understanding, UPR is a double-edged sword. On the one hand, PERK--eIF2a-ATF4 pathway is a dominant UPR arm offering survival advantage under hypoxia. On the other hand, once severe stress persists, UPR will induce ER-stress-relared cell death (apoptosis, autophagy associated programmed death or necrosis). To date, GADD153/CHOP induced by ATF4, has been identified as a pro-apoptosis factor that can activate cascades of caspases, mediating type I programmed cell death (known as apoptosis). It remains to be determined by what mechanisms the UPR induces autophagic death and necrosis.

3.3 Factors expressed paradoxically under hypoxia

3.3.1 HIF-1α

HIFs are core factors regulating oxygen and energy supplies of the tumor bulk, by which tumor cells adapt to hypoxia through inducing expressions of related genes to overcome such an unfavorable low-oxygen condition. HIFs are members of bHLH-PAS protein family including HIF-α and HIF-β subunit, the former of which also includes HIF-1α, HIF-2α and HIF-3α. Functionally, HIF-α (HIF-1α, HIF-2α) can be stably sustained in the hypoxic niche. In the event of cell signaling, HIF-α (HIF-1α, HIF-2α) and HIF-β can form a heterodimer that binds to promoters or enhancers of target genes. Hypoxia not only induces the expression of HIF-1α, but also activates many specific biological effects of HIF-1α gene protein, which functions either to acquire the tolerance to hypoxia or to commit the capability of invasion, metastasis and therapeutic resistance: 1) inducing expression of carbonate dehydrates (CAH) to maintain a stable cytoplasmic PH to promote the survival ability of cancer cells in response to apoptosis-inducing factors; 2) upregulating the expression of MDR gene and its product, P-gp, resulting in resistance to multiple chemotherapeutic agents; 3) mediating the overexpression and activation of DNA kinase (DNA-PK), contributing essentially to the repair of DNA double-strand breaks (DSBs); 4) acting as an upstream regulator of genes encoding vascular endothelial growth factor (VEGF) as well as some key enzymes related to glycolysis, responsible for angiogenesis and glycometabolism within tumors; 5) promoting expressions of anti-apoptosis proteins such as Survivin and XIAP to inhibit the activation of pro-apoptosis proteins Bax and caspases, rendering the tumor cells the ability to escape from apoptosis.

3.3.2 Signal transducer and activator of transcription 3 (STAT3)

STAT3 is an important factor overlapped by many intracellular signal pathways. It can be activated though Janus kinases (JAKs) or tyrosine kinase receptors such as EGFR. Upon phosphorylation at the Tyr705 residue, p-STAT3 translocates to nucleus to bind DNA for inducing the transcription of downstream targets. Emerging reports have demonstrated that STAT3 is associated with poor prognosis in many cancers including HNSCC. STAT3 induces resistance to therapy in tumors via activation of anti-apoptosis factors, such as Bcl-2, Bcl-xl as well as Survivin and downregulation of P53. Recently, a study demonstrated that STAT3 participates in inhibition of apoptosis caused by PIs in HNSCC (C. Li et al, 2009). Under hypoxia, STAT3 can be activated by ROS (Simon et al, 1998). Selvendiran et al (Selvendiran et al, 2009) found that STAT3 can be activated by production of ROS under 1% O_2 in ovarian cancer. In their study, overexpressed STAT3 contributed to similar rate of proliferation as that under normoxia but increased drug resistance under hypoxia. Through blockage of STAT3 using RNAi technique, ovarian tumor cells with defective expression of STAT3 exhibited affected proliferation as well as increased sensitivity to traditional chemotherapeutics under hypoxia. In HNSCCs, STAT3 was also found to be constitutively activated and associated with cervical lymph node metastasis in laryngeal cancer. Silencing STAT3 gene with specific siRNA enhances the sensitivity of Hep-2 human laryngeal carcinoma cells to ionizing radiation both in vitro and in xenotransplanted mice model. (X. Li, et al, 2010a, 2010b)

3.4 Hypoxic dynamic complication in solid tumor

3.4.1 Category of hypoxia

In solid tumor, hypoxia can be categorized as chronic continuing hypoxia and cyclic hypoxia (also called intermittent hypoxia or fluctuating hypoxia) depending on distances of tumor cells from the adjacent vessels. The former is incurred from the condition that tumor cells locating far from vessels result to diffusion-limited and relatively stable delivery of oxygen. On the other hand, the latter characterized by acute hypoxia/reoxygenation is caused by status of nearby vessels that suffer from dynamic changes in blood perfusion not least as a result of the abnormal vasculature and the mechanical instability of microvessel walls caused by proliferating tumor cells and/or circulating blood cells. With regard to insufficiency in blood or oxygen supply, hypoxia is classified as mild hypoxia (PO2: 1-3%), moderate hypoxia (PO2: 0.1-1%) and severe hypoxia (PO2: 0-0.1%) ((Koumenis & Wouters, 2006). Additionally, in term of duration of persistent hypoxic condition, hypoxia is divided into acute hypoxia lasting several minutes to several hours as well as prolonged chronic hypoxia during which cells are exposed to hour-to-day intracellular low PO2. The complex nature of hypoxia and different responses to distinct hypoxia by tumor cells may explain why it is so difficult to antagonize hypoxia-induced therapeutic resistance in HNSCCs.

3.4.2 Chronic versus cyclic

In most lab experiments, there is an important difference ignored by us. That is the parameters of hypoxic condition selected by most investigators are usually simple and fairly stable. However, reoxygenation may occur during manipulation of assorted cells. To date, cyclic hypoxia has been less studied than chronic hypoxia. The setting of cyclic hypoxic condition was not consistent among various studies on cyclic hypoxia. Here we introduce the difference between the two as follows with special emphasis on the importance of cyclic hypoxia. Firstly, cyclic hypoxia confers more potential therapeutic resistance than chronic hypoxia. It has been demonstrated by many studies that increased expression of HIF-1α contributes to cyclic hypoxia-induced resistance. In addition, it has been confirmed that chronically hypoxic tumor cells are more susceptible to ionizing radiation (IR) or DNA-damaging drugs than acutely hypoxic tumor cells because of decreased homologous recombination (HR) function, a main pathway to repair DNA double-strand breaks (DSBs) in the S and G2 phases of the cell cycle. Secondly, cyclic hypoxia induces an enhanced metastasis. It was found that mice bearing melanoma xenografts exposed to cyclic hypoxia suffered from increased incidence of pulmonary metastases (Rofstad et al, 2010). Furthermore, tumor cells treated by cyclic hypoxia up-regulates the expression of VEGF-A, the ligand of VEGFR-1 on bone marrow derived cells confirmed to form "premetastasis niche". Therefore, induction of VEGF-A by hypoxia may be an important promoter of metastasis. Thirdly, cyclic hypoxia enhances metabolism of Tirapazimine (TPZ), an agent with specific hypoxic cytotoxicity, by intratumoral vessels adjacent to the populated tumor cells, which attenuates the effects of TPZ (Cárdenas-Navia et al, 2007). Finally, cyclic hypoxia is pervasive. As early as 1996, Kimura's group (Kimura et al, 1996) measured microvessel red cell flux (RCF) and perivascular PO2 in xenotransplant of R3230Ac mammary carcinomas using intratumoral dorsal flap window chambers. They found that the baseline RCF and PO2 underwent a highly dynamic process, demonstrating that fluctuating hypoxia is a common phenomenon within a tumor. More recently, another group (Cárdenas-Navia et al, 2008) used phosphorescence lifetime imaging to detect fluctuation of vascular PO2 in rat fibrosarcomas, 9L gliomas and R3230 mammary adenocarcinomas transplanted in dorsal skin-fold window chambers. By short interval periodic imaging, they found O2 delivery to tumors is constantly instable. In addition, hypoxia, including acute and chronic hypoxia, causes genomic instability. Cyclic hypoxia mostly induces DNA double-strand breaks (DSBs) by generating reactive oxygen species (ROS). Chronic hypoxia causes genomic instability due to the defective HR ability. Thereby, both types of hypoxia facilitate mutagenesis leading to clonal selection with therapy-resistant, invasive and metastatic phenotype (see Fig. 2).

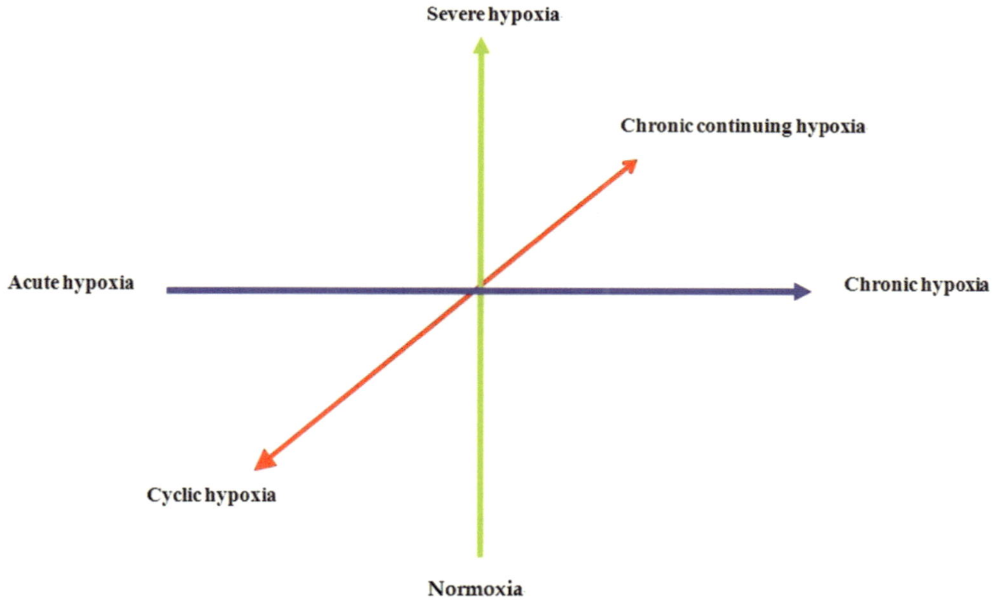

Fig. 2. Dynamic heterogeneity of hypoxia in solid tumor. Distinct hypoxia patterns exist in solid tumor. These patterns may overlap and co-exist in the same tumor bulk, which can be reflected though the 3D axis. Any point of this axis represents a combined type of hypoxia pattern in a tumor.

3.4.3 Hypoxic duration- and/or degree-related responses

The existing status of oxygen level in tumor bulk is very heterogeneous, which is reflected by detected PO_2 ranging from 0% to 100%, namely, from anoxia to normoxia. It is plausible that paradoxical activation of associated factors under hypoxia is also heterogeneous and dynamic in solid tumor, implying that focusing on one single target factor is insufficient to carry out an effective therapy. To date, although HIF-1α has been comprehensively studied under different hypoxic conditions, it is not the case in the study of short period of severe hypoxia as well as chronic moderate hypoxia. This can be partially explained by the fact that regulation of HIF-1α is actually a negative feedback loop via HIF-1α-dependent induction of prolyl hydroxylase enzymes that promote the von Hippel-Lindau (VHL) tumour suppressor protein-mediated HIF-1α degradation by ubiquitin-proteasome system under moderate hypoxia. On the contrary, the induction of prolyl hydroxylase enzymes is inhibited under severe hypoxia. Activation of eIF2α has been indicated as a transient process during severe hypoxia, which is decreased following the prolonged duration of hypoxic status. Under moderate hypoxia, eIF2α exhibits a gradually elevated activation along with elongation of hypoxic time.

4. Role of cancer stem cells (CSCs) in hypoxia-induced therapeutic resistance in HNSCC

4.1 Identification of CSCs in HNSCC

The theory of CSCs, as a milestone of cancer research, has a history of 150 years. The focus of this theory is that there exists a sub-group of tumor cells, like stem cells of normal tissues, with stem traits characterizing growth stasis and self-renewal with specific cell surface markers. This subset of cells within the tumor bulk is known as "cancer stem cells" (CSCs) or "tumor initiating cells (TICs)". Other tumor cells that are considered as progeny of CSCs would face a final differentiation followed by programmed cell death. In term of CSC theory, tumor bulk only originates from CSCs; therapeutic failures in cancer management are a result of insufficient elimination of these heterogeneous subpopulation. In addition, the subset is believed to play important roles in invasion, metastasis and therapeutic resistance in various malignancies. To date, CSCs or CSC like cells have been identified in different cancer including HNSCC. In 2007, a subpopulation of cells with characterized stemness and CD44 marker in HNSCC was first isolated and identified (Prince et al, 2007). It was also demonstrated that $CD133^+$ cells in Hep-2 human squamous laryngeal carcinoma cells have stem cell-like characters (Zhou et al., 2009). Subsequently, other investigators identified a $CD133^+$ CSC-like subset with chemoresistance in oral squamous carcinoma (Zhang et al., 2009). More recently, $CD44^+$ CSCs have also been isolated and identified from human laryngeal squamous carcinoma. All these data confirm the existence of CSCs in HNSCC, which shed light on a novel area to get further insight into the mechanisms of chemo- and radioresistance in HNSCC with respect to SCCs.

4.2 CSCs and microenvironment

4.2.1 "Seeds and soil" theory

The microenvironment of CSCs also called "niche", consists of cellular and non-cellular components surrounding CSCs (Scadden, 2006), including direct cell contacts, cell-matrix contacts, cytokines, blood vessels, mesenchymal cells and so on. It serves to protect CSCs from differentiation and apoptosis, and keeps the status of self-renewing (Iwasaki & Suda, 2009). As a matter of fact, the significance of the niche function is far beyond these, as it affects the physiology of CSCs to a far more great extent. As early as 1889, through analysis of 735 cases of breast cancers, British assistant doctor Stephen Paget (Paget, 1989) found that breast cancer cells preferred liver to settle in rather than spleen that has vascular supply as abundant as liver. Nearly a century later, after the quiescence of the " seeds and soils ", Hart and Fidler (Hart & Fidler, 1980) injected melanoma cells into mice implanted with ovary tissue, kidney tissue and lung tissue in muscle or under the skin, and these implanted tissues had previously established vascular supplies of their own. Finally, they demonstrated that melanoma cells just metastasized to grafted ovary and kidney, suggesting that the formation of tumor is not only influenced by the characters of tumor cells but also depends on the niche. Because CSCs are a kind of cells that can self-renew in malignancy, the niche of CSC must be critical for preserving the property of self-renewal.

Recently, many studies provided evidence for the "seeds and soil" even as they further disclosed the relationship between CSC and its niche. A group attenuated the adhesion between CSCs and some components of the niche, such as hyaluronan, through interfering with CD44, thereby, inhibited the neoplasia of myeloid leukemia (Jin et al, 2006; Krause et al, 2006). Calabrese et al (Calabrese et al, 2007) found that most medulloblastoma stem cells grew by adhering to endothelial cells selectively, and these CD133+ cells could give rise to new tumors only when co-transplanted with endothelial cells. Kaplan et al (Kaplan et al, 2005) introduced a concept of "premetastatic niche", which meant the microenvironment of metastasized organs had been induced to transform into a condition better for the formation of secondary tumor. All of the findings above suggest that targeting the niche will be a very significant approach to eliminate CSCs.

4.2.2 Niche and heterogeneity

Species are selected by adaptation to environmental changes as proven by the earliest dinosaurs to today's diverse biological species. Such is Darwinian evolution, a possible explanation for survival. The development of tumors might be a process of survival of the fittest by the pressure of microenvironment.

It is known to all that cells in various types of tumors are different from each other in many aspects, such as size, appearance, antigen expression, cell membrane composition and sensitivity to different treatment modalities (Ichim & Wells, 2006; Heppner, 1984; Axelson, 2005). There are two explanatory models to the potential heterogeneity of the tumor cells, the stochastic model and the hierarchical model. Firstly, the stochastic model attributes the tumor development to the "genetic instability", through which the ones best adapting to the microenvironment are selected to obtain the advantage of proliferation (Nowell, 1976; Tysnes & Bjerkvig, 2007). This model shows that the tumor parenchyma contains many types of tumor cells with the ability to form tumors in the microenvironment (Bjerkvig, 2009). Secondly, the hierarchical model supports that the initial tumor and the metastatic tumor are both evolved from CSCs, which seems contradicting to the first model.

The two controversial models are currently interpreted by some recent investigations. Odoux et al (Odoux et al, 2008) found that a small number of CSCs subsets with the ability of self-renewal and differentiation exist in liver metastases in patients suffering from colon cancer, and this sub-group of cells are more invasive and expanding than the CSCs in the primary tumor. Surprisingly, as a considered decisive element in the evolution of tumor (Cahill et al, 2009), genetic instability was present in this subset. A recent genomics study found that aberrant stem cells significantly express the regulatory protein molecules which function to adapt to microenvironmental stimuli with respect to the gene expression profile of murine embryonic stem cell lines and its malignant counterpart, murine teratocarcinoma cell lines (Heffron, 2007). Campbell and Polyak (Campbell & Polyak, 2007) integrated the results of their research on breast cancer and a number of related reports, and ended up with that the heterogeneity of tumor cells may be due to the combination of some levels of the stochastic model and the hierarchical model. They found that the origin of breast cancer may initially be normal CD44-expression stem cells or progenitor cells, which undergo self-renewal, differentiation and mutation-driven clonal evolution motivated by the environmental changes and gene mutations, resulting in a bunch of different genotypes and diverse stages of development of tumor cells. This indicates that the hierarchical model in cancer stem cell theory is the extension of the stochastic model. Tumor tissues are evolved through genetic alterations, phenotypic changes and the impacts of micro-environment. So there may be more than one type of stem cell subsets with different characteristics in parenchyma, which exhibits different genetic or epigenetic phenotypes and ability to adapt to microenvironment, and the distinct characteristics of epithelial to mesenchymal transition (Werb & Evans, 2004). Therefore, not all CSCs have the ability to survive and metastasize, only those with the ability to adapt to the microenvironment are selected (Odoux, C et al, 2008; Lagasse, 2008) to do so.

4.2.3 Hypoxia and CSCs

As is known, CSCs are a subpopulation of tumor cells that co-exist with differentiated tumor cells in the same microenvironment, in which hypoxia serves as a necessary component for CSCs growth, self-renewal and differentiation (Keith & Simon, 2007). It has been demonstrated that HIF-1α could induce the expression of some crucial genes related with CSCs' self-renewal and multipotency, including Oct4 and Notch1. Under hypoxia, stable expression of HIF-1α in CSCs can stimulate expressions of Oct4 and Notch1, and activate the associated signaling of critical pathways, promoting specific properties of CSCs and related multipotency. In view of the mentioned above, we can introduce the concept of interaction between tumor hypoxic microenvironment and CSCs. Traditionally, the standard for evaluating the efficacy of a treatment regimen is the sizable contraction of the tumor bulk. However, most tumor relapse after a period of paracmasis, probably because traditional chemo- and radiotherapy only kill tumor cells in rapid proliferation and differentiation rather than CSCs, the latter of which with are in slow divisions and proliferation, conferring therapeutic resistance. The formation of the relapsed tumor is driven by CSCs under proper microenvironment at a certain time after the treatment regimens are completed.

4.2.4 CSC's resistance and related mechanisms

Lots of convincing data showed that CSCs subset displays powerful resistance to traditional chemo- and/or radio-therapy compared with non-CSCs of in same tumor or parent cells in vitro. Currently, the mechanisms of CSCs-related therapeutic resistance have not been well understood. Perhaps, basic principles regarding CSC-caused therapeutic resistance can be categorized as follows.

4.2.4.1 Quiescence

Lots of cytotoxic drugs mostly kill tumor cells with rapid proliferation, which settle in cellular s-phase cycle. However, it is believed that CSCs, like normal stem cells, mostly reside in G_0/G_1 phase, which reduces efficacy of anti-cancer agents.

4.2.4.2 Overexpression of protective genes

Another cause of CSCs-related resistance is that this subset overexpresses some factors that protect CSCs from apoptosis and cytotoxicity. It has been well confirmed that CSCs express high levels of ABC drug transporters. Due to ATP hydrolysis, these proteins function to efflux drugs from tumor cells to protect against cytotoxicity. ABC superfamily includes 7 subfamilies from ABCA to ABCG (ABCB1 is P-gp). Among the superfamily, ABCG2 has been studied most extensively and is believed to be the most critical transporter of drugs. However, in clinic, targeting on ABCG2 alone has a minimal effect in the correction of chemorisistance by cancers, suggesting other ABC components also participate in chemoresistance or CSC's resistance is not determined only by ABC transporters. Liu et al (Liu et al, 2006) isolated CD133-positive tumor cells from glioblastoma and demonstrated that along with ABC transporters, these CSCs overexpressed anti-apoptotic factors, such as BCL-XL, Xiap, Survivin as well as cIAPs and DNA repair protein MGMT, which suggests that powerful repair ability combined with anti-apoptotic features may be partially responsible for CSC's resistance. Through studying CSCs from hepatocellular carcinoma (HCC), Ma et al (Ma et al, 2008) demonstrated that HCC CSCs confer chemorestistance via preferential induction of AKT/PKB and BCL-2 survival pathways. Using specific AKT1 inhibitors, survival of HCC CSCs can be abolished.

5. How to cope with the therapeutic resistance induced by hypoxia

5.1 Targeting genes related with hypoxia

Based on the mentioned above, it is evident that blockage of paradoxical activation of genes by transgenic techniques or improvement of hypoxic status in tumor microenvironment could overcome hypoxia-induced therapeutic resistance and relapse in HNSCC. Gene therapy mostly pointing to some critical target genes and associated gene products in HIF-1α, UPR and mTOR pathways and some activators and regulators of HIF-1α in alternative pathways such as EGFR and STAT3 pathways offers hope in this regard. However, transgenic techniques using either viral or non-viral vectors have limitations for application in human body. As previously described, dynamic hypoxic heterogeneity exists in solid tumors. It is difficult to determine the specificity and effectiveness of a single-gene targeted therapy to hypoxic cells in a huge tumor bulk. Therefore, there should be a long-term exploration before gene therapy can be used as an efficient method of modifying therapeutic resistance in HNSCC. It is likely that a strategy targeting multiple genes would be a potential solution to CSC-associated therapeutic resistance under the condition that hypoxic status in each individual tumor is evaluated objectively.

5.2 Targeting CSCs and hypoxic microenvironment

As stated, only CSCs can facilitate tumorigenesis and confer therapeutic resistance, which is the major cause of therapeutic failure. Therefore, successful targeting on CSCs is expected to provide a chance of cure for cancers. To date, targeting on CSCs has been faced with difficulties, because mechanisms underlying CSC-related therapeutic resistance have not been well understood. Although Notch, Oct-4, Wnt, Bmi and other stemness related factors were demonstrated to play a critical role in CSCs physiology, it is difficult to target them specifically in CSCs among the huge population of cancer cells. It is interesting to note that the clinical course of anti-ABCG-2 drugs in cancer treatment mirrors that of anti-bacterial agents in the control of infection. Based on this observation, some scholars believe that CSCs also experience evolutionary processes, and the driving force for these processes, selection stress by microenvironment, should be the target for cancer therapy. Although more CSCs markers have been identified in cancers, CSCs isolated by these markers are in minority, approximately 2-5%. However, increasing evidence has revealed that CSCs are not rare when isolated based on stem traits, which suggests that CSC markers are limited and not all CSCs express the same markers. Therefore, it is possible that CSCs are existing in separate subpopulations with distinct biological features, which are affected by their niche, and what is worse, these features are in constant change. Given that targeting CSCs is a putative approach, it would be much more important to concentrate on the manipulation of niche as the direct target in curing cancers. For example, we can resort to approaches to maintain the homeostasis of the niche by manipulating non-cellular components, especially fluctuating hypoxia. Consistent with this idea, traditional Chinese medicine (TCM) is to cure the disease by rectifying imbalance in body environment and re-establish the homeostasis of the human body, which may offer some hope in this regard. And intriguingly, lots of herbs have been identified as antioxidant compounds. Cai et al (Cai et al, 2004) have demonstrated that 112 traditional chinese medicinal plants used as anti-cancer herbs have a more powerful antioxidant activity compared with common vegetables and fruits which are considered as good natural sources of dietary antioxidants. Tang et al (Tang et al, 2004) also identified the antioxidant function of TCM extracts. These pieces of evidence implicate that TCM is a promising strategy capable of targeting on ROS-induced evolution of CSCs. Indeed, data from several reports have provided direct evidence that some herbs in TCM could target CSCs. Observations made by Jiang et al (Jiang et al, 1983) demonstrated that camptothecin and harringtonin could inhibit the clonal formation of human stem cells. Furthermore, anti-tumor and therapeutic resistance-reversing effects of some phytochemicals such as Curcumin have been confirmed and proven to be prospective, which exhibit the capability of targeting side population cells (Fong et al, 2010). More recently, high inhibitory effect on breast cancer cells was acquired by combining stealthy liposomes from vinorelbine and parthenolide (Liu et al, 2008). Taken together, chemotherapy combined with TCM may dominate anti-cancer treatment if the niche is properly manipulated to overcome the chemoresisitance of CSCs resulting from genetic instability.

5.3 Inducing UPR pro-death arms

As is known, UPR is a double-edged sword. On the one side, it can help tumor cells relieve hypoxic stress； On the other hand, UPR can induce apoptosis or autophagy-related cell death under severe stress. Induction of UPR pro-death arms may be a promising modality to reverse hypoxia-induced resistance to traditional therapy. At this point, some agents, such as PIs, which can enhance ER overload, represent a promising perspective. PIs inhibit proteasome to reduce ERAD, which can intensify ER-stress caused by accumulation of unfolded protein. Recently, Fels et al (Fels et al, 2008) found that PIs can effectively enhance UPR responses of hypoxic tumor cells and ameliorating ER-stress can reverse PIs effects. They demonstrated that hypoxic tumor cells treated by PIs underwent apoptosis, autophagy and necrosis. Intriguingly, some groups reported that tumor cells can activate STAT3 to resist PIs therapy in HNSCC (C. Li et al, 2009). Therefore, PIs combined with STAT3 inhibition could achieve potential efficiency.

5.4 Chopping off hypoxia from the "root"

For strategies used to improve local hypoxia, some groups have tried using inhalation of Carbogen（95%O2 and 5%CO2）and hyperbaric oxygen chambers to improve local hypoxic condition within tumors, and thus therapeutic resistance, but the results are not as satisfactory. In this regard, it is necessary to modify traditional approaches and to explore a new way of oxygen delivery to rectify the intratumoral hypoxic condition. It is a common sense that vascular structure of tumor is very different from its counterpart of normal tissue, the former of which exhibits architectural distortion, higher permeability and irregular infuse, facilitating fluctuating hypoxia and providing specific target strategy. Vascular disrupting agents (VDAs) serve as a novel type of anti-cancer target agent. In contrast with angiogenesis inhibitors (AIs) that mostly prevent neoformation of vascular structure, VDAs directly block or damage existing blood vessels in tumor bulk to commit necrosis. To date, VDAs have been in phase of clinic trails, and small molecular VDAs have been mostly studied. The mechanisms of VDAs action include: 1) induce TNF-α secretion by tumor cells to cause apoptosis of endothelial cells constituting microvessels; 2) through binding to microtubule protein, VDAs facilitate disaggregation of microtubules to damage cell skeleton of vascular endothelium. VDAs have been believed to cause intratumoral necrosis, leaving the remaining periphery to be oxygenated. Therefore, combination of VDAs may cut both fluctuating and continuous hypoxia from the "boot".

Although improvement of tumor hypoxia has been achieved, imaging results are not always consistent with changes of endogenous markers of hypoxia, indicating that the improvement of intratumor hypoxia as observed by imaging does not represent the thorough rectification of intracellular hypoxic metabolisms of the cancer cells. Therefore, it is highly likely that there exist a "time gap" between improvement of intratumor hypoxia and thorough rectification of intracellular hypoxic metabolisms. Currently, length of this window phase is unclear. It is of paramount importance for hypoxic cells to gain thorough recovery of the intracellular oxygenation using this compensation time and become more susceptible to chemoratiation.

6. Future directions

Up till now, the impact of hypoxia on CSCs in HNSCC and its relation between chemo- and radiotherapeutic resistance is largely unknown. To further elucidate the causes of chemo- and radiotherapeutic resistance and post-treatment relapse in HNSCC with respect to effects of tumor microenvironment on tumor cells, the first step is to study how hypoxic microenvironment regulates CSCs in HNSCC. Through establishment of HIF-1α knock-down cell lines (HIF-1α$^{-/-}$), the correlation between induction of HIF-1α and related gene expressions associated with self-renewal as well as multipotency of CSCs is to be observed. Meanwhile, the differential expression of these genes between CD133^{+} and CD133^{-} cells must be documented. Furthermore, the proliferative activity of CD133^{+} CSCs should be measured by culturing HIF-1α$^{+/+}$ and HIF-1α$^{-/-}$ cells under normal or hypoxic conditions, thereby to understand whether hypoxic microenvironment modulates the differentiation and proliferation of CSCs by regulation of HIF-1α in HNSCC.

The established concept of interaction between tumor hypoxic microenvironment and CSCs helps us to further understand the mechanisms behind the therapeutic resistance in HNSCC. If CSCs are taken as anti-cancer targets, the strategies by focusing on tumor microenvironment will be promising for purposely intervention of CSCs (Iwasaki & Suda, 2009). It can be inferred that CSCs are the critical element responsible for therapeutic resistance in HNSCC. Improving hypoxic conditions and regulating CSCs-related signaling pathways during chemo- and radiotherapy of HNSCC offers hope for reversion of therapeutic sensitivity in HNSCC and elimination of therapeutic resistance and relapse, aiming at improving outcomes of HNSCC.

7. References

Al-Sarraf, M. (1987). Chemotherapeutic management of head and neck cancer. Cancer and Metastasis Reviews, Vol 6, No. (3), pp. 181–98. ISSN 0167-7659

Argiris, A., Karamouzis, MV., Raben, D. & Ferris, RL. (2008). Head and neck cancer. Lancet, Vol 371, No. (9625), pp. 1695–1709. ISSN 0140-6736

Axelson, H., Fredlund, E., Ovenberger, M., Landberg, G. & Pahlman S. (2005). Hypoxia-induced dedifferentiation of tumor cells—a mechanism behind heterogeneity and aggressiveness of solid tumors. Seminars in Cell & Developmental Biology, Vol. 16 No. (4-5), pp. 554-563. ISSN 1084-9521

Bjerkvig, R., Johansson, M., Miletic, H. & Niclou, SP. (2009). Cancer stem cells and angiogenesis. Seminars in Cancer Biology, Vol. 19 No. (5), pp. 279–284. ISSN 1044-579X

Cahill, DP., Kinzler, KP., Vogelstein, B. & Lengauer, C. (1999). Genetic instability and darwinian selection in tumours. Trends in Cell Biology, Vol, 9 No. (12), pp. 57–60. ISSN 0962-8924

Cai, Y., Luo, Q., Sun, M. & Corke, H. (2004). Antioxidant activity and phenolic compounds of 112 traditional Chinese medicinal plants associated with anticancer. Life Sciences, Vol 74, No. (17), pp. 2157–2184. ISSN 0024-3205

Calabrese, C., Poppleton, H., Kocak, M., Hogg, TL., Fuller, C., Hamner, B., Oh, EY., Gaber, MW., Finklestein, D., Allen, M., Frank, A., Bayazitov, IT., Zakharenko, SS., Gajjar, A., Davidoff, A. & Gilbertson, RJ. (2007). A perivascular niche for brain tumor stem cells. Cancer Cell, Vol. 11 No. (1), pp. 69–82. ISSN 1535-6108

Campbell, LL. & Polyak, K. (2007). Breast Tumor Heterogeneity - Cancer Stem Cells or Clonal Evolution? Cell Cycle, Vol. 6 No. (19), pp. 2332–2338. ISSN 1538-4101

Cárdenas-Navia, LI., Secomb, TW., & Dewhirst, MW. (2007). Effects of fluctuating oxygenation on tirapazamine efficacy: Theoretical predictions. International Journal of Radiation Oncology Biology Physics, Vol 67, No. (2), pp. 581–586. ISSN 0360-3016

Cárdenas-Navia, LI., Mace, D., Richardson, RA., Wilson, DF., Shan, S. & Dewhirst MW. (2008). The pervasive presence of fluctuating oxygenation in tumors. Cancer Research, Vol 68, No. (14), pp. 5812–5819. ISSN 0008-5472

Cohen, EE., Lingen, MW. & Vokes, EE. (2004). The expanding role of systemic therapy in head and neck cancer. Journal of Clinical Oncology, Vol 22, No.(9), pp: 1743–1752. ISSN 0732-183X

Fels, DR., Ye, J., Segan, AT., Kridel, SJ., Spiotto, M., Olson, M., Koong, AC. & Koumenis, C. (2008). Preferential cytotoxicity of bortezomib toward hypoxic tumor cells via overactivation of endoplasmic reticulum stress pathways. Cancer Research, Vol 68, No. (22), pp. 9323–9330. ISSN 0008-5472

Fong, D., Yeh, A., Naftalovich, R., Choi, TH. & Chan, MM. (2010). Curcumin inhibits the side population (SP) phenotype of the rat C6 glioma cell line: towards targeting of cancer stem cells with phytochemicals. Cancer Letters, Vol 293, No. (1), pp. 65–72. ISSN 0304-3835

Hart, IR. & Fidler, IJ. (1980) Role of organ selectivity in the determination of metastatic patterns of B16 melanoma. Cancer Research, Vol. 40 No. (7), pp. 2281–2287. ISSN 0008-5472

Heffron, CC., Gallagher, MF., Guenther, S., Sherlock, J., Henfrey, R., Martin, C., Sheils, O. & O'Leary, JJ. (2007). Global mRNA analysis to determine a transcriptome profile of cancer stemness in a mouse model. Anticancer Research, Vol. 27 No. (3A), pp. 1319–1324. ISSN 0250-7005

Heppner, GH. (1984). Tumor heterogeneity. Cancer Reserch, Vol. 44 No. (6), pp. 2259–2265. ISSN 0008-5472

Ichim, CV. & Wells, RA. (2006). First among equals: The cancer cell hierarchy.Leukemia & Lymphoma, Vol. 47 No. (10), pp. 2017–2027. ISSN 1042-8194

Iwasaki, H. & Suda, T. (2009). Cancer stem cells and their niche. Cancer Science, Vol 100, No. (7), pp. 1166–1174. ISSN 1347-9032

Jiang, TL., Salmon, SE. & Liu, RM. (1983). Activity of camptothecin, harringtonin, cantharidin and curcumae in the human tumor stem cell assay. European Journal of Cancer & Clinical Oncology, Vol 19, No (2), pp. 263-270. ISSN 1078-8956

Jin, L., Hope, KJ., Zhai, Q., Smadja-Joffe, F. & Dick, JE. (2006). Targeting of CD44 eradicates human acute myeloid leukemic stem cells. Nature Medicine, Vol. 12 No. (10), pp. 1167–1174. ISSN 1078-8956

Kaplan, RN., Riba, RD., Zacharoulis, S., Bramley, AH., Vincent, L., Costa, C., MacDonald, DD., Jin, DK., Shido, K., Kerns, SA., Zhu, Z., Hicklin, D., Wu, Y., Port, JL., Altorki, N., Port, ER., Ruggero, D., Shmelkov, SV., Jensen, KK., Rafii, S. & Lyden, D. (2005). VEGFR1-positive haematopoietic bone marrow progenitors initiate the pre-metastatic niche. Nature, Vol. 438 No. (7069), pp. 820–827. ISSN 0028-0836

Keith, B. & Simon, MC. (2007). Hypoxia-inducible factors, stem cells, and cancer. Cell, Vol 129, No (3), pp. 465-472. ISSN 0092-8674

Kimura, H., Braun, RD., Ong, ET., Hsu, R., Secomb, TW., Papahadjopoulos, D., Hong, K. & Dewhirst, MW. (1996). Fluctuations in red cell flux in tumor microvessels can lead to transient hypoxia and reoxygenation in tumor parenchyma. Cancer Research, Vol 56, No (23), pp. 5522-5523. ISSN 0008-5472

Koumenis, C. & Wouters, BG. (2006). "Translating" tumor hypoxia: unfolded protein response (UPR)-dependent and UPR-independent pathways. Molecular Cancer Research, Vol 4, No. (7), pp. 423–436. ISSN 1541-7786

Krause, DS., Lazarides, K., von Andrian, UH. & Van Etten, RA. (2006). Requirement for CD44 in homing and engraftment of BCR-ABL-expressing leukemic stem cells. Nature Medicine, Vol. 12 No. (10), pp. 1175–1180. ISSN 1078-8956

Lagasse, E. (2008). Cancer stem cells with genetic instability: the best vehicle with the best engine for cancer. Gene Therapy, Vol. 15 No. (2), pp. 136–142. ISSN 0969-7128

Lavaf, A., Genden, EM., Cesaretti, JA., Packer, S. & Kao, J. (2008). Adjuvant radiotherapy improves overall survival for patients with lymph node-positive head and neck squamous cell carcinoma. Cancer. Vol. 112, No. (3), pp. 535–543. ISSN 0008-543X

Li, C., Zang, Y., Sen, M., Leeman-Neill, RJ., Man, DS., Grandis, JR. & Johnson, DE. (2009). Bortezomib up-regulates activated signal transducer and activator of transcription-3 and synergizes with inhibitors of signal transducer and activator of transcription-3 to promote head and neck squamous cell carcinoma cell death. Molecular Cancer Therapeutics, Vol 8, No (8), pp. 2211-2220. ISSN 1535-7163

Li, X., Di, B., Shang, Y., Zhou, Y., Cheng, J. & He, Z. (2009). Clinicopathologic risk factors for distant metastases from head and neck squamous cell carcinomas. European Journal Surgical Oncology, Vol 35, No 12, () pp. 1348-1358. ISSN 0748-7983

Li, X., Wang, H., Lu, X. & Di, B. (2010a). Stat3 blockade with shRNA enhances radiosensitivity in Hep-2 human laryngeal squamous carcinoma cells. Oncology Reports, Vol 23, No (2), pp. 345-353 ISSN 1021-335X

Li, X., Wang, H., Lu X. & Di, B. (2010b). Silencing STAT3 with short hairpin RNA enhances the radiosensitivity of xenograft human laryngeal squamous cell carcinoma in vivo. Experimental and Therapeutic Medicine, Vol 1, No (6), pp. 947-953 ISSN 1792-0981

Liu, G., Yuan, X., Zeng, Z., Tunici, P., Ng, H., Abdulkadir, IR., Lu, L., Irvin, D., Black, KL. & Yu, JS. (2006). Analysis of gene expression and chemoresistance of $CD133^+$ cancer stem cells in glioblastoma. Molecular Cancer, Vol 5, No (67), pp. ISSN 1476-4598

Liu, Y., Lu, WL., Guo, J., Du, J., Li, T., Wu, JW., Wang, GL., Wang, JC., Zhang, X. & Zhang, Q. (2008). A potential target associated with both cancer and cancer stem cells: a combination therapy for eradication of breast cancer using vinorelbine stealthy liposomes plus parthenolide stealthy liposomes. Journal of Controlled Release, Vol 129, No (1), pp. 18-25. ISSN 0168-3659

Ma, S., Lee, TK., Zheng, BJ., Chan, KW. & Guan, XY. (2008). CD133+ HCC cancer stem cells confer chemoresistance by preferential expression of the Akt/PKB survival pathway. Oncogene, Vol 27, No (12), pp. 1749-1758 ISSN 0950-9232

Nowell, PC. (1976). The clonal evolution of tumor cell populations. Science, Vol. 194 No. (4260), pp. 23–28. ISSN 0036-8075

Odoux, C., Fohrer, H., Hoppo, T., Guzik, L., Stolz, DB., Lewis, DW., Gollin, SM., Gamblin, TC., Geller, DA. & Lagasse, E. (2008). A Stochastic Model for Cancer Stem Cell Origin in Metastatic Colon Cancer. Cancer Research, Vol. 68 No. (17), pp. 6932–6941. ISSN 0008-5472

Prince, ME., Sivanandan, R., Kaczorowski, A., Wolf, GT., Kaplan, MJ., Dalerba, P., Weissman, IL., Clarke, MF. & Ailles, LE. (2007). Identification of a subpopulation of cells with cancer stem cell properties in head and neck squamous cell carcinoma. Proceedings of the National Academy of Sciences of the United States of America, Vol. 104, No. (3), pp. 973–978. ISSN 0027-8424

Paget, S. (1989). The distribution of secondary growths in cancer of the breast. Cancer and Metastasis Reviews, Vol. 8 No. (2), pp. 98–101. ISSN 0167-7659

Rofstad, EK., Gaustad, JV., Egeland, TA., Mathiesen, B. & Galappathi K. (2010). Tumors exposed to acute cyclic hypoxic stress show enhanced angiogenesis, perfusion and metastatic dissemination. International Journal of Cancer, Vol. 127, No. (7), pp. 1535–1546. ISSN 0020-7136

Scadden, DT. (2006). The stem-cell niche as an entity of action. Nature, Vol. 441 No. (7097), pp. 1075–1079. ISSN 1078-8956

Selvendiran K, Bratasz A, Kuppusamy ML, Tazi MF, Rivera BK & Kuppusamy P. (2009). Hypoxia induces chemoresistance in ovarian cancer cells by activation of signal transducer and activator of transcription 3. International Journal of Cancer, Vol. 125, No. (9), pp. 2198–2204. ISSN 0020-7136

Shrime, MG., Gullane, PJ., Dawson, L., Kim, J., Gilbert, RW., Irish JC, Brown DH & Goldstein DP. (2010). The impact of adjuvant radiotherapy on survival in T1-2N1 squamous cell carcinoma of the oral cavity. Archives of Otolaryngolgoy Head & Neck Surgery, Vol. 136, No. (3), pp. 225–228. ISSN 0886-4470

Simon, AR., Rai, U., Fanburg, BL. & Cochran, BH. (1998). Activation of the JAK-STAT pathway by reactive oxygen species. American Journal of Physiology, Vol. 275, No. (6 pt 1), pp. c1640-1652. ISSN 0002-9513

Tang, SY., Whiteman, M., Peng, ZF., Jenner, A., Yong, EL. & Halliwell, B. (2004). Characterization of antioxidant and antiglycation properties and isolation of active ingredients from traditional chinese medicines. Free Radical Biology and Medicine, Vol. 36, No. (12), pp. 1575–1587. ISSN 0891-5849

Tobias, JS., Monson, K., Gupta, N., Macdougall, H., Glaholm, J., Hutchison, I., Kadalayil, L., Hackshaw, A. & UK Head and Neck Cancer Trialists' Group. (2010). Chemoradiotherapy for locally advanced head and neck cancer: 10-year follow-up of the UK Head and Neck (UKHAN1) trial. Lancet Oncology, Vol. 11, No. (1), pp. 66–74. ISSN 1470-2045

Tysnes, BB. & Bjerkvig, R. (2007). Cancer initiation and progression: involvement of stem cells and the microenvironment. Biochimica et Biophysica Acta, Vol. 1775 No. (2), pp. 283–297. ISSN 0006-3002

Vokes, EE., Weichselbaum, RR., Lippman, SM. & Hong, WK. (1993). Head and neck cancer. New England Journal of Medicine, Vol. 328, No. (3), pp: 184–94. ISSN 0028-4793

Werb, Z. & Evans, G. (2004). Oncogenes and cell proliferation: maintenance of genomic integrity, tumor stem cells, and the somatic microenvironment. Current Opinion in Genetics and Development, Vol. 14 No. (2), pp. 1–3. ISSN 0959-437X

Zhang, Q., Shi, S., Yen, Y., Brown, J., Ta, JQ. & Le, AD. (2009). A subpopulation of CD133(+) cancer stem-like cells characterized in human oral squamous cell carcinoma confer resistance to chemotherapy. Cancer Letters, Vol. 289 No. (2), pp. 151–160. ISSN 0304-3835

Zhou, L., Wei, X., Cheng, L., Tian, J. & Jiang, JJ. (2007). CD133, one of the markers of cancer stem cells in Hep-2 cell line. Laryngoscope, Vol. 117 No. (3), pp. 455–460. ISSN 0023-852X

14

New Therapeutic Strategies in Small Cell Lung Cancer: The Stem Cell Target

Guadalupe Aparicio Gallego[1], Vanessa Medina Villaamil[1],
Guillermo Alonso Curbera[2] and L. Antón Aparicio[1,2,3]
[1]*Biomedical Research Institute INIBIC. Coruña University Hospital. A Coruña*
[2]*Medical Oncology Service. A Coruña University Hospital. A Coruña*
[3]*Medicine Department. University of A Coruña*
Spain

1. Introduction

In 1889, Sir S. Paget introduced the *soil and seed* hypothesis of metastasis to medicine and credited the idea to Fuchs. In Paget´s study, he concluded that the distribution of metastases cannot be due to chance alone and that different tissues provide optimal conditions for the growth of specific cancers. In the *soil and seed* metaphor, the *soil* refers to the secondary site of tumour growth and development and perhaps the chemical signals produced in the microenvironment at the sites of metastasis. The *seed* is the ostensible stem cell or tumour-initiating cell from the primary tumour. These tumour-initiating cells are the tumorigenic force behind tumour initiation, growth, metastasis, drug resistance, and relapse. In a variation of this idea, called the *homing* hypothesis, a secondary signal secreted by cells at the future metastatic sites "calls" the tumour cells to the site and permits them to proliferate in the new environment. In this hypothesis, the *seed* produces cell surface receptors that are able to recognise the site demarcated by the *soil*. Although the mechanisms that define tissue specificity remain obscure, researchers have focused on small messenger molecules as attractants and larger cell surface receptors that guide the tumour-initiating cells. Based on the hypothesis introduced by Paget, other groups have focused on chemokines and their receptors as viable candidates for *soil and seed* signalling and have proposed a "spatial and temporal code" composed of specific combinations of such molecules, while other molecules are responsible for neovascularisation, metastasis, and immunosurveillance avoidance. Lung cancers result from complex genetic and epigenetic changes and are characterised by stepwise malignant progression of cancer cells with an associated accumulation of genetic alterations. This process, referred to as multistep carcinogenesis, develops through the clonal evolution of initiated lung cells. Initiation consists of the acquisition of defined genetic alterations in a small number of genes that confer a proliferative advantage and facilitate progression towards invasive neoplasia. Although many of these genetic changes occur independently of histological type, their frequency and timing of occurrence with respect to cancer progression differ between small cell lung carcinomas (SCLC), which may originate from epithelial cells with neuroendocrine features, and non-SCLCs, which originate from bronchial, bronchiolar or alveolar epithelial cells. Furthermore, a number of genetic and epigenetic differences have been identified between squamous cell carcinoma (SCC), which arises from bronchial epithelial cells through a squamous metaplasia/dysplasia process, and adenocarcinoma (ADC), which is derived from alveolar or bronchiolar epithelial cells. Hence, lung tumours have been classified according to tumour morphology, but classification is complicated by the fact that a number of different histologic tumour characteristics frequently exist within the same neoplasm. In the 1990s, SCLC accounted for approximately one-quarter of all lung cancers, but a recent Surveillance Epidemiology and End Results (SEER) database analysis found that the incidence has since decreased to approximately 13%. SCLC now accounts for 15% of all newly diagnosed lung cancers and 60% to 70% of patients present with extensive stage (ES) tumours. For patients with limited-stage (LS)-SCLC, standard treatment has consisted of chemotherapy combined with radiotherapy (RT), while chemotherapy alone has been the standard for ES-SCLC patients. Despite a high initial rate of response to chemotherapy, most patients die from rapid recurrence. The median range of survival time after diagnosis for patients with ES-SCLC is 8 to 10 months, and only 5% to 10% of patients survive for as long as 2 years. Although chemotherapy is an essential component in the treatment of SCLC, improvements in survival in the past two decades have primarily been achieved through the appropriate application of radiotherapy. The standard treatment for patients outside of clinical trials is as follows: LS-SCLC patients receive combination chemotherapy, which generally consists of cisplatin and etoposide, with concurrent thoracic radiotherapy; and ES-SCLC patients receive combination chemotherapy (etoposide and cisplatin or carboplatin). The current standard treatment for most cancers involves some combination of chemotherapy, hormonal therapy, radiation treatment, and a growing list of molecularly targeted therapeutics, depending on the tumour characteristics and stage. Following treatment, tumour regression is normally used as an indicator of therapeutic success. To better treat cancer, the new ideas regarding CSCs must be integrated into our strategies for clinical intervention. One approach to inhibit cancer stem cells is to target the proteins that are essential for the growth and maintenance of stem cells, such as the growth regulatory pathways that function in embryonic cells. One pathway, controlled by the Hedgehog (Hh) signalling molecule, contains several genes that function as either tumour suppressor genes or oncogenes. Other pathways that are critical to embryonic development and are potentially important in cancer have also been described, including the Wnt and Notch pathways. These pathways are also subjects of drug development for the treatment of a number of conditions.

2. Development of the airway

The respiratory system is an outgrowth of the ventral wall of the foregut, and the epithelium of the larynx, trachea, bronchi, and alveoli originates in the endoderm. The cartilaginous, muscular, and connective tissue components arise in the mesoderm. In the fourth week of development, the tracheo-oesophageal septum separates the trachea from the foregut, dividing the foregut into the lung bud anteriorly and the oesophagus posteriorly. Lungs are composed of two primary tissue layers, namely epithelium and mesenchyme. Previous investigations have demonstrated that mutual interactions between these two tissues are essential for the sequential events of organogenesis, determination, growth, morphogenesis, and cytodifferentiation. This mutual interaction is defined as embryonic induction. The morphogenesis and cytodifferentiation of embryonic lung epithelial components are modulated by surrounding mesenchymal components. In embryonic organs that are formed by a process of progressive branching of the epithelium, such as the lung, the mesenchyme plays a determining role in the formation of the characteristic morphology of the organ. Increasing evidence has suggested that the formation of the tracheo-bronchial tree and alveoli results from heterogeneity of the epithelial-mesenchymal interactions along the developing respiratory tract. Genetic data have supported this idea and shown that this heterogeneity is likely the result of activation of distinct networks of signalling molecules along the proximal-distal axis. Among these signals, fibroblast growth factors, retinoids, Sonic hedgehog and transforming growth factors appear to play prominent roles. Variable levels of FGFs, Shh, TGFβ, EGF, retinoid receptors, and other signals that play a role in lung morphogenesis have been reported in the adult lung. Increasing genetic evidence has suggested that the Gli genes play multiple roles during prenatal development, particularly in the lung. All three genes are widely expressed during embryonic development in distinct but sometimes overlapping domains. The extent to which these regulators are expressed during adult life to mediate cellular activities in processes such as post-injury repair and compensatory lung growth is currently unclear. Lung bud initiation has been well-established to be regulated by the Sonic hedgehog (Shh) signalling pathway, by fibroblast growth factor (FGF) receptor signalling, and likely by retinoid-related signalling. Branching morphogenesis is a dichotomous branching process that involves defining the proximal-distal structure of the conducting airway prior to the saccular stage and is dependent on the integrated effects of the conducting airway prior to the saccular stage. Several growth factors have been implicated in branching morphogenesis. Epidermal growth factor (EGF) and transforming growth factor (TGFα) are expressed in embryonic murine lung; both factors influence growth and branching morphogenesis. During early lung branching, the EGF protein is present in bronchial epithelial cells, whereas the EGF mRNA is localised to the mesenchyme; this discordance between the location of the protein and mRNA suggests that EGF is produced by the mesenchyme and acts on the epithelium. EGF receptors (EGFR) have been found in epithelial cells and in the mesenchyme surrounding the branching epithelium of the mouse lung. These data are compatible with the notion that EGF acts in an autocrine and paracrine fashion. Retinoic acid (RA) and glucocorticoid signalling pathways have long been appreciated as major contributors to prenatal and postnatal lung maturation, and some evidence exists for their coordination or antagonism during lung development. Retinoic acid also plays an important role in morphogenesis. RA stimulates lung epithelial branching activity via an epithelial-mesenchymal interaction that, in part, involves the up-regulation of the expression of EGFR, Insulin-like Growth Factors (IGF), basic Fibroblast Growth Factor (bFGF-2), and PDGF.

3. The airway stem cells

For several years, a consensus has been achieved that various types of stem cells exist, differing according to their position within the pulmonary tree, and that the stem cells often form pools that are ready to proliferate in response to injury and effect local repair. The classical subdivision of the airway tree into regions with individual stem cell harbours was accepted many years ago. Thus, the local repopulating cells of the trachea (basal, mucous secretory), bronchus (basal, mucous secretory), bronchiole (Clara) and alveolus (type II peneumocytes) remain, for the most part, the first reserve of airway stem cells. Stem cell research in the lung has progressed rather slowly due to the anatomical and functional complexities associated with the numerous distinct cell types. This organ must be divided into various anatomical regions when considering multipotent progenitor or stem cells. Evidence has clearly suggested that multipotent progenitors of the conducting airway epithelium and gas-exchange alveolar regions are derived from different populations of stem cells that are anatomically separated in the lung. Stem cell niches in the conducting airways must also be uniquely divided between the proximal and distal regions. Bronchial airways harbour at least two distinct progenitor cell populations. Both basal and non-ciliated secretory cell types of the bronchial airways have been shown to exhibit proliferative capacity. The disparity between bronchial and bronchiolar airways is consistent with a mechanism in which the activity of distinct progenitor cell pools accounts for the regional differences both in lineage specifications during lung development and in the cellular composition of tracheo-bronchial and bronchiolar airways (Table 1).

Tissue	Epithelial stem cell niche	Daughter cells
Lung proximal	Tracheal basal cell	Mucous, ciliated, neuroendocrine
	Tracheal mucus-gland duct cell	Mucous, ciliated, neuroendocrine
	Tracheal secretory cell	Mucous, ciliated, neuroendocrine
	Bronchiolar Clara cell	Mucous, ciliated (Type I/II pneumocyte)
Distal	Alveolar type II pneumocyte	Type I and II pneumocytes (Clara cells),
	Neuroendocrine	PNEC (and Clara cells)

Table 1. Stem or progenitor cell characteristics in the airway

Epithelial cell composition and zone boundaries depend on both the species and the individual animal history. In normal mice, a renewing cell system encompassing a gland-containing, pseudostratified epithelium with Clara cells and few goblet cells is present in the upper trachea. In rats, a similar system, but with more goblet cells and no Clara cells, is present in the entire trachea, whereas this zone in humans penetrates many bronchial generations. Distally, the airway epithelium becomes glandless and cuboidal. This region is dominated by a Clara cell based lineage system before its transformation into a type II cell-based system in the alveoli. Stem cell niches in the airway have been characterised through experiments with rodent models. Stem cells in the proximal mouse trachea reside in the submucous gland duct, whereas those from the bronchi and bronchioles come from a subset of cells expressing a Clara-cell-specific protein located near neuroendocrine bodies and bronchoalveolar-duct junctions.

4. Stem cells and lung cancer

Stem cells give rise to a number of different cell types that can be classified into three groups: fully differentiated cells, transit-amplifying cells, and stem cells. The fully differentiated cells are mitotically inactive cells. These cells are at the end stages of cellular differentiation and will never re-enter the active cell cycle. The transit-amplifying (TA) cells are fast growing cells that are not fully differentiated. TA cells are able to proliferate for several generations, but they eventually terminally differentiate and must be replenished by the SC. Pluripotency is the ability of a SC to differentiate into the heterogeneous population of cells that comprise a tissue or, in the case of cancer stem cells (CSCs), a tumour. There is growing evidence that some, if not all, tumours are derived from cells with the stem cell properties of self-renewal, multilineage potential, and proliferative capacity. Stem cells are candidates as the "cell of origin" for cancer because they have a pre-existing capacity for self-renewal and unlimited replication. In addition, stem cells are relatively long-lived compared to other cells within tissues. They therefore have a greater opportunity to accumulate the multiple additional mutations that may be required to increase the rate of cell proliferation and produce clinically significant cancers. Recent work has suggested that a subpopulation of cancer cells with stem-cell-like properties may be critical for triggering tumour development. Insights into the function and characteristics of CSCs offer a novel approach to understanding the progression of metastasis. Given that a single cancer cell can drive the formation of a metastatic tumour, CSCs are likely responsible for distant tumourigenesis and primary tumour formation. Thus, research focussed on the role of CSCs in primary lesions has led to discovery that CSCs can drive tumour formation in leukaemia and various solid tumours. While little work has been done to elucidate the role of CSCs in metastasis, properties of CSCs, such as self-renewal and differentiation, make them logical candidates as metastatic colonisers. To facilitate the discussion of CSCs with different metastatic ability, a distinction should be made when referring to two potential subtypes of CSCs: primary tumour cancer stem cells (pCSCs) and metastatic cancer stem cells (mCSCs). The first, pCSCs, constitute the original population of tumorigenic cells that initiate the formation of haematopoietic and solid tumours and are the centre of most CSC. The second group, mCSCs, represent a distinct population of cells with the intrinsic properties to disseminate from the primary site and generate the distant metastases. Although other cell subpopulations may break free of the primary tumour and invade the blood stream, mCSCs, like their pCSCs counterparts, are solely responsible for the initiation of tumours. mCSCs are related to pCSCs in the essential properties of self-renewal and differentiation that are needed for the propagation of the bulk of the tumour, but the two cell types differ in key ways. Unlike pCSCs, mCSCs disseminate from the tumour, colonise foreign tissue, and likely have additional alterations (whether mutational, epigenetic, or adaptive) that allow survival and propagation in secondary sites. The key to developing effective future therapies thus seems to be the identification and characterisation of these cancer stem cells and the development of drugs that specifically target these cells. Classically, the stem/progenitor cells of the pulmonary epithelium have been considered the basal cells in the proximal airways, Clara cells in the bronchioles and type II pneumocytes in the alveoli. There is evidence that the basal and parabasal cells are stem cells in the human lung. Clara cells have been shown to be the progenitors of themselves and of ciliated cells in the bronchioles. Recent research has established that a subset of Clara cells fulfils the criteria of adult, niche-specific stem cells. Pools of stem cells have been discovered that express Clara cell secretory protein (CCSP) but are not typical Clara cells. These variant CCSP-expressing (or vCE) cells show multipotent differentiation. The vCE cells are located in discrete pools in neuroepithelial bodies and at the broncho-alveolar duct junction. In the trachea and bronchi, the basal cells are widely believed to be stem cells. The basal cells and the parabasal cells that lie just above them certainly form a pluripotential reserve cell that, unlike the surrounding epithelium, usually survives injury. Procedures that involve denuding the trachea have demonstrated the capacity of basal cells to produce all of the major cell phenotypes found in the trachea, including basal, ciliated, goblet and granular secretory cells. Controversially, pulmonary neuroendocrine cell (PNEC) populations have been suggested to be able to proliferate and serve as a reservoir of progenitor/stem cells that are capable of epithelial regeneration.

Stem/progenitor	Daughter	Lineage progression
Basal	Basal	
	Mucous	Ciliated
	Secretory	Ciliated
	PNEC	
Tracheal	Basal	
Gland duct	Mucous	
	Ciliated	
Clara	Clara	
	Ciliated	
	PNEC	
	Type II?	
Type II	Type II	
	Type I	
	PNEC	
	Clara	
PNEC	Clara	

Table 2. Possible lung cell lineages. Adapted from Otto WRJ. Pathol. 2002.

5. Small cell lung cancer

SCLC is the most common lung tumour in the spectrum of pulmonary neuroendocrine malignancies, which include typical carcinoid (TC), atypical carcinoid (AC), large-cell neuroendocrine carcinoma (LCNEC), and small-cell lung carcinoma (SCLC). The histological classification of SCLC has evolved substantially over the past several decades

	WHO (1967)	WHO (1981)	IASLC (1988)
Oat cell	Lymphocyte-like	Oat cell	Small-cell carcinoma
Polygonal	Polygonal	Intermediate	Small-cell carcinoma
	Fusiform		Mixed small-cell/large-cell carcinoma
	Other	Combined oat cell carcinoma	Combine small-cell carcinoma

WHO: World Health Organization
IALSC: International Association for the Study of Lung Cancer

Table 3. Classification of small-cell lung carcinoma

Interestingly, a large proportion of SCLC contains a component of NSCLC. Approximately 5% to 10% of patients diagnosed with SCLL will have mixed tumours, meaning that other pathologies, such as adenocarcinoma or squamous cell carcinoma, can be found within the pathologic specimen. The WHO classification of SCLC includes only one variant, combined small cell carcinoma, an SCLC with a mixed non-small-cell component (adenocarcinoma, squamous cell carcinoma, large cell carcinoma, or spindle cell or giant cell carcinoma). Although various synonyms are in the current clinical terminology (anaplastic small-cell carcinoma, small-cell undifferentiated carcinoma, small-cell neuroendocrine carcinoma, oat cell carcinoma, and mixed small-cell/large-cell carcinoma), the use of these terms is discouraged to avoid confusion. Although the precise cell of origin is not known for SCLC, there is probably a pluripotent bronchial precursor cell that can differentiate into each of the major histologic types of lung cancer. However, within the spectrum of neuroendocrine tumours, a closer morphologic and genetic similarity exists between large cell neuroendocrine carcinoma and small cell carcinoma than either typical or atypical carcinoid. Although classified as a neuroendocrine (NE) tumour, the biological origins of this cancer have remained a matter of conjecture. Recently, SCLC has been shown to be dependent on the activation of Hedgehog signalling, an embryonic pathway implicated in the regulation of stem cell fates. This finding sheds new light on the potential histogenesis of SCLC. SCLC and carcinoid tumours both show high-level expression of neuroendocrine genes. Only a few markers are shared between SCLC and carcinoids, whereas a distinct group of genes defines carcinoid tumours, suggesting that carcinoids are highly divergent from malignant lung tumours, as has been reported. Recent studies have shown that the most useful neuroendocrine markers for SCLC in formalin-fixed, paraffin-embedded tissue sections are chromogramin A, synaptophysin, Leu-7, and certain neural cell adhesion molecules (NCAMs). Bombesin or gastrin-related peptide (GRP), keratin (AE1/AE3) and membrane antigen (EMA). DNA analysis of SCLC reveals a high percentage of aneuploidy in up to 85% of cases. Finally, the expression of proliferative markers, such as PCNA, thymidylate synthase, MCM2 and MCM6, is highest in SCLC, which is known to be the most rapidly dividing lung tumour.

6. Targeted agents that have been evaluated in SCLC

Various chemotherapy schemes have been evaluated for SCLC, but the combination of cisplatin and etoposide is widely considered the standard, with observed response rates of 80-85% and approximately 25% of patients obtaining a complete response. However, most patients experience disease relapse, and neither maintenance chemotherapy nor dose-intensive chemotherapy regimens have led to improved outcomes.

6.1 Topoisomerase I and II inhibitors

A topoisomerase I inhibitor, Topotecan, has shown response rates of 14% to 38% in chemosensitive patients, but the response rates in patients with chemorefractory disease are lower. Irinotecan, another topoisomerase I inhibitor, has demonstrated 10% partial response and 22% stable disease in refractory or relapsed SCLC. Etoposide-containing regimens currently remain the standard first line therapy in North America, while irinotecan-containing regimens are used in Japan. Thus, the combination of carboplatin and irinotecan may be a viable alternative to etoposide-containing regimens. Novel topoisomerase I and II inhibitors appear to continue to exhibit activity in patients with SCLC and warrant further investigation in this disease (particularly in non-Asian populations). However, whether these agents will be more active than etoposide remains to be determined.

6.2 Alkylating agents

The results are similar to those seen with other regimens.

6.3 Picoplatin

The role of picoplatin in SCLC is still not well defined and should be further explored in the future.

6.4 Antimetabolites

Pemetrexed has been shown to have minimal activity as a second-line agent in the treatment of patients with SCLC. Elevated thymidylate synthase expression in SCLC tumours has been proposed as one of the reasons for the observed lack of efficacy.

6.5 Antiangiogenic agents

Bevacizumab combined with standard first line therapy of cisplatin plus etoposide has shown a 64% response rate (RR), 4.7 months of progression-free survival (PFS), 30% of PFS at 6 months and 10.9 months of overall survival (OS). Upon employing bevacizumab to cisplatin plus irinotecan, the RR, PFS and OS were similar to those in the study conducted by ECOG. Another trial has reported an 84% overall RR, with PFS of 9.1 months and OS of 12.1 months. The importance of maintenance bevacizumab following combined modality treatment in patients with LD-SCLC is questionable; the response rate and OS are similar to what is seen with traditional chemotherapy with cisplatin, etoposide and radiation alone. Cediranib, a potent inhibitor of both VEGFR-1 and VEGFR-2, also has activity against c-kit, platelet derived growth factor beta (PDGFR-β), and FMS-like tyrosine kinase 4 (Flt-4). The response rate for Cediranib in recurrent SCLC that had progressed following platinum-based chemotherapy did not meet the predefined target. Vandetanib is an oral inhibitor of angiogenesis that targets VEGFR-2 and VEGFR-3 and inhibits tumour growth through activity against RET and EGFR/HER1. No difference in PFS or OS exists in vadetanib-treated patients compared with placebo-treated patients. Sorafenib, an oral multi-kinase inhibitor that targets both tumour proliferation via inhibition of Raf, stem cell factor receptor (KIT), and Flt-3 and angiogenesis by targeting VEGFR-2, VEGFR-3, and PDGFR-β, has been recommended for further evaluation in SCLC. Sunitinib is a novel, multi-targeted, small-molecule inhibitor of VEGFR-1, -2, and -3, PDGFR-α and –β, Flt-3, c-kit, the receptor encoded by the rearranged during transfection (*ret*) proto-oncogene, and Flt3. Thalidomide initially appeared to be a promising drug, but inclusion of this drug has ultimately failed to show any benefit in OS. Thalidomide in combination with chemotherapy in patients with SCLC shows, contrary to the results of the prior study, no significant difference between the thalidomide-treated patients and placebo-treated patients in OS. Based on the results of these trails, the role of anti-angiogenic therapy in the treatment of patients with SCLC remains to be determined. All agents studied to date appear to produce similar response rates and OS that are similar to the results achieved with chemotherapy alone (in most cases). Maintenance therapy with these agents does not appear to be beneficial in patients with SCLC.

6.6 MMP inhibitors

Many trials with MMPIs in SCLC have been equally disappointing. Of the multiple MMPs elevated in SCLC, marimistat targets MMP-1, MMP-2, MMP-9 and MMP-12 at low concentrations, while BAY 12-9566 targets MMP-2 at low concentrations.

6.6.1 mTOR inhibitors

At this time, mTOR inhibitors do not appear to be beneficial in the treatment of patients with SCLC.

6.7 Kit inhibition

Imatinib appears not to be beneficial in SCLC, even in patients with known c-kit mutations.

6.8 B cell leukaemia/lymphoma-associated gene 2 (Bcl-2)

Despite these discouraging results, a new class of oral BCL-2 antagonists is currently being developed and evaluated in patients with SCLC.

7. Signalling pathways that drive cancer stem cells

In cancer tissues, homeostasis is tightly regulated to ensure the generation of mature cancer cells throughout life without a depletion of the cancer stem cell pools. Each tissue is composed of a cellular hierarchy including stem cells able to generate all progeny, committed progenitors, and terminally differentiated cells. The stem cells in each tissue are believed to communicate with their microenvironment or surrounding stroma to maintain their homeostasis. Thus, the pathways that control stem cell self-renewal and the microenvironment in which the cancer stem cells (CSCs) reside may both play roles in targeted therapies

7.1 Hedgehog (Hh)

The Hh gene family encodes several secreted glycoproteins, including Indian Hedgehog (Ihh), Desert Hedgehog (Dhh), and Sonic Hedgehog (Shh). These proteins mediate signalling in embryogenesis and development through activation of the Gli family transcription factors. The Hh pathway is somewhat unique in that the signals serve to relieve a series of repressive interactions. The receptor for Hh, the transmembrane protein Patched 1 (Ptch), normally binds and inhibits smoothened (Smoh), a G-protein-coupled receptor that is related to Frizzled (Frz). When secreted Hh binds both Ptch and Hedgehog-interacting protein (Hip), Smoh initiates a transcriptional response. Specifically, Smoh activates the serine/threonine kinase Fused (Fu) to release Gli from sequestration by Suppressor of Fused (SuFu). Subsequently Gli proteins are able to translocate to the nucleus and regulate transcription of cyclin D and E, c-myc, and other genes involved in cell proliferation and differentiation. Shh is one among several important factors derived from the lung endoderm and is required for proliferation, differentiation, and patterning of the mesenchyme. Shh regulates pattern formation of a variety of developing structures, including the formation of the primary lung bunds. However, Shh is expressed in the ventral foregut endoderm. Shh is subsequently expressed in a gradient fashion (in the developing lung epithelium) with the highest levels in cells at the tips. In turn, most components of the Shh pathway, including Shh target genes and its receptor Ptch1, are found in the mesenchyme. Shh signalling is initiated upon binding to Ptch1 and results in activation of Shh target genes by Gli transcription factors. Ptch expression in the lung follows the proximal-distal gradient of Shh. Gli1, 2, and 3 are expressed in overlapping but distinct domains in the lung mesenchyme. The proximal-distal gradient is evident in Gli1, which together with Ptch, is transcriptionally upregulated by Shh and is expressed in the subepithelial mesenchyme. All three Gli genes are expressed in the lung mesenchyme during the pseudoglandular stage of development, and mutations in the Gli genes give rise to various lung and foregut defects. Shh signalling has been implicated in the regulation of Gli genes, notably in Gli1 and Gli3 transcription in the lung. Gli2 has also been implicated in the regulation of Ptch1 and Gli1 components of the Shh signalling cascade in the lung. Thus, Shh is part of an epithelial network of regulators that restricts fibroblast growth factor 10 (FGF-10) expression. Shh-FGF-10 interaction supports a model in which the growing epithelial bud, which expresses high levels of Shh, interacts with a chemotactic source (FGF-10) in the distal mesenchyme for its elimination. This model supports the idea that not only the presence of FGF-10, but also its correct spatial distribution, is necessary for patterning. If FGF-10 signals are diffuse rather than localised, direct clues are lost and branching is disrupted. Importantly, the data suggest that under normal conditions, Shh plays a role in controlling FGF-10 expression in the distal lung. Expression of Shh and Ptch does not seem to be influenced by FGF-10; however, both genes are down-regulated by FGF-7 in lung explant cultures.

7.2 Gli genes

The vertebrate Gli gene family currently consists of three members, Gli1, 2 and 3, which are orthologous to Drosophila cubitus interruptus and encode DNA-binding proteins with five zinc fingers.

7.3 BMP-4

Bone Morphogenetic Protein (BMP) belongs to the TGFβ superfamily of growth factors, and at least three members (BMP-4, -5 and -7) are present in the developing lung. BMP-4 is an important regulator of epithelial proliferation and proximal-distal cell fate during lung morphogenesis. During branching morphogenesis, BMP-4 is dynamically expressed in the distal epithelium of branching airways. BMP-4 stimulates distal lung formation but might preferentially induce alveolar type I cell fate.

7.4 TGFβ-1

TGFβ-1 is a member of a sub-family of peptides having at least two other members, all expressed in the developing lung. TGFβ signalling is mediated by serine-threonine kinase receptors (type I and II) and Smad transcription factors. TGFβ-1 transcripts are uniformly expressed in the sub-epithelial mesenchyme. TGFβ-1 protein accumulates later at sites of cleft formation and along proximal airways. TGFβ-1 promotes the synthesis of the extra-cellular matrix, which, when deposited in the epithelial-mesenchymal interface, is thought to prevent local branching.

8. Perspectives and future directions in therapy for SCLC

The recurrence of tumours after initial tumour regression by conventional therapies is also frequent. One potential reason for this recurrence is the failure of current therapies to target CSCs. The design and development of new cancer treatments is therefore necessary to target stem cell properties, i.e., self-renewal and differentiation. If the malignancy results from a blocked ontogeny, the treatment of cancer by inducing differentiation should be possible. These strategies have had variable success. In addition to inducing differentiation, a number of stem cell self-renewal pathways have been targeted for the treatment of various human tumours. If most solid tumours are composed of a minor population of self-renewing (stem) cells and a large fraction of non-renewing cells, cancer therapy failure following radiation and chemotherapy treatment is not the result of a rare cell evolving from within the tumour but the result of regrowth of the cancer stem cells. Of course, tumour stem cells could accumulate genetic changes that render them even more drug resistant, radiation resistant, or aneuploid. Because cures are achieved for many types of cancer, the cancer stem cells must be eliminated by a given therapeutic strategy. Regardless of which therapeutic paradigm turns out to be most effective, SCLC will clearly have to be treated with a "targeted medicine" approach if chemotherapy is to be widely successful in the clinic. This approach requires that each patient be segregated into a specific treatment group according to the constellation of molecular alterations that define his or her disease. The remarkable variation in genetic profiles across patients suggests that each tumour represents a distinct disease state that can only be effectively treated with precision therapy that targets the specific signalling pathway that is unique to each tumour. An important molecular mechanism that promotes cell differentiation is signal transduction. Signal transduction pathways ensure the reception of the concentration gradients of morphogens and their transformation into the differentiation of cells within tissues and organs. Hence, the key molecular rearrangements at the molecular level may be assumed to be related to changes in genes that participate in signal transduction pathways. In some contexts, these signals may be independently responsible for distinct aspects of tissue self-renewal, such as survival, proliferation and inhibition of differentiation. In other cases, the various signalling cascades may act in a hierarchy and regulate each other. Studies in which pathways are antagonised by treatment with pharmacological agent antagonists and/or agonists of Hh pathway signalling further demonstrate an ongoing requirement for pathway activity in the growth of additional cancer types. As a specific Smo antagonist, cyclopamine may be generally useful in the treatment of such cancers and represents a therapeutic strategy that may be further supported by the absence of observable toxicity in cyclopamine-treated animals. Cyclopamine inhibits Hh pathway activation by binding directly to Smo. This binding interaction is localised in the heptahelical bundle. Moreover, the binding influences the Smo protein conformation. Cyclopamine binding is also sensitive to Ptch function and provides biochemical evidence for an effect of Ptch on the structure of Smo. Cyclopamine appears to interfere with these signalling events by influencing Smo function; cyclopamine antagonises Hh pathway activity in a Ptch-independent manner and exhibits attenuated potency toward an oncogenic, constitutively active form of Smo. Pharmacologic inhibition of the Hh pathway has been necessary as a research tool to understand Hh pathway biology and is an attractive mechanism to evaluate antitumour activity. The first evidence that Smo could be antagonised came with the isolation of compounds called cyclopamine and jervine from corn lilies, which caused teratogenic effects (including cyclopia) in lambs. Significant new therapeutic strategies in SCLC will result from a deep understanding of the biology of response and resistance to targeted therapy. These approaches are in development to block embryonic pathways that play a role in cancer stem cells, including the Notch, Hh, and Wnt pathways.

9. Conclusions

The introduction of effective targeted agents for SCLC has lagged behind that for non-small-cell lung cancer. However, the number of agents now being tested has increased and includes agents that have shown some anti-tumour activity against other types of cancer, such as inhibitors of the Hh signalling pathway. This activity has prompted the development of agents that can inhibit Hh signalling. If the cancer stem cells that are responsible for driving the growth of cancer types associated with Hh pathway activation indeed come from stem cells trapped in a state of active renewal by pathway activities, then a logical therapeutic approach for these cancers would be to impose a state of pathway blockade. As we look towards the future, an important area of investigation will clearly involve analysing how the Hh pathway exerts its effect and whether shared molecular targets are involved in influencing self-renewal in the context of stem cells and cancer. Additionally, Hh probably integrates with other niche-derived signals, such as BMP (Bone Morphogenic Protein), Wnt and Notch. By understanding the molecular events governing CSCs, the development of therapeutics aimed at targeting these cells will become possible. The development of such therapeutics is of paramount importance because CSCs may mediate the resistance to current treatment and the relapse of the most aggressive tumours. This resistance may in part result in the reactivation of several signalling cascades, such Hh, Wnt, Notch, and EGF, in the CSCs combined with an increase in DNA repair mechanisms and ABC transporter-mediated multi-drug resistance.

10. References

10.1 Introduction

Chung LW, Baseman A, Assikis V, et al. Molecular insights into prostate cancer progression: the missing link of tumor microenvironment. J Urol 2005; 173:10-20.

Dean M, Fojo T, Bates S. Tumour stem cells and drug resistance. Nat Rev Cancer 2005; 5:275-284.

Ettinger DS, Aisner J. Changing face of small-cell lung cancer: real and artifact. J Clin Oncol 2006; 24:4526-4527.

Fuchs E. Das Sarkom des Uvealtractus. Graefe´s Arch Ophthalmol 1182; XII:233.

Govindan R, Page N, Morgensztern D, et al. Changing epidemiology of small-cell lung cancer in the United States over the last 3o years: analysis of the surveillance, epidemiologic, and end results database. J Clin Oncol 2006; 24:4539-4544.

Hewitt RE, McMarlin A, Kleiner D, et al. Validation of a model of colon cancer progression. J Pathol 2000; 192:446-454.

Hinson JA, Jr, Perry MC. Small cell lung cancer. CA Cancer J Clin 1993; 43:216-225.

Langley RR, Fidler IJ. Tumor cell-organ microenvironment interactions in the pathogenesis of cancer metastasis. Endocr Rev 2007;28:297-321.

Muller A, Homey B, Soto H, et al. Involvement of chemokine receptors in breast cancer metastasis. Nature 2001;410:50-56.

Murphy PM. Chemokines and the molecular basis of cancer metastasis. N Engl J Med 2001;345:833-835.

Pardal R, Clarke FM, Morrison SJ. Applying the principles of stem cell biology to cancer. Nat Rav Cancer 2003;3:895-902.

Paget S. The distribution of secondary growths in cancer of the breast. Lancet 1889; 133: 571-573

Roy M, Pear WS, Aster JC. The multifaceted role of Notch in cancer. Curr Opin Gene Dev 2007;17:52-59.

Setler-Stevenson WG. The role of matrix metalloproteinases in tumor invasion metastasis, and angiogenesis. Surg Oncol Clin North Am 2001; 10:383-392.

Simon GR, Turrisi A. Management of small cell lung cancer: ACCP evidence-based clinical practice guidelines. (2nd edition). Chest 2007; 132:324S-339S.

Slotman BJ, Suresh S. Radiotherapy in small-cell lung cancer:Lessons learned and future directions. Int J Radiat Oncol Biol Phys 2011; 79:998-1003.

Strieter RM. Chemokines: not just leukocyte chemoattractans in the promotion of cancer. Nat Immunol 2001; 2:285-286.

10.2 Development of airway

Cardoso WV. Transcription factors and pattern formation in the developing lung. Am J Physiol 1995; 269:L429-L442.

Dameron F. L´influence de divers mesenchymes sur la differentiation de l´epithelium pulmonaire de l´embryon de poulet en culture in vitro. J Embryol Exp Morphol 1961; 9:628-633.

Duan DY, Yue E, Zhou B, et al. Submucosal gland development in the airway is controlled by Lymphoid Enhancer Binding Factor 1 (LEF1). Development. 1999; 126:4441-4453.

Hackett BB, Brody SL, Liang M, et al. Primary structure of hepatocyte nuclear factor/forkhead homologue 4 and characterization of gene expression in the developing respiratory system and reproductive epithelium. Proc Natl Acad Sci USA. 1995; 92:4249-4253.

Han VKM, Hill DJ, Strain A, et al. Identification of somatomedin/insulin-like growth factor immunoreactive cells in the human fetus. Pediatr Res. 1987; 22:254-249.

Klempt M, Hutchins A-M, Gluckman PD, et al. IGF binding protein-2 gene expression and location of IGF-I and IGF-II in fetal rat lung. Development. 1992;115:765-772.

Metzger RJ, Krasnow MA. Genetic control of branching morphogenesis. Science 1999;284:1635-1639.

Nogawa H, Ito T. Branching morphogenesis of embryonic mouse lung epithelium in mesenchyme-free culture. Development 1995;121:1015-1022.

Offield MF, Jetton TL, Labosky RA, et al. PDX-1 is required for pancreatic outgrowth and differentiation of the rostral duodenum. Development 1996;122:983-995.

Roman J, McDonald JA. Expression of fibronectin, the integrin alpha 5, and alpha-smooth muscle actin in heart and lung development. Am J Respir Cell Mol Biol 1992;6:472-480.

Schruger L, Varani J, Killen PD, et al. Laminin expression in the mouse lung increases with development and stimulates spontaneous organotypic rearrangement of mixed lung cells. Dev Dyn 1992;195:43-44.

Spooner BS, Wessels NK. Mammalian lung development: interactions in primordium formation and bronchial morphogenesis. J Exp Zool 1070;175:445-454.

Ten Have-Opbroek AA. The development of lung in mammals: an analysis of concepts and findings. Am J Anat 1981;162:201-219.

Ten Have-Opbroek AA. Lung development in the mouse embryo. Exp Lung Res 1991;17:111-130.

Wessels NK. Mammalian lung development: interactions in formation and morphogenesis of tracheal buds. J Exp Zool 1979;175:445-460.

10.3 The airway stem cells

Borthwick DW, Shahbazian M, Krantz QT, et al. Evidence for stem-cell niches in the tracheal epithelium. Am J Respir Cell Mol Biol 2001;24:662-670.

Cotsarelis GS, Cheng Z, Dong G, et al. Existence of slow-cycling limbal epithelial basal cells that can be preferentially stimulated to proliferate: implications on epithelial stem cell. Cell 1989;57:201-209.

Engelhart JF, Schlossberg H, Yankaskas JR, et al. Progenitor cells of the adult human airway involved in submucosal gland development. Development 1995;121:2031-2046.

Evans MJ, Cabral-Anderson LJ, Freeman G. Role of the Clara cell in renewal of the bronchiolar epithelium. Lab Invest 1978;38:648-655.

Giangreco A, Reynolds SD, Stripp BR. Terminal bronchioles harbour a unique airways stem cell population that lo calices to the bronchoalveolar duct junction. Am J Pathol 2002;161:173-182.

Hong KU, Reynolds SD, Giangreco A, et al. Clara cell secretory protein-expressing cells of the airway neuroepithelial body microenvironment include a label-retaining subset and are critical for epithelial renewal after progenitor cell depletion. Am J Respir Cell Mol Biol 2001;24:671-681.

Hoyt RF Jr, McNelly NA, McDowell EM, et al. Neuroepithelial bodies stimulate proliferation of airway epithelium in fetal hamster lung. Am J Physiol 1991;260:L234-L240.

Hoyt RF Jr, Sorkin SP, McDowell EM, et al. Neuroephithelial bodies and growth of the airway ephitelium in developing hamster lung. Anat Rec 1993;236:15-22.

Peake JL, Reynolds SD, Stripp BR, et al. Alteration of pulmonary neuroendocrine cells during epithelial repair of naphthalene-induced airway injury. Am J Pathol 2000;156:279-286.

Reynolds SD, Giangreco A, Power JH, et al. Neuroepithelial bodies of pulmonary airways serve as a reservoir of progenitor cells capable of epithelial regeneration. Am J Pathol 2000;156:269-278.

Reynolds SD, Hong UK, Giangreco A, et al. Conditional clara cell ablation reveals a self-renewing progenitor function of pulmonary neuroendocrine cells. Am J Physiol 2000;278:L1256-L1263.

Van Lommel A, Lauweryns JM, Berth-Ovd HR. Pulmonary neuroepithelial bodies are inervated by vagal afferent nerves: an investigation with in vivo anterograde DiI tracing and confocal microscopy. Anat Hubryol 1998; 197:325-330.

Van Lommel, A., Bolle T, Fannes W, et al. The pulmonary neuroendocrine system: the past decade. Arch Histol Cytol 1999; 62:1-16.

10.4 Stem cells and lung cancer

Adamson IY, Bowden DH. The type 2 cell as progenitor of alveolar epithelial regeneration. A cytodynamic study in mice after exposure to oxygen. Lab Invest 1974;30:35.

Adamson IY, Bowden DH, Cote MG, et al. Lung injury induce by butylated hydroxytoluene: cytodynamic biochemical studies in mice. Lab Invest 1977;36:26.

Adamson IY, Bowden DH. Bleomycin-induced injury and metaplasia of alveolar type 2 cells. Relationship of cellular responses to drug presence in the lung. Am J Pathol 1979;96:531.

Aguayo SM, Miller YE, Waldron JA, et al. Brief report: idiopathic diffuse hyperplasia of pulmonary neuroendocrine cells and airways disease. N Engl J Med 1999;327:1285-288.

Belinsky SA, Deverenx TR, Foley JF, et al. The role of the alveolar type II cell in the development and progression of pulmonary tumors in the A/J. Cancer Res 1992;52:3164-3173.

Bishop AE. Pulmonary epithelial stem cells. Cell Prolif 2003;37:89-96.

Boers JE, Ambergen AW, Thumissen FB. Number and proliferation of Clara Cell in normal human airway epithelium. Am J Resp Crit Care Med 1999;159:1585.

Boers JE, Ambergen AW, Thunnissen FB. Number and proliferation of basal and parabasal cells in normal airway epithelium. Am J Respir Crit Care Med 1998;157:2000.

Daly RC, Transtek VF, Pairolero PC, et al. Bronchoalveolar Carcinoma: factors affecting survival. Ann Thorac Lurg 1991;51:368-376.

Donnelly GM, Haack DG, Heird CS. Tracheal epithelium: Cell kinetios and differentiation in normal rat tissue. Cell Tissue Kinet 1982;15:119.

Emura E. Stem cells of the respiratory epithelium and their in vitro cultivation. In Vitro Cell Dev Biol Anim 1997;33:3-14.

Emura E. Stem cells of the respiratory tract. Paediatr Respir Rev 2002;3:36.

Evans MJ, Cabral Anderson LJ, Freeman G. Role of the Clara cell in renewal of the bronchiolar epithelium. Lab Invest 1978;38:648.

Evans MJ, Cabral LJ, Stephens RJ, et al. Transformation of alveolar type II cells to type I cells following exposure to nitrogen dioxide. Exp Mol Pathol 1975;22:145.

Evans MJ, Johnson LV, Stepehns RJ, et al. Renewal of the terminal bronchiolar epithelium in the rat following exposure to NO2 or O3. Lab Invest 1976;35:246.

Fong KM, Zimmerman PV, Smith PJ. Lung pathology: The molecular genetics of non-small cell lung cancer. Pathology 1995;27:295-301.

Gazdar AF, Linnoila TR, Foley JF. Peripheral airway cell differentiation in human ung cancer cell lines. Cancer Res.1990;50:5481-5487.

Giangreco A, Reybolds SD, Stripp BR. Terminal bronchioles harbour a unique irway stem cell population that localizes to the bronchoalveolar junction. Am J Pathol 2002;161:173-112.

Gosbey JR. Pulmonary neuroendocrine cell system in pediatric and adult lung disease. Microsc. Res Techn 1997;37:107.

Gupta WD, Bernhard EJ, Muschel RJ, et al. Oververview of cell cycle and apoptosis. In: Pass HI et al. Principles and Practice. Philadephia PA: Lippincott Williams Wilkins; 2000. p.67-81.

Hong KV, Reynolds SD, Giangreco A, et al. Clara cell secretory protein-expressing cells of the airway neuroepithelial body microenvironment include a label-retaining subset and are critical for epithelial renewal after progenitor cell depletion. Am J Resp Cell Mol Biol 2001;24:671-681.

Inayama Y, Hook GE, Brody AR, et al. In vitro and in vivo growth and differentiation of clones of tracheal basal cells. Am J Pathol 1989;134:539.

Inayama Y, Hook GE, Brody AR, et al. The differentiation potential of tracheal basal cells. Lab Invest 1988;58:706.

Kim CFB, Jackson EL, Woolfenden AE, et al. Identification of bronchioalveolar stem cells in normal lung and lung cancer. Cell 2005;121:823-835.

Kitamura H, Kameda Y, Ito T, et al. Atypical adenomatous hyperplasia of the lung. Implications for the pathogenesis of peripheral lung adenocarcinoma. Am J Clin Pathol 1999;111:610-622.

Linnoila RI, Jensen SM, Steinberg SM, et al. Peripheral airway cell marker expression in non-small cell lung carcinoma. Am J Clin Pathol 1992;97:233-243.

Linnoila RI, Mulshine Jl, Steinberg SM, et al. Neuroendocrine differentiation in endocrine and nonendocrine lung carcinomas. Am J Clin Pathol 1988;90:641-652.

Linnoila RI. Effects of diethylnitrosamine on lung neuroendocrine cells. Exp Lung Res 1982;3:225.

Linnolia RI, Aisner SC. Pathology of lung cancer: exercise in classification. Lung Cancer. Current Clinical Oncology. Edited by BE Johnson, DH Johnson. New York: John Wiley & Sons; 1994; p.73-95.

Liu JY, Nettesheim P, Randall SH. Growth and differentiation of tracheal epithelial progenitor cells. Am J Physiol 1994;266:296.

Liu X, Driskel RR, Engelhardt JF. Airway glandular development and stem cells. Current Topics Develop Biol 2004;64:33-55.

Lobo NA, Shimono Y, Qian D, et al. The biology of cancer stem cells. Annu Rev Cell Dev Biol 2007;23:675-699.

McDowell EM, Trump BF. Pulmonary small cell carcinoma showing tripartite differentiation in individual cells. Hum Pathol 1981;12:296-224.

Moran CA, Hochholzer L, Fishback N, et al. Mucinons (so-called colloid) carcinomas of lung. Mod Pathol 1992;5:634-638.

Nettesheim P, Jetten AM, Inayama Y, et al. Pathways of differentiation of airway epithelial cells. Environ Health Perspect 1990;85:317.

Petersen I, Petersen S. Towards a gentic-based classification on human lung cancer. Anal Cell Pathol 2001;22:111-121.

Plopper CG, Dungworth DL. Structure, function, cell injury and cell renewal of bronchiolar and alveolar epithelium. In: McDowell EM, ed. Lung carcinomas. New York: Churchill Livingstone; 1987. p.94-128.

Reddy R, Buckley S, Doerken M, et al. Isolation of a putative progenitor subpopulation of alveolar epithelial type 2 cells. Am J Physiol Lung Cell Mol 2004;286:L658-L667.

Reynolds SD, Giangreco A, Power JHT, et al. Neuroepithelial bodies of pulmonary airways serve as a reservoir of progenitor cells capable of epithelial regeneration. Am J Pathol 2000;156:269.

Reynolds SD, Hong KU, Giangreco A, et al. Conditional Clara cell ablation reveals a self-renewing progenitor function of pulmonary neuroendocrine cells. Am J Physiol Lung Cell Mol Physiol 2000;278:L1256.

Sekido Y, Fong KM, Minna JD. Progress in understanding the molecular pathogenesis of human lung cancer. Biochim Biophys Acta 1998;1378:F21-F59.

Stingl J, Caldas C. Molecular heterogenicity of breast carcinomas and the cancer stem cell hypothesis. Nat Rev Cancer 2007;7:791-799.

Sunday Me, Willett CG, Patikar K, et al. Modulation of oncogenes and tumor suppressor gene expression in a hamster model of chronic lung injury with varying degrees of pulmonary neuroendocrine cell hyperplasia. Lab Invest 1994;70:875.

Sunday ME, Willett CG. Induction and spontaneous regression of interval pulmonary neuroendocrine cell differentiation in a model of prenoplastic lung injury. Cancer Res 1992;82:2677s-2686s.

Sunday ME, Willett CG. Induction and spontaneous regression of intense pulmonary neuroendocrine cell differentiation in a model of preneoplastic lung injury. Cancer Res 1992;52:2677S.

Taipale J, Beachy PA. The hedgehog and Wnt signalling pathways in carcer. Nature 2001:441;349-354.

Ten Have-Opbroek AA, Benfield JR, van Krieken JH, Dijkman JH. The alveolar type II cell is a pluripotential stem cell in the genesis of human adenocarcinomas and squamous cell carcinomas. Histal Histopathol 1997;12:319-336.

Travis WD, Colby TV, Corrin B, et al. Histological Typing of Lung and Pleural Tumors (Springer, Berlin) 1999.

Travis WD, Linder J, Mackay B. Classification, histology, cytology and electron microscopy. In: Pass HI et al. Lung Cancer. Principles and Practice Philadephia PA: Lippincott Williams Wilkins; 2000. p.453-496.

Watkins DN, Berman DM, Burkholder SG, et al. Hedgehog Signalling Within Airway Epithelial Progenitors and in Small Cell Lung Cancer. Nature 2003; 422:313-317.

Witschi H. Proliferation of type II alveolar cells: a review of common response in toxic lung injury. Toxicology 1976;5:267-277.

Yang A, Schweizer R, Sun, D, et al. p63 is essential for regenerative proliferation in limb, craniofacial and epithelial development. Nature 1999; 398; 714-718.

Zakowski MF. Pathology of small cell lung cancer. Semin Oncol 2003; 30:3-8.

10.5 Smal cell lung cancer

Magnum MD, Greco FA, Hainsworth JD, et al. Combination small-cell and non-small-cell lung cancer. J Clin Oncol 1989;7:607-618.

McCue PA, Finkel GC. Smal-cell lung carcinoma:an evolving histopathologic spectrum. Semin Oncol 1993;20:153-162.

Nicholson SA, Beasley MB, Brambilla E, et al. Small cell lung carcinoma (SCLC): a clinicopathologic study of 100 cases with surgical specimens. Am J Surg Pathol 2002;26:1184-1197.

Travis WD, Brambilla E, Muller-Hermelink HK, et al. World Health Organization Classification of Tumors: Tumors of the Lung, Pleura, Thymus and Heart. IARC Press, Lyon, 2004:31-34.

Travis WD. Lung tumors with neuroendocrine differentiation. Eur J Cancer 2008;45:suppl 1:251-266.

10.6 Targeted agents that has been evaluated in smal-cell lung cancer

Ahmad T, Eisen T. Kinase inhibitionwith BAY 43-9006 in renal cell carcinoma. Clin Cancer Res 2004; 10:6388S-63892S.

Ardizzoni A, Hansen H, Dombernowsky P, et al. Topotecan, a new active drug in the second-line treatment of small-cell lung cancer: a phase II study in patients with refractory and sensitive disease. The European Organization ofr Research and Treatment of Cancer Early Clinical Studies Group and New Drug development Office, and the Lung cancer Cooperative Group. J Clin Oncol 1997;15:2090-2096.

Evans Wk, Shepherd F, Feld R, et al. VP-16 and cisplatin as first-line therapy for small-cell lung cancer. J Clin Oncol 1985;3:1471-1477.

Gitlitz BJ, Glisson BS, Moon J, et al. Sorafenib in patients with platinum (plat) treated extensive stage small cell lung cancer (E- SCLC): a SWOG (S0435) phase II trial. J Clin Oncol (ASCO meeting abstracts) 2008;26:8039.

Goodman GE, Crowley JJ, Blasko JC, et al. Treatment of limited small-cell lung cancer with etoposide and cisplatin alternating with vincristine, doxorubicin, and cyclophosphamide versus concurrent etoposide, vincristine, doxorubicin, adncyclophosphamide and cest radiotherapy: a Southwest Oncology Group Study. J Clin Oncol 1990;8:39-47.

Growen HJ, Fokkema E, Biesma B, et al. Pacltaxel and cqwrboplatin in the treatment of small-cell lung cancer patients resistant to cyclophosphamide, doxorubicin, and etoposide: a non-cross-resistant schedule. J Clin Oncol 1999;17:927-932.

Hanna N, Bunn PA Jr, Langer C, et al. Raandomized phase III trial comparing irinotecan/cisplatin with etoposide/cisplatin in patients with previosuly untreated extensice-stage disease small-cell lkung cancer. J Clin Oncol 2006;24:2038-2043.

Horn L, Dalhberg SE, Sandler AB, et al. Phase II study of cisplatin plus etoposide and bevacizumab for previously untreated, extensive-stage small-cell lung cancer: Eastern Cooperative Oncology Group Study E3501. J Clin Oncol 2009;27:6006-6011.

Johnson DH, Bass D, Einhorn LH, et al. Combination chemotherapy with or without thoracic radiotherapy in limited-stage small-cell lung cancer: a randomized trial of the Southeastern Cancer Study Group. J Clin Oncol 1993;11:1223-1229.

Lara PN Jr, Natale R, Crowley J, et al. Phase III trial of irinotecan/cisplatin compared with etoposide/cisplatin in extensive-stage small-cell lung cancer:clinical and pharmacogenomic results from SWOG So124. J Clin Oncol 2009;27:2530-2535.

Nelson AR, Fingleton B, Rothenberg ML, et al. Matrix metalloproteinases: biologic activity and clinical implications. J Clin Oncol 2000;18:1135-1149.

Lucchi M, Mussi A, Fontanini G, et al. Small cell lung carcinoma (SCLC): the angiogenic phenomenon. Eur J Cardiothorac Surg 2002;21:1105-1110.

Patton JF, Spigel DR, Greco FA, et al. Irinotecan (I), carboplatin (C), and radiotherapy (RT) followed by maintenance bevacizumab (B) in the treatment (tx) of limited-stage small cell lung cancer (LS- SCLC): update of a phase II trial of the Minnie Pearl Cancer Research Network. J Clin Oncol (ASCO meeting abstracts) 2006;24:7085.

Ramalingam SS, Mack PC, Vokes EE, et al. Cediranib (AZD2171) for the treatment of recurrent small cell lung cancer (SCLC): a California Consortium phase II study. Meeting abstracts. J Clin Oncol 2008;26:8078.

Ready N, Dudek AZ, Wang XF, et al. CALGB 30306: a phase II study of cisplatin ©, irinotecan (I) and bevacizumab (B) for untreated extensive stage small cell lung cancer (ES- SCLC). J Clin Oncol 2007;25:7563.

Sculier JP, Klastersky J, Liberet P, et al. Cycplophosphamide, doxorubicin and vincristine with amphotericin B in sonicated liposomes as salvage therapy for small cell lung cancer. Ur J Cancer 1990;26:919-921.

Shepherd FA, Giaccone G, Seymour L, et al. Prospective, randomized, double-blind, placebo-controlled trial of marimastat after response to first-line chemotherapy in patients with small-cell lung cancer: a trial of the National Cancer Institute of Canada-Clinical Trials Group and the European Organization for Research and Treatment of Cancer. J Clin Oncol 2002;20:4434-4439.

Shepherd FA, Ginsberg RJ, Haddad R, et al. Importance of clinical staging in limited small-cell lung cancer: a valuable system to separate prognostic subgroups. The University of Toronto Lung Oncology Group. J Clin Oncol 1993;11:1592-1597.

Spigel DR, Hainsworth JD, Yardley DA, et al. Phase II trial of irinotecan, carboplatin, and bevacizumab in patients with extensive-stage small cell lung cancer. Meeting abstracts. J Clin Oncol 2007;25:18130.

Sundstron S, Bremmes RM, Kaasa S, et al. Cisplatin and etoposide regimen is superior to cyclophosphamide, epirubicin, and vincristine regimen in small-cell lung cancer: results from a randomized phase III trial with 5 years' follo-up. J Clinc Oncol 2002;20:4665-4672.

Von Pawel J, Schiller JH, Shepherd FA, et al. Topotecan versus cyclophosphamide, doxorubicin, and voincristine for the treatment of recurrent small-cell lung cancer. J Clin Oncol 1999; 17:658-667.

Wilhelm SM, Carter C, Tang L, et al. BAY 43-9006 exhibits broad spectrum oral antitumor activity and targets the RAF/MEK/ERK pathway and receptor tyrosine kinases involved in tmor progression and angiogenesis. Cancer Res 2004; 64:7099-7109.

10.7 Signaling pathways driving cancer stem cells

Cardoso WV. Molecular regulation of lung development. Annu Rev Physiol. 2001; 63: 471-494

Clevidence DR, Overdier DG, Peterson RS, et al. Members of the HnF3/forkhead family of transcription factors exhibit distinct cellular expression patterns in lung and regulate the surfactant protein B promoter. Dev Biol. 1994; 166:195-209.

Grindley JC, Bellusci S, Perkins D, Hogan BLM. Evidence for the involvement of the Gli gene family in embryonic mouse lung development. Dev Biol. 1997; 188: 337-348.

Litingtung Y, Lei L, Westphal H, Chiang C. Sonic hedgehog is essential to foregut development. Nat Genet. 1998; 20: 58-61.

Mendelson CR. Role of transcription factors in fetal lung development and surfactant protein gene expression. Annu Rev Physiol. 2000; 62: 875-915.

Pepicelli CV, Lewis PM, McMahon AP. Sonic hedgehog regulates branching morphogenesis in the mammalian lung. Curr Biol. 1998; 8: 1083-1086.

Sera R, Pelton RW, Moses HL. TGFβ1 inhibits branching morphogenesis and N-myc expression in lung bud organ cultures. Development. 1994; 120: 2153-2161.

10.8 Perspective and future directions in therapy for SCLC

Antón Aparicio LM, García Campelo R, Alonso Curbera G. Small-cell lung carcinoma: What is new in therapy? Cancer & Chemotherapy 2007;2:168-174.

Borzillo GV, Lippa B. The Hedgehog signaling pathway as a target for anticancer drug discovery. Curr Top Med Chem 2005;5:147-157.

Chen JK, Taipale J, Young KE, et al. Small molecule modulation of smoothened activity. Proc Natl Acad Sci USA 2002;99:14071-14076.

Frank-Kamenetsky M, Zhang XM, Bottega S, et al. Small-molecule modulators of hedgehog signaling: Identification and characterization of smoothened agonists and antagonists. J Biol 2002;1:10.

Incardona JP, Gaffield W, Kapur RP, et al. The teratogenic Veratrum alkaloid cyclopamine inhibits sonic hedgehog signal transduction. Development 1998; 125:3553-3562.

Mahindroo N, Punchihewa C, Fujii N. Hedgehog-Gli signaling pathway inhibitors as anti-cancer agents. J Med Chem 2009;52:3829-3845.

Taipale J, Chen JK, Cooper MK, et al. Effects of oncogenic mutations in Smoothened and Patched can be reversed by cyclopamine. Nature 2000;406:1005-1009.

Tremblay MR, Nesler M, Weatherhead R, et al. Recent patents for Hedgehog pathway inhibitors for the treatment of malignancy. Expert Opin Ther Pat 2009;19:1039-1056.

Watkins DN, Berman DM, Burkholder SG, et al. Hedgehog signaling within airway epithelial progenitors and in SCLC. Nature 2003;422:313-317.

Watkins DN, Berman DM, Burkholder SG, et al. Hedgehog signaling within airway epithelial progenitors and in small cell cancer. Nature 2003;422:313-317.

Watkins DN, Berman DM, Burkholder SG, et al. Hedgehog signaling progenitor phenotype in SCLC. Cell Cycle 2003;2:196-198.

Williams JA, Guicherit OM, Zaharian BI, et al. Identification of a small molecule inhibitor of the hedgehog signaling pathway: Effects on basal cell carcinoma-like lesions. Proc Natl Acad Sci USA 2003;100:4616-4621.

Part 6

Genetic Manipulation and Its Possible Clinical Implications for Squamous Cell Carcinoma

15

MicroRNA Dysregulation in Squamous Cell Carcinoma of Head and Neck

Thian-Sze Wong, Wei Gao, Wai-Kuen Ho, Jimmy Yu-Wai Chan, William Ignace Wei and Raymond King-Yin Tsang
The University of Hong Kong
Hong Kong SAR,
China

1. Introduction

Head and neck cancers refers to cancer arising in the head or neck regions including parnasal sinuses, nasal cavity, nasopharynx, oral cavity, salivary gland, oropharynx, pharynx, hypopharynx, larynx, and lymph node. Histologically, squamous cell carcinoma is the predominant form. The cancer progenitor cells are premalignant cells in the mucosa layer of head and neck. Cumulative genetic and epigenetic alterations lead to behavioural changes from hyperplasia to invasive carcinoma. Head and neck squamous cell carcinoma (HNSCC) is the sixth most common cancer worldwide. It is the 4th most common cancer among men in the European Union (Black et al., 1997). In United State, over 12,000 patients died from HNSCC every year (Altekruse et al., 2008). Globally, there are approximately 650,000 new cases of HNSCC and 350,000 patients dying from HNSCC annually (Parkin et al., 2005). Most patients will develop local-regional disease with cervical lymph node involvements. HNSCC is heterogeneous in nature. Early disease might not have any symptoms. Further, the inconspicuous locations of some HNSCC make it difficult to be identified at the early stages. Thus, patients arrive at the clinic by large present late and have poor prognosis. The overall survival rate of HNSCC patients is about 50% (Stell, 1989; Argiris et al, 2004). Development of local recurrence, distant metastasis and secondary primary tumor is also common in HNSCC. Despite the advances of cancer treatment in last several decades, the overall survival rate of HNSCC did not have much improvement (Stell, 1989; Argiris and Eng, 2003).

HNSCC is a multifactorial disease. Major risk factors are alcohol consumption and tobacco use (Jaber et al., 1999). HNSCC is particularly common in countries with high alcohol and tobacco consumption e.g. southern Africa, Australia, Brazil, France, India, The Netherlands, Papua-New Guinea and Switzerland (Parkin et al., 2005). Smoking and drinking habit is associated with early onset of HNSCC (Farshadpour et al., 2007). Patients with alcohol and tobacco use generally have poor prognosis and poor survival rate (Farshadpour et al., 2011). Other risk factors of HNSCC include age, environmental exposures (including UV exposure and viral infection such as Epstein-Barr Virus and Human Papilloma Virus), sex, hygiene, industrial inhalants, and gender (Argiris et al., 2003). Regional lymph node involvement is also an indicator of poor prognosis. About 20–50% N0 patients will develop nodal metastasis. The overall survival rate reduced to 50% in case if lymph node metastasis is observed (von Buchwald et al., 2002).

Management of HNSCC is based primarily on the tumor locations and stages (Akervall, 2005). For early HNSCC (stage I and II) surgical resection together with radiotherapy is the primary treatment regime. For advanced disease (stage III and IV) multidisciplinary treatment including surgery, radiation and chemotherapy is adopted (Posner, 2010). For loco-regionally advanced HNSCC, concurrent chemo-radiotherapy is used in case where the tumor is unresectable or adverse functional loss will be resulted from the operation (Wong et al., 2011). For oral squamous cell carcinoma, surgical excision of the primary tumor and/or selective neck dissection is the major treatment (Bilde et al., 2006). For pharyngeal and laryngeal SCC, radiotherapy and/or concomitant chemotherapy are commonly used (Lajer et al., 2011). It has been shown that the use of concomitant chemo- and radio-therapy is more effective in advanced HNSCC (Robbins, 2005).

2. MicroRNA

MicroRNA are small non-protein-coding RNA, which regulate mRNA at post-transcriptional level. MicroRNA are small epigenetic regulators usually about 19–22 or 19–25 nucleotides long (Ambrose, 2004). They are highly conserved molecules among different species including nematode, drosophila, vertebrate, and human indicating its significance in cellular functions. MicroRNA was first discovered in 1993 in nematode *Ceanorhabditis elegans* (*C. elegans*) (Lee et al., 1993). Later, the tumor suppressing microRNA let-7 was identified in *C. elegans* and mammalian models. By then, it was proposed that microRNA had a trans-regulatory role through direct binding to the target mRNA. Computational prediction suggested that microRNA are regulating about 30% of human genes (Lewis et al., 2005). Up till now (1 July 2011), 16,772 microRNA are reported in the miRBase (see miRBase at http://www.mirbase.org, Release 17) at which 8.9% (1,492) are human microRNA. MicroRNA could bind to the target mRNA in a partial or complete complementary manner. They regulate gene expression by promoting target mRNA degradation and/or hindering mRNA translation (Bushati and Cohen, 2007).

MicroRNA are transcribed in genomic DNA. The genes encoding microRNA are located throughout the human genome in intron, exon, coding / non-coding genes (Lee et al., 2002). MicoRNA are first transcribed by RNA polymerase II into long precursor microRNA. This long RNA will be cleaved by Dorsha (RNase III-type nuclease in the nucleus) generating primary microRNA (60–70 nucleotides hairpin molecules). The primary microRNA are later exported into the cytoplasma by Exportin-5 (a Ras-GTP-dependent dsRNA-binding protein). Primary microRNA will be further processed by Dicer (RNase complex) and TRBP [TAR (transactivation-responsive RNA of HIV-1) RNA-binding protein] forming an asymmetric microRNA:microRNA* intermediate duplex (microRNA* is usually functionless and are degraded subsequently). This duplex molecule is then incorporated with Argonaute-containing RNA-induced silencing (RISC) complex forming a functional post-transcriptional regulator (Bartel, 2004). This functional complex usually bind to the 3′ untranslated region of the target mRNA (Lim et al., 2005; Wightman et al., 1993). The complementary binding between microRNA and the target mRNA is not necessary perfect in order to carry out it function as negative regulator. The binding of seed sequence (2-7 nucleotides on the mature microRNA) of the microRNA with the target mRNA would suffice to induce mRNA destabilization and degradation (Filipowicz et al., 2008).

So far, microRNA were identified as negative regulator of specific mRNA (Lim et al., 2005). However, recent findings suggested that microRNA might also act as gene activator. Vasudevan *et al.* demonstrated that miR369-3 could activate translation (Vasudevan et al., 2007). Later, Place *et al.* observed that miR-373 could induce E-cadherin expression in prostate cancer cells (Place et al., 2008). MicroRNA Let-7 can induce upregulation of gene involved in cell cycle arrest (Vasudevan et al., 2007). Although such activating mechanisms are not yet clear, it revealed that many remain to be explored if we want to uncover the exact functions of microRNA in human cells.

3. MicroRNA and cancers

In comparison with the normal counterparts, cancer displays a differential microRNA expression patterns (Lu et al., 2005). Association between human cancers and microRNA dysregulation was first observed in leukemia. Downregulation of miR-15 and miR-16 was first discovered in peripheral blood of chronic lymphocytic leukemia (Calin et al, 2002). For HNSCC, study on individual microRNA was first performed by Jiang *et al.* in 2005 (Jiang et al., 2005). Later, *Tran et al.* performed microRNA expression profiling on head and neck cancer cell lines (Tran et al., 2007).

The microRNA profile of nasopharyngeal carcinoma, oral tongue carcinoma, and laryngeal carcinoma are emerging in the subsequent years (Li et al., 2010; Li et al., 2011; Liu et al., 2009; Rentoft et al., 2011; Scapoli et al., 2010). The underlying mechanism concerning microRNA dysregulation in head and neck cancers is not yet clear although it has been reported that the microRNA processing machinery is upregulated in head and neck cancers (Zhang et al., 2009). Zhang noticed that the microRNA processing enzymes Dicer and Drosha are overexpressed in salivary gland tumor (Zhang et al., 2009). Expression of Dorsha (micoRNA processor) will affect the phenotype of squamous epithelial cells (Muralidhar et al., 2011).

4. Mechanisms of MicroRNA dysregulation in head and neck cancers

4.1 Chromosomal rearrangement

Chromosomal abnormalities are associated with the development of head and neck caners (Akervall, 2005; Gollin et al., 2001). Common chromosomal gains in HNSCC include 3q, 5p, 7p, 8q, 9q, 11q13, and 20q. In comparison, losses of chromosomal region were frequently detected on 3p, 9p, 5q, 8p, 13q, 18q, and 21q. Cromer *et al.* reported that genes related to tumorigenesis and metastasis of hypopharyngeal carcinoma were located on 3q27.3, 17q21.2-q21.31, 7q11.22-q22.1and 11q13.1-q13.3. Chromosomal rearrangement (e.g. deletion or translocation) will result in dysregulation of the gene on the abbreviated loci (Akervall, 2005).

About 50% of the microRNA are located in minimal deleted regions, minimal amplified regions, and breakpoint regions involved in human cancers (Calin et al., 2004). Recently, Persson *et al.*, has shown that t(6;9)(q22–23;p23–24) will lead to fusion of MYB oncogene to the transcription factor gene NFIB in head and neck cancers (Persson et al., 2009). As the 3′-

UTR of MYB is targeted by miR-15a/16, the chromosomal translocation allows the cancer cells to escape control by miR-15a/16. Lee *et al.*, identified that miR-204 located in 9q21.1-22.3, a cancer genomic-associated region of head and neck cancers, is linked to progression of HNSCC (Lee et al., 2010). Loss of heterozygosity (LOH) in these loci are common in HNSCC (Bauer et al., 2008; Spafford et al., 2001).

4.2 DNA hypermethylation

DNA hypermethylation is usually found in the CpG island of tumor suppressor genes. Methylation of the clustered CpG dinucleotides in the CpG island would result in transcriptional silencing of the genes. It is now known that the methylated CpG dinucleotide could also link to the regulation of microRNA expression. Promoter methylation will affect binding of the transcriptional machinery (Zhang et al., 2011). Demethylation treatment of the nasopharyngeal carcinoma cells with demethylating agents would result in let-7 upregulation indicating the involvement of DNA methylation in regulating let-7 expression in nasopharyngeal carcinoma cells (Wong et al., 2011). Kozaki *et al.* identified that DNA methylation is linked to the transcriptional silencing of miR-137 and miR-193a, both of which are tumor suppressing microRNA associated with oral SCC (Kozaki et al, 2008). Apart from microRNA, the methylated microRNA promoter can also be used as a biomarker for HNSCC patients. Langevin *et al.* reported that methylated miR-137 promoter is associated with the clinical pathological characteristic of HNSCC patients (Langevin et al., 2010)

4.3 Genetic polymorphism of microRNA-encoding region

Similar to mRNA, microRNA are also encoded by genomic DNA. Theoretically, any variation in genomic materials will affect the biogenesis and final sequence of the mature microRNA (the seed sequence especially) and affect the specificity of microRNA to their target mRNA. Thus, any genetic variation in the microRNA biogenesis pathway gene, primary microRNA, precursor microRNA or mature microRNA sequence will eventually affect the microRNA regulatory pathways (Slaby et al., 2011)

4.3.1 Single nucleotide polymorphism (SNP) of microRNA-encoding genes

The association between microRNA and SNP has been demonstrated recently (Duan et al., 2007). It has already been demonstrated that SNP will affect the processing of pre-microRNA (Yu et al., 2007). In HNSCC, SNP of miRNA-146a (rs2910164; guanine to cytosine), miR-149 (rs2292832; guanine to thymine), miR-196a2 (rs11614913), and miR-499 (rs3746444; adenine to guanine) are associated with the risk of developing HNSCC (Liu et al 2010). Christensen *et al.* confirmed the association of SNP in miR-196a2 (rs11614913, C/T) with HNSCC. They demonstrated that miR-196a2 polymorphism is associated with the risk of HNSCC (Christensen et al., 2010).

4.3.2 Single nucleotide polymorphism (SNP) of microRNA-targeted genes

Apart from microRNA itself, SNP on microRNA target genes will also affect the binding efficacy of microRNA. Zhang *et al.* demonstrated that SNP associated with microRNA biogenesis pathway genes and microRNA-targeted genes are associated with the prognosis of HNSCC patients (Zhang et al., 2010). They proposed that microRNA-related genetic polymorphisms might be used as predicative markers for secondary primary and/or recurrence in early HNSCC patients (Zhang et al., 2010).

4.4 MicroRNA dysregulation by candidate oncogene

MicroRNA expression could be controlled by oncogene such as myc. He *et al.* reported that the miR-17-92 cluster is transactivated by myc (He et al., 2007). In addition, p53 is also shown to be involved in microRNA dysregulation through inducing miR-34 expression (Chang et al., 2008; He et al., 2005; Melo and Estella, 2011; Suzuki et al., 2009).

5. MicroRNA as molecular markers in circulation and body fluids in HNSCC

With the advance of molecular techniques and understanding in cancers, molecular markers are now considered as an effective auxiliary test in conjunction to histological examination in assisting clinical decision making (Hui et al., 2010). The existence of differential microRNA patterns between cancer and the normal counterparts opens up the possibility of using the differential expressed microRNA in monitoring cancers (Krutovskikh et al., 2010). In view of the myriad of functions of microRNA in cancers, de Planell-Saguer and Rodicio suggested that microRNA is potentially useful as biomarkers for cancer onset, prognosis, risk of diseases and cancer classification (de Planell-Saguer and Rodicio, 2011).

MicroRNA is suitable cancer marker as it is highly stable and is resistant to degradation (Li et al., 2007). Significant amount of extracellular microRNA had been detected in peripheral blood, urine, saliva and semen (Mitchell et al., 2008; Hanke et al., 2009; Park et al., 2009; Zubakov et al., 2010) making it a candidate biomarker for detection and surveillance of HNSCC in a non-invasive manner. In addition, it could be extracted in formalin-fixed paraffin-embedded tissues (Li et al., 2007). Circulating microRNA have been found to be significantly elevated in the peripheral blood of head and neck cancer patients. However, there is no direct evidence showing that primary tumor is the only source of the circulating microRNA. Reduction of the circulating microRNA after removal of the primary tumor suggested that primary tumor is one of the major sources of circulating microRNA (Iguchi et al., 2010; Kosaka et al., 2010).

Peripheral blood has high RNase activity, however, circulating microRNA could still exist in cell-free form and remain stable in the blood (Mitchell et al., 2008). Circulating microRNAs are existed in membrane-bound vesicles (about 50 nm to 1 um) and are released from the cancer cells through exocytosis (Février & Raposo, 2004; Heijnen et al., 1999; Hunter et al., 2008). Recently, Turchinovich *et al.* performed physical analysis on the characteristics of the circulating microRNA. They noticed that circulating microRNA could exist independently without the vesicle provided that they are bound to the Ago2 protein (Turchinovich et al., 2011).

6. Examples of microRNA dysregulation in HNSCC

Depending on the functions, the dysregulated microRNA could be classified into oncogenic microRNA (onco-miR) and tumor suppressing microRNA (Kozaki et al., 2008; Iorio et al., 2005). Identifying the dysregulated microRNA patterns in HNSCC is useful in selecting suitable microRNA biomarkers for use in HNSCC monitoring (Chang et al., 2008; Ferdin et al., 2010). We here performed a review on the potential oncogenic microRNA and tumor suppressing microRNA identified in HNSCC.

6.1 Let-7 Family

Human let-7 has multiple isoforms. They are let-7a-1[Mature sequence: 6 - ugagguaguagguuguauaguu - 27 (MI0000060)], let-7a-2 [Mature sequence: 5 - ugagguaguagguuguauaguu - 26 (MI0000061)], let-7a-3 [Mature sequence: 4 - ugagguaguagguuguauaguu - 25 (MI0000062)], let-7b [Mature sequence: 6 - ugagguaguagguugugugguu - 27 (MI0000063)], let-7c [Mature sequence: 11 - ugagguaguagguuguaugguu - 32 (MI0000064)], let-7d [Mature sequence: 8 - agagguaguagguugcauaguu - 29 (MI0000065), let-7e (Mature sequence: 8 - ugagguaggagguuguauaguu - 29 (MI0000066), let-7f-1 [Mature sequence: 7 - ugagguaguagauuguauaguu - 28 (MI0000067)], let-7f-2 [Mature sequence: 8 - ugagguaguagauuguauaguu - 29 (MI0000068)], let-7g (Mature sequence: 5 - ugagguaguaguuuguacaguu - 26 (MI0000433)], and let-7i [Mature sequence: 6 - ugagguaguaguuugugcuguu - 27 (MI0000434).

In human cancers, expression of let-7 family is usually reduced suggesting its tumor-suppressing role. In comparison with the normal nasopharyngeal cells, let-7 levels were significantly decreased in the nasopharyngeal carcinoma. Reduced expression levels of let-7 (-a, -b, -d, -e, -g, and -i) were detected in nasopharyngeal carcinoma cells compared to normal nasopharyngeal cells. Ectopic expression of let-7 in nasopharyngeal carcinoma cells reduced cell proliferation (Wong et al., 2011). Moreover, c-Myc expression was inhibited in NPC cells transfected with precursor let-7 (Wong et al., 2011). Association of let-7 with cell proliferation was also observed in oral cancer cells (Jakymiw et al. 2010). Let-7a microRNA expression was inhibited in both laryngeal squamous cancer tissues and in laryngeal cancer cell lines (Hep-2 and BEAS-2B). Let-7a could inhibit proliferation and induce apoptosis in laryngeal carcinoma cells (Long et al., 2009). In Hep-2 cells, overexpression of let-7a could also suppress RAS and c-MYC protein expression (Long et al., 2009). It was demonstrated that up-regulated RAS and c-MYC protein levels had inverse correlation with the down-regulated let-7a levels in cancer tissues (Long et al., 2009). Further, let-7a could enhance the chemosensitivity of head and neck cancer cells and might link to the stemness gene expression pathway (Yu et al., 2011).

6.2 MiR-15a [Mature sequence: 14 - uagcagcacauaaugguuugug - 35 (MI0000069)]

Regulation of miR-15a is altered in head and neck cancer cells (Persson et al. 2009). Expression of miR-15a was inversely correlated with protein kinase C which was usually overexpressed in primary HNSCC (Cohen et al., 2009). It has been shown that overexpression of miR-15a suppressed cyclin E protein expression and inhibition of miR-15a enhanced cyclin E protein expression in laryngeal cancer cell line. Precursor miR-15a could also affect DNA synthesis in laryngeal carcinoma cells but the related mechanisms are not yet identified (Cohen et al., 2009). These results indicated that miR-15a might function as a tumor suppressor through regulating the gene associated with the proliferation pathways of cancer cells (Cohen et al., 2009).

6.3 MiR-21 [Mature sequence: 8 - uagcuuaucagacugauguuga - 29 (MI0000077)]

Overexpression of miR-21 was first reported in human glioblastoma and miR-21 is now recognized as an potent anti-apoptotic factor (Fu et al., 2011). Upregulation of miR-21 is observed in multiple human cancers including breast, cervical, colon, leukemia, liver, lung, ovarian, pancreas, prostate, stomach and thyroid as well as head & neck (Krichevsky et al., 2009; Volinia et al., 2006). Elevated expression of miR-21 is observed in tongue squamous cell carcinomas. Suppressing miR-21 in tongue SCC cell lines (SCC-15 and CAL27) reduced cell survival and induced apoptosis (Li et al., 2009). It has been found that the expression level of miR-21 was reversely correlated with TPM1. The observation suggested that miR-21 may inhibit cell apoptosis partly via silencing the expression of TPM1 (Li et al., 2009). Furthermore, it has been shown that miR-21 expression was an independent prognostic factor associated with survival rate (Li et al., 2009). Moreover, repeated injection of miR-21 antisense oligonucleotide could inhibit tumor formation in nude mice (Li et al., 2009). Laryngeal cancer cell line (JHU-O11) transfected with miR-21 displayed enhanced cell growth (Chang et al., 2008).

6.4 MiR-29 [Mature sequence: 54 - uagcaccauuugaaaucgguua – 75 (MI0000735)]

MiR-29c expression was suppressed in nasopharyngeal carcinomas in comparison with normal healthy nasopharyngeal epithelia (Sengupta et al., 2008). The function of miR-29c is not yet clear. In HeLa cells, transfection of miR-29c precursor could suppress expression of collagen 3A1, 4A1, 15A1, laminin, and thymine-DNA glycosylase (TDG) linking to tumor cell invasiveness and metastatsis (Sengupta et al., 2008).

6.5 MiR-100 [Mature sequence: 13 - aacccguagauccgaacuugug - 34 (MI0000102)] and miR-125b [Mature sequence: 15 - ucccugagacccuaacuuguga - 36 (MI0000446)]

Suppression of both miR-100 and miR-125b were reported in HNSCC. Expression levels of miR-125b and miR-100 were decreased in oral squamous cell carcinoma cell lines and tumors of alveolar ridge, buccal mucosa, floor of mouth, retromolar trigone and tongue (Henson et al., 2009). Overexpression of miR-100 and miR-125b inhibited cell proliferation in buccal mucosa cell lines (Henson et al., 2009). Suppressed expression of miR-100 and miR-125b in oral cancer cells may lead to cancer progression and loss of sensitivity to ionizing radiation (Henson et al., 2009).

6.6 MiR-133 family

MiR-133 has 2 isoforms: miR-133a [Mature sequence: 53 - uuugguccccuucaaccagcug – 74 (MI0000450)] and miR-133b [Mature sequence: 66 - uuugguccccuucaaccagcua – 87 (MI0000822)]. Downregulation of miR-133 had been reported in HNSCC including tongue SCC (Child et al., 2009). Decreased expression of miR-133a and miR-133b was observed in tongue SCC cells. Tongue SCC cell lines (Cal27, HN21B and HN96) transfected with miR-133a and miR-133b precursors showed reduced proliferation rate and elevated apoptosis rate (Wong et al., 2008a). Overexpression of miR-133a and miR-133b reduced the expression of pyruvate kinase type M2 (PKM2) in tongue SCC cell lines (Wong et al., 2008a). The elevated expression of PKM2 in tongue SCC tissues was associated with the down-regulated expression of miR-133a and miR-133b (Wong et al., 2008a).

6.7 MiR-137 [Mature sequence: 59 - uuauugcuuaagaauacgcguag – 81 (MI0000454)]

Expression of mir-137 was downregulated in tongue carcinoma cells. Ectopic expression of miR-137 could inhibit cell growth cell growth in tongue SCC cell line HSC-6 and HSC-7 (Kozaki et al., 2008). MiR-137 is essential to cell cycle control of HNSCC. MiR-137 mimics enhanced the accumulation of G0-G1 phase cells, suggesting that it was associated with cell cycle arrest at the G1-S checkpoint (Kozaki et al., 2008). Expression of CDK6, E2F6, and NCOA2/TIF2 was suppressed by miR-137 in tongue SCC cell lines (Kozaki et al., 2008). Apart from the microRNA itself, the methylation status of miR-137 promoter has potential clinical value. Methylated miR-137 is a potential prognostic marker in HNSCC and is associated with survival (Langevin et al., 2011).

6.8 MiR-138 [Mature sequence: 23 - agcugguguugugaaucaggccg - 45 (MI0000476)]

MiR-138 is linked to cell invasion, cell cycle arrest and apoptosis of HNSCC (Liu et al. 2009). Reduced expression of miR-138 was reported in oral tongue cell lines UM1, UM2, Cal27, SCC1, SCC4, SCC9, SCC15, SCC25 (Liu et al., 2009). High level of miR-138 could reduce migration and invasion rate of tongue cancer cell UM1 and UM2 (Jiang et al., 2010). It has been demonstrated that overexpression of miR-138 could reduce expression of two key genes in the Rho GTPase signaling pathway, RhoC and ROCK2, leading to the reorganization of the stress fibers (Jiang et al., 2010). In contrast, inhibition the expression of miR-138 increased RhoC and ROCK2, contributing to an elongated cell morphology and enhanced cell migration and invasion (Jiang et al., 2010). The expression level of miR-138 was inhibited in hypopharyngeal carcinoma cell line (1386Tu) and oropharyngeal carcinoma cell line (686Tu) compared to non-tumorigenic cells (OKF4-E6/7 and NHOK) (Liu et al., 2009)

6.9 MiR-141 [Mature sequence: 59 - uaacacugucugguaaagaugg – 80 (MI0000457)]

Dysregulation of miR-141 was observed in head and neck cancer. However, its role in the pathogenesis remains unknown. Enhanced miR-141 expression was observed in NPC specimens in comparison with normal nasopharyngeal epithelium. Suppression of miR-141 affected cell cycle, apoptosis, cell growth, migration and invasion in NPC cells (Zhang et al., 2010). It has been shown that miR-141 directly targeted BRD3, UBAP1 and PTEN that are involved in NPC carcinogenesis (Zhang et al., 2010). Furthermore, inhibition of miR-141 affected the expression levels of some important molecules in the Rb/E2F, JNK2 and AKT pathways (Zhang et al., 2010). In contrast, Nurul-Syakima *et al.* demonstrated that miR-141 was downregulated in HNSCC and the results were different from those observed in NPC (Nurul-Syakima et al., 2011). Further studies are warranted to elucidate the role of miR-141 in head and neck cancers.

6.10 MiR-184 [Mature sequence: 53 - uggacggagaacugauaagggu – 74 (MI0000481)]

MiR-184 was overexpressed in early oral SCC (Cervigne et al., 2009). Cervigne *et al.* demonstrated that miR-184 was upregulated during the progression of progressive dysplasia and oral SCC suggesting that miR-184 might potentially be used as a biomarker for malignant transformation. In tongue SCC, primary tumor has higher level of miR-184 in comparison with the paired normal epithelial cells. Inhibition of endogenous miR-184 in tongue SCC cell lines (Cal27, HN21B, and HN96) resulted in reduced cell proliferation rate and enhanced apoptotic rate (Wong et al., 2008b). The observations that miR-184 levels were increased in the plasma before operation and decreased significantly after surgical treatment suggested that plasma miR-184 levels might serve as biomarker in oral tongue SCC patients (Wong et al., 2008b).

6.11 MiR-193a [Mature sequence 21 - ugggucuuugcgggcgagauga – 42 (MI0000487)]

The expression of miR-193a was inhibited in buccal mucosa cell line HO-1-N-1 cell line. Furthermore, HO-1-N-1 cell line transfected with miR-193a mimics displayed suppressed cell growth and induced apoptosis (Kozaki et al., 2008). In addition, miR-193a mimics reduced the protein levels of E2F6 and PTK2/FAK (Kozaki et al., 2008).

6.12 MiR-204 [Mature sequence 33 - uucccuuugucauccuaugccu – 54 (MI0000284)]

The expression of miR-204 was suppressed in tongue SCC cell lines (SCC58, SCC61, SCC151) and hard palate cell line SCC135 (Lee et al., 2010). Overexpression of miR-204 inhibited migration, adhesion and invasion of HNSCC cell (Lee et al., 2010). MiR-204 expression was reduced in NPC cell lines JSQ3 (Nasal cavity) and SQ38 (pyriform sinus) compared to samples of pooled normal buccal mucosa. NPC cell lines transfected with miR-204 mimics displayed suppressed cell-matrix interaction, motility and invasiveness (Lee et al., 2010).

6.13 MiR-205 [Mature sequence: 34 - uccuucauuccaccggagucug – 55 (MI0000285)]

MiR-205 is associated with the epithelial-mesenchymal transition of head and neck carcinoma (Zidar et al., 2011). It was proposed that high expression levels of miR- 205 can be used to detect HNSCC positive lymph nodes (Fletcher et al., 2008).

6.14 MiR-222 [Mature sequence: 69 - agcuacaucuggcuacugggu – 89 (MI0000299)]

MiR-222 is associated with the aggressiveness of tongue cancer cell lines (Liu et al., 2009b). Overexpression of miR-222 in UM1 resulted in reduced cell invasion (Liu et al., 2009b). It has been shown that miR-222 directly targeted metalloproteinase 1 (MMP1) and manganese superoxide dismutase 2 (SOD2) and suppressed their expression in oral tongue SCC cell lines (Liu et al., 2009b). These results indicated that miR-222 may serve as a novel therapeutic target for oral tongue SCC patients (Liu et al., 2009b).

6.15 Others microRNA dysregulation

It was recently shown that the expression levels of miR-221 to miR-375 could be used to distinguish tumor from normal tissue with high specificity and sensitivity (Avissar et al., 2009). The expression levels of miR-196b, miR-138, miR-155, miR-142-3p, and miR-18a were elevated and expression levels of miR-204, miR-449a, miR-34c-3p, miR-143, and miR-145 were reduced in NPC samples in comparison with normal nasopharyngeal tissues (Chen et al., 2009). Several biological pathways including TGF-Wnt pathways, G1-S cell cycle progression, VEGF signaling pathways, apoptosis and survival pathways, and IP3 signaling pathways are targeted by these down-regulated microRNA (Chen et al., 2009).

Tumor sites	Sub-sites	MicroRNA	Dysregulation	Related functions	References
oral cavity carcinoma	alveolar ridge	miR-100	down-regulated	proliferation	(Henson et al., 2009)
		miR-125b	down-regulated	proliferation	(Henson et al., 2009)
	buccal mucosa	miR-100	down-regulated	proliferation	(Henson et al., 2009)
		miR-125b	down-regulated	proliferation	(Henson et al., 2009)
		miR-193a	down-regulated	growth	(Kozaki et al., 2008)
	floor of mouth	miR-100	down-regulated	proliferation	(Henson et al., 2009)
		miR-125b	down-regulated	proliferation	(Henson et al., 2009)
		miR-138	down-regulated	migration, invasion	(Jiang et al., 2010; Liu et al., 2009a)
	hard palate	miR-204	down-regulated	migration, invasion	(Lee et al., 2010)
	retromolar trigone	miR-100	down-regulated	proliferation	(Henson et al., 2009)
		miR-125b	down-regulated	proliferation	(Henson et al., 2009)
	tongue	miR-100	down-regulated	proliferation	(Henson et al., 2009)
		miR-125b	down-regulated	proliferation	(Henson et al., 2009)
		miR-138	down-regulated	migration,	(Henson et al., 2009;
		miR-184	up-regulated	invasion	Liu et al., 2009a)
		miR-204	down-regulated	apoptosis,	(Wong et al., 2008b)
		miR-222	down-regulated	proliferation	(Lee et al., 2010)
		miR-21	up-regulated	migration,	(Liu et al., 2009b)
		miR-133a	down-regulated	invasion	(Li et al., 2009)
		miR-133b	down-regulated	invasion	(Wong et al., 2008a)
		miR-137	down-regulated	apoptosis,	(Wong et al., 2008a)
				survival	(Kozaki et al., 2008)
				proliferation,	
				apoptosis	
				proliferation,	
				apoptosis	
				growth	
naso pharyngeal carcinoma		miR-196b	up-regulated		(Chen et al., 2009)
		miR-138	up-regulated	proliferation	(Chen et al., 2009)
		miR-155	up-regulated	metastasis	(Chen et al., 2009)
		miR-142-3p	up-regulated	apoptosis,	(Chen et al., 2009)
		miR-18a	up-regulated	invasion	(Chen et al., 2009)
		miR-204	down-regulated	migration,	(Chen et al., 2009)
		miR-449a	down-regulated	invasion	(Chen et al., 2009)
		miR-34c-3p	down-regulated		(Chen et al., 2009)
		miR-143	down-regulated		(Chen et al., 2009)
		miR-145	down-regulated		(Chen et al., 2009)
		let-7 family	down-regulated		(Wong et al., 2011)
		miR-29c	down-regulated		(Sengupta et al., 2008)
		miR-141	up-regulated		(Zhang et al., 2010)
		miR-204	down-regulated		(Lee et al., 2010)

Tumor sites	Sub-sites	MicroRNA	Dysregulation	Related functions	References
pharyngeal carcinoma	oropharynx	miR-138	down-regulated		(Liu et al., 2009a)
	hypo pharynx	miR-138	down-regulated		(Liu et al., 2009a)
laryngeal carcinoma		miR-let-7a miR-204 miR-21 miR-15a	down-regulated down-regulated up-regulated down-regulated	Proliferation, apoptosis migration, invasion growth proliferation	(Long et al., 2009) (Lee et al., 2010) (Chang et al., 2008) (Cohen et al., 2009)

Table 1. MicroRNA dysregulation in HNSCC

7. The role of viral-encoded microRNA in head and neck cancers

7.1 Epstein-Barr Virus (EBV)

EBV is a member of gamma-Herpes virus and is closely associated with the progression of undifferentiated nasopharyngeal carcinoma (Wei and Sham, 2005). EBV is the first identified oncogenic virus. Expression of EBV-encoded oncoproteins are linked to epithelial-mesenchymal transition of metastatic nasopharyngeal carcinoma (HoriKawa et al., 2011). EBV could alter somatic gene expression by controlling the microRNA biogenesis machinery of the host cells. Li *et al.* observed that LMP1 could induce expression of miR-10b and promote metastasis of nasopharyngeal carcinoma cells (Li et al., 2010). Du *et al.* reported that EBV oncoprotein LMP1 and LMP2A could activate miR-155 expression in nasopharyngeal carcinoma cells which is associated with the nodal status and metastasis of nasopharyngeal carcinoma patients (Du et al., 2011).

Apart from the viral oncoprotein, the microRNA encoded by EBV virus itself is also playing a part in pathogenesis of nasopharyngeal carcinoma cells. EBV-encoded microRNA was first discovered in 2004 (Pfeffer et al., 2004). At present, 25 precursors and 44 mature microRNA were identified (Sanger database Release 16). The identified EBV microRNA are encoded in 2 major clusters: BHRF1 cluster and BART cluster (Lung et al., 2009). Barth *et al.* demonstrated that EBV-BART2 could target EBV DNA polymerase BALF5 hindering the lytic replication of EBV (Barth et al., 2008). EBV-encoded microRNA could regulate the activity of EBV and enhance the survival of the host cells (Lo et al., 2007). For example, BART5-5p could target pro-apoptotic gene PUMA contributing to the resistance to apoptotic agents (Choy et al., 2008).

As mentioned above, expression of the EBV oncoprotein LMP1 (Key viral oncoprotein linked to the pathogenesis of nasopharyngeal carcinoma) is critical in the pathogenesis of nasopharyngeal carcinoma. LMP1 act as tumor necrosis factor receptor (TNFR). It is the activator in multiple cancer-related pathways and could enhance proliferation, migration, and cell cycle progression in nasopharyngeal carcinoma cells (Kung et al., 2011). It is now known that LMP1 expression is partly controlled by the EBV-encoded microRNA. Lo *et al.* demonstrated that BART1-5p, BART16-5p and BART17-5p are involved in the regulation of LMP1 in nasopharyngeal carcinoma cells (Lo et al., 2007). In addition, LMP1 can suppress somatic gene expression by inducing somatic microRNA expression (Anastasiadou et al., 2011; Motsch et al., 2007).

7.2 Human Papilloma Virus (HPV)

HPV is a DNA virus and could infect squamous epithelial cells (Muno et al., 2003; Tran et al., 2007). HPV infection was closely associated with cervical cancer and account for 70% of the cervical cancers (No et al., 2011). Recent data suggested that it could also play a role in HNSCC. In general, HPV could be found in about 30% of the HNSCC. According to Heller and Münger, HPV is associated with 24% oral cavity cancer and 36% in oropharynx cancer (Hellner and Münger, 2011). HPV infection has also been reported in nasopharyngeal carcinoma (Lo et al., 2010). Increasing evidence suggested that HPV is closely associated with tonsillar cancer with prevalence ranged from 50-100% (Hammarstedt et al., 2006; Nasman et al., 2009; Syrjanen, 2004). Alcohol and tobacco consumption is linked to the risk of HPV infection (Chaturvedi et al., 2008; Tran, 2007). HPV status greatly influences the clinical features and prognosis of head and neck cancer patients (Lajer and Buchwald, 2010). The viral-encoded oncoprotein is a sensitive and specific marker for identifying tonsillar carcinoma patients (Hellner and Münger, 2011).

HPV-infected HNSCC cells had a different microRNA expression pattern in comparison with the HPV-negative counterpart (Wald et al., 2011; Wang et al., 2008). It is now clear that HPV could affect the host microRNA expression patterns resulting in the distinct clinical features (Lajer and Buchwald, 2010). Similar to EBV, HPV-encoded microRNA could modulate the microRNA expression machinery of the host (Wang et al., 2009). Lajer *et al.* reported that HPV infection is closely associated with the alteration of miR-127-3p and miR363 in oral and pharyngeal SCC (Lajer et al., 2011). By interfering the E6-p53 and E7-pRb pathways, HPV E6 and E7 oncoproteins could control expression of miR-15/16 cluster, miR-17-92 family, miR-21, miR-23b, miR-34a, and miR-106b/93/25 cluster in the host cells (Zheng and Wang, 2011).

By the time of writing, there is still no HPV-encoded microRNA reported and its role is largely unknown. In addition, the oncogenic role of HPV is affected by geographic factors (Lajer et al., 2010). The prevalence of HPV-associated HNSCC varies between different geographic regions. Low prevalence is reported in Asia, Central Europe, and Latin America (Kreimer et al., 2005; Ribeiro et al., 2011). HPV is nearly undetectable in tonsillar carcinoma of the Chinese patients (Li et al., 2003). The data suggested that HPV infection is a risk factor for a subset of HNSCC and the molecular pathways associated with HPV-negative HNSCC remain to be elucidated.

8. Methods used in microRNA detection

Similar to gene expression patterns, head and neck cancers had specific microRNA expression patterns. With microRNA profiling, Lu *et al.* could distinguish poorly differentiated carcinoma from the rest (Lu et al., 2005). Thus, there is a need to develop molecular techniques to (1) detect and quantify known microRNA; and (2) identify novel microRNA; and (3) perform global and high throughput microRNA profiling. Since identification of the first microRNA in *C. elegan*, the technologies employed to examine microRNA are fast evolving. The following session will briefly describe the common methods used in microRNA research. Among all the method, northern blotting is nearly the first use to detect and quantify specific microRNA expression (Lau et al., 2001). To date, this technique is largely replaced by others in detecting and quantifying microRNA. *In situ* hybridization detection is used to monitor the cellular and subcellular distribution of microRNA (Wienholds et al., 2005). *In situ* hybridization could be used on both frozen section and on archival formalin-fixed paraffin-embedded (FFPE) allowing localization of microRNA in clinical specimens. Real-time quantitative PCR is now the most commonly used technique in detecting and quantifying microRNA of interest. With the growing number of microRNA sequence published in the miRBase, real-time quantitative PCR primers and probe set could be designed to amplify specific microRNAs. For high throughout microRNA profiling, different form of microRNA array are commercially available. The oligo-nucleotide arrays allow detection of the whole miRBase library in a single run and are very suitable to use in examining the expression patterns of samples (Liu et al., 2008). Recently, next generation sequencing (deep sequencing) is employed to identify novel microRNA. The technique allows sequencing of the whole genome within weeks. In addition, deep sequencing can be used to identify posttranscriptional modifications in mature microRNAs. Initial studies have suggested that these post-transcriptionally modified, so-called isomiRs, might be evidence of tissue-specific or even tumor-specific distribution (Lee et al., 2010; Kunchenbauer et al., 2008). Commonly used system for microRNA identification includes Solexa (Illumina), SOLiD (ABI), and 454 (Roche) which allows detection of microRNA in low abundance (Fridlander et al., 2008).

9. MicroRNA and epigenetic therapies

MicroRNA could target multiple gene transcripts making it a good choice for systemic therapy of cancers. The rationale of microRNA-based therapy is similar to siRNA-based therapy. Based on the gene sequence, the microRNA/siRNA of a target gene could be synthesized chemically and delivered to the cancer patients. Synthetic microRNA can be used to restore the levels of basal tumor suppressing microRNA in cancer cells. In addition, microRNA antagonist (partially or completely complementary to specific microRNA sequences) can be designed based on the mature microRNA sequence to inhibit the overexpressed oncogenic microRNA in cancer cells (Krutzfeldt et al., 2005). The therapeutic microRNA could be packed into microvesicles and delivered to the cancer sites directly or through the circulation system (Skog et al., 2008). Cancer cell could take up the microvesicles at high efficiency as the constituent of microvesicle are similar to the plasma membrane (Thery et al., 2002). Elmén *et al.* tested this idea using mouse models and non-human primate models [African green monkeys (*Chlorocebus aethiops*)] (Elmén et al., 2008). They synthesized the miR-122 antagonist and delivered it into the animal model. MiR-122 is related to the cholesterol mechanisms in liver cells. The miR-122 antagonist could be taken by the liver cells resulting in decreased plasma cholesterol levels without any toxicity. Similar to drug treatment, the major challenge of microRNA-based therapy is the efficiency to deliver the therapeutic microRNA to cancer tissues as microvesicle in circulation is actively cleaned up by macrophage and kidney. Further, large microvesicles are difficult to pass through the capilliary endothelium and extracellular matrix of head and neck tissues (Bader et al., 2011). Advances in the microRNA delivery system are necessary in order to put microRNA-based therapy into clinical practice.

10. Concluding remarks

HNSCC is a complex disease caused by accumulating genetic, epigenetic and proteomic alterations. MicroRNA is a potent regulator controlling multiple biological processes including cell growth, differentiation, cell death, development and immune responses (Flynt et al., 2008; Stefani et al., 2008; Lodish et al., 2008). With emerging data supporting that microRNA plays a central role in gene dysregulation in human malignancies, unraveling the microRNA expression patterns in different HNSCC is essential and critical if we want to develop better diagnostic and prognostic system for our patients. On the other hand, gaining better insight into the regulatory mechanisms of microRNA would allow us to design therapeutic regime, which targets the disease with better outcome. We could anticipate that our knowledge to HNSCC will be changed with the increase in understanding of microRNA in the coming decades. Translating our knowledge into clinical management will be a beneficial to the treatment and prognosis of our patients.

11. References

Akervall, J. (2005). Gene profiling in squamous cell carcinoma of the head and neck. *Cancer Metastasis Reviews*, Vol.24, No.1, (January 2005), pp. 87–94, ISSN 0167-7659

Altekruse SF, Kosary CL, Krapcho M, Neyman N, Aminou R, Waldron W, Ruhl J, Howlader N, Tatalovich Z, Cho H, Mariotto A, Eisner MP, Lewis DR, Cronin K, Chen HS, Feuer EJ, Stinchcomb DG, Edwards BK: *SEER Cancer Statistics Review 1975-2007*. National Cancer Institute. Bethesda, MD. Available from: http://www.seer.cancer.gov/csr/1975_2008/index.html

Ambros, V. (2004). The functions of animal microRNAs. *Nature*, Vol.431, No. 7006, (September 2004), pp. 350-355, ISSN 0028-0836

Anastasiadou, E., Boccellato, F., Vincenti, S., Rosato, P., Bozzoni, I., Frati, L., Faggioni, A., Presutti, C., and Trivedi, P. (2010). Epstein-Barr virus encoded LMP1 downregulates TCL1 oncogene through miR-29b. *Oncogene*, Vol.29, No.9, (March 2010), pp. 1316–1328, ISSN 0950-9232

Argiris, A., and Eng, C. (2003). Epidemiology, staging, and screening of head and neck cancer. *Cancer treatment and research*, Vol.114, (Jan 2003) pp. 15-60, ISSN 0927-3042

Argiris, A., Brockstein, B. E., Haraf, D. J., Stenson, K. M., Mittal, B. B., Kies, M. S., Rosen, F. R., Jovanovic, B., and Vokes, E. E. (2004). Competing causes of death and second primary tumors in patients with locoregionally advanced head and neck cancer treated with chemoradiotherapy. *Clinical Cancer Research*, Vol.10, No.6, (March 2004), pp. 1956-1962, ISSN 1078-0432

Avissar, M., Christensen, B. C., Kelsey, K. T., and Marsit, C. J. (2009). MicroRNA expression ratio is predictive of head and neck squamous cell carcinoma. *Clinical Cancer Research*, Vol. 15, No. 8, (April 2009), pp. 2850–2855, ISSN 1078-0432

Bader, A. G., Brown, D., Stoudemire, J., and Lammers, P. (2011). Developing therapeutic microRNAs for cancer. *Gene Therapy*, (June 2011), ISSN 0969-7128

Bartel, D. P. (2004). MicroRNAs: genomics, biogenesis, mechanism, and function. *Cell*, Vol.116, No.2, (Jan 2004) pp. 281-97, ISSN 0092-8674

Barth, S., Pfuhl, T., Mamiani, A., Ehses, C., Roemer, K., Kremmer, E., Jäker, C., Höck, J., Meister, G., and Grässer, F. A. (2008). Epstein-Barr virus-encoded microRNA miR-

BART2 down-regulates the viral DNA polymerase BALF5. *Nucleic Acids Research*, Vol.36, No.2, (Feb 2008), pp. 666-675, ISSN 0305-1048

Bauer, V. L., Braselmann, H., Henke, M., Mattern, D., Walch, A., Unger, K., Baudis, M., Lassmann, S., Huber, R., Wienberg, J., et al. (2008). Chromosomal changes characterize head and neck cancer with poor prognosis. *Journal of Molecular Medicine*, Vol.86, No.21, (December 2008), pp. 1353–1365, ISSN 0946-2716

Bilde, A., Buchwald, von, C., Johansen, J., Bastholt, L., Sørensen, J. A. H. M., Marker, P., Krogdahl, A., Hansen, H. S., Specht, L., Kirkegaard, J., et al. (2006). The Danish national guidelines for treatment of oral squamous cell carcinoma. *Acta Oncologica* (Stockholm, Sweden), Vol. 45, No.3, (January 2006), pp. 294-299, ISSN 1651-226X

Black, R. J., Bray, F., Ferlay, J., and Parkin, D. M. (1997). Cancer incidence and mortality in the European Union: cancer registry data and estimates of national incidence for 1990. *European Journal of Cancer* (Oxford, England : 1990), Vol.33, No.7, (June 1997), pp. 1075-1107, ISSN 0959-8049

Buchwald, von, C., Bilde, A., Shoaib, T., and Ross, G. (2002). Sentinel node biopsy: the technique and the feasibility in head and neck cancer. *ORL J. Otorhinolaryngoly Related Specialities*, Vol.64, No.4, (June 2002), pp. 268–274. ISSN 0301-1569

Bushati, N., and Cohen, S. M. (2007). microRNA functions. *Annual Review of Cell and Developmental Biology*, Vol. 23, (January 2007), pp. 175-205, ISSN 1081-0706

Calin, G. A., Dumitru, C. D., Shimizu, M., Bichi, R., Zupo, S., Noch, E., Aldler, H., Rattan, S., Keating, M., Rai, K., et al. (2002). Frequent deletions and down-regulation of micro-RNA genes miR15 and miR16 at 13q14 in chronic lymphocytic leukemia. *Proceedings of the National Academy of Sciences of the United States of America*, Vol.99, No.24, (November 2002), pp. 15524-15529, ISSN 0027-8424

Calin, G. A., Sevignani, C., Dumitru, C. D., Hyslop, T., Noch, E., Yendamuri, S., Shimizu, M., Rattan, S., Bullrich, F., Negrini, M., et al. (2004). Human microRNA genes are frequently located at fragile sites and genomic regions involved in cancers. *Proceedings of the National Academy of Sciences of the United States of America*, Vol.101, No.9, (March 2004), pp.2999–3004, ISSN 0027-8424

Cervigne, N. K., Reis, P. P., Machado, J., Sadikovic, B., Bradley, G., Galloni, N. N., Pintilie, M., Jurisica, I., Perez-Ordonez, B., Gilbert, R., et al. (2009). Identification of a microRNA signature associated with progression of leukoplakia to oral carcinoma. *Human Molecular Genetics*, Vol.18, No.24, (December 2009), pp. 4818-4829, ISSN 0964-6906

Chang, S. S., Jiang, W. W., Smith, I., Poeta, L. M., Begum, S., Glazer, C., Shan, S., Westra, W., Sidransky, D., and Califano, J. A. (2008). MicroRNA alterations in head and neck squamous cell carcinoma. *International Journal of Cancer*, Vol.123, No.12, (December 2008), pp. 2791-2797, ISSN 0020-7136

Chang, T.-C., Yu, D., Lee, Y.-S., Wentzel, E. A., Arking, D. E., West, K. M., Dang, C. V., Thomas-Tikhonenko, A., and Mendell, J. T. (2008). Widespread microRNA repression by Myc contributes to tumorigenesis. *Nature Genetics*, Vol.40, No.1, (January 2008), pp. 43–50, ISSN 1061-4036

Chaturvedi, A. K., Engels, E. A., Anderson, W. F., and Gillison, M. L. (2008). Incidence trends for human papillomavirus-related and -unrelated oral squamous cell carcinomas in the United States. *Journal of Clinical Oncology*, 2008 vol. 26 (4) pp. 612-619, ISSN 0732-183X

Chen, H. C., Chen, G. H., Chen, Y. H., Liao, W. L., Liu, C. Y., Chang, K. P., Chang, Y. S., and Chen, S. J. (2009). MicroRNA deregulation and pathway alterations in nasopharyngeal carcinoma. *British Journal of Cancer*, Vol.100, No.6, (March 2009), pp. 1002-1011, ISSN 0007-0920

Childs, G., Fazzari, M., Kung, G., Kawachi, N., Brandwein-Gensler, M., McLemore, M., Chen, Q., Burk, R. D., Smith, R. V., Prystowsky, M. B., et al. (2009). Low-level expression of microRNAs let-7d and miR-205 are prognostic markers of head and neck squamous cell carcinoma. *The American Journal of Pathology*, Vol.174, No.3, (March 2009), pp. 736-745, ISSN 0002-9440

Choy, E. Y.-W., Siu, K.-L., Kok, K.-H., Lung, R. W.-M., Tsang, C.-M., To, K.-F., Kwong, D. L.-W., Tsao, S.-W., and Jin, D.-Y. (2008). An Epstein-Barr virus-encoded microRNA targets PUMA to promote host cell survival. *The Journal of Experimental Medicine*, Vol.205, No.11, (Oct 2008), pp. 2551-2560, ISSN 2551–2560

Christensen, B. C., Avissar-Whiting, M., Ouellet, L. G., Butler, R. A., Nelson, H. H., McClean, M. D., Marsit, C. J., and Kelsey, K. T. (2010). Mature microRNA sequence polymorphism in MIR196A2 is associated with risk and prognosis of head and neck cancer. *Clinical Cancer Research*, Vol.16, No.14, (July 2010), pp. 3713-3720, ISSN 3713–3720.

Cohen, E. E. W., Zhu, H., Lingen, M. W., Martin, L. E., Kuo, W.-L., Choi, E. A., Kocherginsky, M., Parker, J. S., Chung, C. H., and Rosner, M. R. (2009). A feed-forward loop involving protein kinase Calpha and microRNAs regulates tumor cell cycle. *Cancer Research*, Vol.69, No.1, (January 2009), pp. 65-74, ISSN 0008-5472

de Planell-Saguer, M., and Rodicio, M. C. (2011). Analytical aspects of microRNA in diagnostics: A review. *Analytica Chimica Acta*, Vol.699, No.2, (August 2011), pp. 134-152, ISSN 0003-2670

Du, Z.-M., Hu, L.-F., Wang, H.-Y., Yan, L.-X., Zeng, Y.-X., Shao, J.-Y., and Ernberg, I. (2011). Upregulation of MiR-155 in nasopharyngeal carcinoma is partly driven by LMP1 and LMP2A and downregulates a negative prognostic marker JMJD1A. *PLoS ONE*, Vol.6, No.4, (2011), ISSN 1932-6203

Duan, R., Pak, C., and Jin, P. (2007). Single nucleotide polymorphism associated with mature miR-125a alters the processing of pri-microRNA. *Human Molecular Genetics*, Vol.16, No.9, (May 2007), pp. 1124-1131, ISSN 0964-6906

Elmén, J., Lindow, M., Schütz, S., Lawrence, M., Petri, A., Obad, S., Lindholm, M., Hedtjärn, M., Hansen, H. F., Berger, U., et al. (2008). LNA-mediated microRNA silencing in non-human primates. *Nature*, Vol.452, No.7189, (April 2008), pp. 896–899, ISSN 0028-0836

Farshadpour, F., Hordijk, G. J., Koole, R., and Slootweg, P. J. (2007). Non-smoking and non-drinking patients with head and neck squamous cell carcinoma: a distinct population. *Oral Disease*, Vol.13, No.2, (March 2007), pp. 239–243, ISSN 1354-523X

Farshadpour, F., Kranenborg, H., Calkoen, E. V. B., Hordijk, G. J., Koole, R., Slootweg, P. J., and Terhaard, C. H. (2011). Survival analysis of head and neck squamous cell carcinoma: influence of smoking and drinking. *Head & Neck*, Vol.33, No.6, (June 2011) pp. 817-823, ISSN 1043-3074

Ferdin, J., Kunej, T., and Calin, G. A. (2010). Non-coding RNAs: identification of cancer-associated microRNAs by gene profiling. *Technology in Cancer Research & Treatment*, Vol.9, No.2, (April 2010), pp. 123–138, ISSN:1533-0346

Février, B., and Raposo, G. (2004). Exosomes: endosomal-derived vesicles shipping extracellular messages. *Current Opinion in Cell Biology*, Vol.16, No.4, (August 2004), pp. 415–421, ISSN 0955-0674

Filipowicz, W., Bhattacharyya, S. N., and Sonenberg, N. (2008). Mechanisms of post-transcriptional regulation by microRNAs: are the answers in sight? *Nature Reviews Genetics*, Vol.9, No.2, (Feburary 2008), pp. 102–114, ISSN:1471-0056

Fletcher, A. M., Heaford, A. C., and Trask, D. K. (2008). Detection of metastatic head and neck squamous cell carcinoma using the relative expression of tissue-specific mir-205. *Translational Oncology*, 2008 vol. 1 (4) pp. 202-208, ISSN 1936-5233

Flynt, A. S., and Lai, E. C. (2008). Biological principles of microRNA-mediated regulation: shared themes amid diversity. *Nature Reviews Genetics*, Vol.9, No.11, (November 2008), pp. 831–842, ISSN 1471-0056

Friedländer, M. R., Chen, W., Adamidi, C., Maaskola, J., Einspanier, R., Knespel, S., and Rajewsky, N. (2008). Discovering microRNAs from deep sequencing data using miRDeep. *Nature Biotechnology*, Vol.26, No., 4, (April 2008), pp. 407–415, ISSN 1087-0156

Fu, X., Han, Y., Wu, Y., Zhu, X., Lu, X., Mao, F., Wang, X., He, X., Zhao, Y., and Zhao, Y. (2011). Prognostic role of microRNA-21 in various carcinomas: a systematic review and Meta-analysis. *European Journal of Clinical Investigation*, (April 2011), ISSN 0014-2972

Gollin, S. M. (2001). Chromosomal alterations in squamous cell carcinomas of the head and neck: window to the biology of disease. *Head & Neck*, Vol. 23, No.3, (March 2001), pp. 238–253, ISSN 1043-3074

Hammarstedt, L., Lindquist, D., Dahlstrand, H., Romanitan, M., Dahlgren, L. O., Joneberg, J., Creson, N., Lindholm, J., Ye, W., Dalianis, T., et al. (2006). Human papillomavirus as a risk factor for the increase in incidence of tonsillar cancer. *International Journal of Cancer*, Vol.119, No.11, (December 2006), pp. 2620–2623, ISSN 0020-7136

Hanke, M., Hoefig, K., Merz, H., Feller, A. C., Kausch, I., Jocham, D., Warnecke, J. M., and Sczakiel, G. (2010). A robust methodology to study urine microRNA as tumor marker: microRNA-126 and microRNA-182 are related to urinary bladder cancer. *Urologic Oncology*, Vol.28, No.6, (October 2010), pp. 655–661, ISSN 1078-1439

He, L., He, X., Lim, L. P., de Stanchina, E., Xuan, Z., Liang, Y., Xue, W., Zender, L., Magnus, J., Ridzon, D., et al. (2007). A microRNA component of the p53 tumour suppressor network. *Nature*, Vol.447, No. 7148, (June 2007), pp. 1130–1134. ISSN 0028-0836

He, L., Thomson, J. M., Hemann, M. T., Hernando-Monge, E., Mu, D., Goodson, S., Powers, S., Cordon-Cardo, C., Lowe, S. W., Hannon, G. J., et al. (2005). A microRNA polycistron as a potential human oncogene. *Nature*, Vol.435, No.7043, (June 2005), pp. 828–833, ISSN 0028-0836

Heijnen, H. F., Schiel, A. E., Fijnheer, R., Geuze, H. J., and Sixma, J. J. (1999). Activated platelets release two types of membrane vesicles: microvesicles by surface shedding and exosomes derived from exocytosis of multivesicular bodies and alpha-granules. *Blood*, Vol.94, No.11, (December 1999), pp. 3791–3799, ISSN 0006-4971

Hellner, K., and Münger, K. (2011). Human papillomaviruses as therapeutic targets in human cancer. *Journal of Clinical Oncology*, Vol.29, No.13, (May 2011), pp. 1785–1794, ISSN 0732-183X

Henson, B. J., Bhattacharjee, S., O'Dee, D. M., Feingold, E., and Gollin, S. M. (2009). Decreased expression of miR-125b and miR-100 in oral cancer cells contributes to malignancy. *Genes Chromosomes & Cancer*, Vol.48, No.7, (July 2009), pp. 569–582, ISSN 1045-2257

Horikawa, T., Yoshizaki, T., Kondo, S., Furukawa, M., Kaizaki, Y., and Pagano, J. S. (2011). Epstein-Barr Virus latent membrane protein 1 induces Snail and epithelial-mesenchymal transition in metastatic nasopharyngeal carcinoma. *British Journal of Cancer*, Vol.104, No.7, (March 2011), pp. 1160–1167, ISSN 0007-0920

Hui, A. B. Y., Lenarduzzi, M., Krushel, T., Waldron, L., Pintilie, M., Shi, W., Perez-Ordonez, B., Jurisica, I., O'Sullivan, B., Waldron, J., et al. (2010). Comprehensive MicroRNA profiling for head and neck squamous cell carcinomas. Clinical *Cancer Research*, Vol.16, No.4, (Feb 2010) pp. 1129-39

Hunter, M. P., Ismail, N., Zhang, X., Aguda, B. D., Lee, E. J., Yu, L., Xiao, T., Schafer, J., Lee, M.-L. T., Schmittgen, T. D., et al. (2008). Detection of microRNA expression in human peripheral blood microvesicles. *PLoS ONE*, Vol.3, No.11, (November 2008), pp. e3694, ISSN 1932-6203

Iguchi, H., Kosaka, N., and Ochiya, T. (2010). Secretory microRNAs as a versatile communication tool. *Communicative & Integrative Biology*, Vol.3, No.5, (September 2010), pp. 478–481, ISSN 1942-0889

Iorio, M. V., Ferracin, M., Liu, C.-G., Veronese, A., Spizzo, R., Sabbioni, S., Magri, E., Pedriali, M., Fabbri, M., Campiglio, M., et al. (2005). MicroRNA gene expression deregulation in human breast cancer. *Cancer Research*, Vol.65, No.16, (August 2005), pp. 7065–7070. ISSN 0008-5472

Jaber, M. A., Porter, S. R., Gilthorpe, M. S., Bedi, R., and Scully, C. (1999). Risk factors for oral epithelial dysplasia--the role of smoking and alcohol. *Oral Oncology*, Vol.35, No.2, (March 1999), pp. 151–156, ISSN 1368-8375

Jakymiw, A., Patel, R. S., Deming, N., Bhattacharyya, I., Shah, P., Lamont, R. J., Stewart, C. M., Cohen, D. M., and Chan, E. K. L. (2010). Overexpression of dicer as a result of reduced let-7 MicroRNA levels contributes to increased cell proliferation of oral cancer cells. *Genes Chromosomes & Cancer*, Vol.49, No.6, (June 2010), pp. 549–559, ISSN 1045-2257

Jiang, J., Lee, E. J., Gusev, Y., and Schmittgen, T. D. (2005). Real-time expression profiling of microRNA precursors in human cancer cell lines. *Nucleic Acids R*esearch, Vol.33, No.17, (September 2005), pp. 5394–5403, ISSN 0305-1048

Jiang, L., Liu, X., Kolokythas, A., Yu, J., Wang, A., Heidbreder, C. E., Shi, F., and Zhou, X. (2010). Downregulation of the Rho GTPase signaling pathway is involved in the microRNA-138-mediated inhibition of cell migration and invasion in tongue squamous cell carcinoma. *International Journal of Cancer*, Vol.127, No.3, (August 2010), pp. 505–512, ISSN 0020-7136

Kosaka, N., Iguchi, H., and Ochiya, T. (2010). Circulating microRNA in body fluid: a new potential biomarker for cancer diagnosis and prognosis. *Cancer Science*, Vol.101, No.10, pp. 2087–2092, ISSN 1347-9032

Kozaki, K.-I., Imoto, I., Mogi, S., Omura, K., and Inazawa, J. (2008). Exploration of tumor-suppressive microRNAs silenced by DNA hypermethylation in oral cancer. *Cancer Research*, Vol.68, No.7, (April 2008), pp. 2094–2105, ISSN 0008-5472

Kreimer, A. R., Clifford, G. M., Boyle, P., and Franceschi, S. (2005). Human papillomavirus types in head and neck squamous cell carcinomas worldwide: a systematic review. *Cancer Epidemiology Biomarkers Prevention*, Vol.14, No.2, (February 2005), pp. 467–475, ISSN 1055-9965

Krichevsky, A. M., and Gabriely, G. (2009). miR-21: a small multi-faceted RNA. *Journal of Cellular Molecular Medicine*, Vol.13, No.1, (January 2009), pp. 39–53, ISSN 1582-1838

Krutovskikh, V. A., and Herceg, Z. (2010). Oncogenic microRNAs (OncomiRs) as a new class of cancer biomarkers. *BioEssays*, Vol.32, No.10, (October 2010), pp. 894–904, ISSN 0265-9247

Krützfeldt, J., Rajewsky, N., Braich, R., Rajeev, K. G., Tuschl, T., Manoharan, M., and Stoffel, M. (2005). Silencing of microRNAs in vivo with 'antagomirs'. *Nature*, Vol. 438, No.7068, (December 2005), pp. 685–689, ISSN 0028-0836

Kuchenbauer, F., Morin, R. D., Argiropoulos, B., Petriv, O. I., Griffith, M., Heuser, M., Yung, E., Piper, J., Delaney, A., Prabhu, A.-L., et al. (2008). In-depth characterization of the microRNA transcriptome in a leukemia progression model. *Genome Research*, Vol.18, No.11, (November 2008), pp. 1787–1797, ISSN 1088-9051

Kung, C.-P., Meckes, D. G., and Raab-Traub, N. (2011). Epstein-Barr virus LMP1 activates EGFR, STAT3, and ERK through effects on PKCdelta. *Journal of Virology*, Vol.85, No.9, (May 2011), pp.4399–4408, ISSN 0022-538X

Lajer, C. B., and Buchwald, von, C. (2010). The role of human papillomavirus in head and neck cancer. *APMIS : acta pathologica, microbiologica, et immunologica Scandinavica*, Vol.118, No.6-7, (June 2010), pp. 510-519, ISSN 0903-4641

Lajer, C. B., Nielsen, F. C., Friis-Hansen, L., Norrild, B., Borup, R., Garnæs, E., Rossing, M., Specht, L., Therkildsen, M. H., Nauntofte, B., et al. (2011). Different microRNA signatures of oral and pharyngeal squamous cell carcinomas: a prospective translational study. *British Journal of Cancer*, Vol.104, No.5, (March 2010), pp. 830–840, ISSN 0007-0920

Langevin, S. M., Stone, R. A., Bunker, C. H., Grandis, J. R., Sobol, R. W., and Taioli, E. (2010). MicroRNA-137 promoter methylation in oral rinses from patients with squamous cell carcinoma of the head and neck is associated with gender and body mass index. *Carcinogenesis*, Vol.31, No.5, (May 2010), pp. 864–870, ISSN 0143-3334

Langevin, S. M., Stone, R. A., Bunker, C. H., Lyons-Weiler, M. A., Laframboise, W. A., Kelly, L., Seethala, R. R., Grandis, J. R., Sobol, R. W., and Taioli, E. (2011). MicroRNA-137 promoter methylation is associated with poorer overall survival in patients with squamous cell carcinoma of the head and neck. *Cancer*, Vol.117, No.7, (April 2011), pp. 1454–1462, ISSN 0008-543X

Lau, N. C., Lim, L. P., Weinstein, E. G., and Bartel, D. P. (2001). An abundant class of tiny RNAs with probable regulatory roles in Caenorhabditis elegans. *Science*, Vol.294, No.5543, (October 2001), pp. 858–862, ISSN 0036-8075

Lee, L. W., Zhang, S., Etheridge, A., Ma, L., Martin, D., Galas, D., and Wang, K. (2010). Complexity of the microRNA repertoire revealed by next-generation sequencing. *RNA*, Vol.16, No.11, (November 2010), pp. 2170–2180, ISSN 1355-8382

Lee, R. C., Feinbaum, R. L., and Ambros, V. (1993). The C. elegans heterochronic gene lin-4 encodes small RNAs with antisense complementarity to lin-14. *Cell*, Vol.75, No.5, (December 1993), pp. 843–854, ISSN 0092-8674

Lee, Y., Jeon, K., Lee, J.-T., Kim, S., and Kim, V. N. (2002). MicroRNA maturation: stepwise processing and subcellular localization. *The EMBO Journal*, Vol.21, No.17, (September 2002), pp. 4663–4670, ISSN 0261-4189

Lee, Y., Yang, X., Huang, Y., Fan, H., Zhang, Q., Wu, Y., Li, J., Hasina, R., Cheng, C., Lingen, M. W., et al. (2010). Network modeling identifies molecular functions targeted by miR-204 to suppress head and neck tumor metastasis. *PLoS Computional Biology*, Vol.6, No.4, pp. e1000730, ISSN 1553-734X

Lewis, B. P., Burge, C. B., and Bartel, D. P. (2005). Conserved seed pairing, often flanked by adenosines, indicates that thousands of human genes are microRNA targets. *Cell*, Vol.120, No.1, (January 2005), pp. 15–20, ISSN 0092-8674

Li, G., Wu, Z., Peng, Y., Liu, X., Lu, J., Wang, L., Pan, Q., He, M.-L., and Li, X.-P. (2010). MicroRNA-10b induced by Epstein-Barr virus-encoded latent membrane protein-1 promotes the metastasis of human nasopharyngeal carcinoma cells. *Cancer Letter*, Vol.299, No.1, (December 2010), pp.29–36, ISSN 0304-3835

Li, J., Huang, H., Sun, L., Yang, M., Pan, C., Chen, W., Wu, D., Lin, Z., Zeng, C., Yao, Y., et al. (2009). MiR-21 indicates poor prognosis in tongue squamous cell carcinomas as an apoptosis inhibitor. *Clinical Cancer Research*, Vol. 15, No.12, (June 2009), pp. 3998–4008, ISSN 1078-0432

Li, J., Smyth, P., Flavin, R., Cahill, S., Denning, K., Aherne, S., Guenther, S. M., O'Leary, J. J., and Sheils, O. (2007). Comparison of microRNA expression patterns using total RNA extracted from matched samples of formalin-fixed paraffin-embedded (FFPE) cells and snap frozen cells. *BMC Biotechnolology*, Vol.7, (June 2007) pp. 36-41, ISSN 1472-6750

Li, L., Zhang, Z.-M., Liu, Y., Wei, M.-H., Xue, L.-Y., Zou, S.-M., Di, X.-B., Han, N.-J., Zhang, K.-T., Xu, Z.-G., et al. (2010). DNA microarrays-based microRNA expression profiles derived from formalin-fixed paraffin-embedded tissue blocks of squammous cell carcinoma of larynx. *Zhonghua Bing Li Xue Za Zhi*, Vol.39, No.6, (June 2010), pp. 391–395. ISSN 0529-5807

Li, T., Chen, J.-X., Fu, X.-P., Yang, S., Zhang, Z., Chen, K.-H., and Li, Y. (2011). microRNA expression profiling of nasopharyngeal carcinoma. *Oncology Report*, Vol.25, No.5, (May 2011), pp. 1353–1363, ISSN 1021-335X

Li, W., Thompson, C. H., Xin, D., Cossart, Y. E., O'Brien, C. J., McNeil, E. B., Gao, K., Scolyer, R. A., and Rose, B. R. (2003). Absence of human papillomavirus in tonsillar squamous cell carcinomas from Chinese patients. *The American Journal of Pathology*, Vol.163, No.6, (December 2003), pp. 2185–2189, ISSN 0002-9440

Lim, L. P., Lau, N. C., Garrett-Engele, P., Grimson, A., Schelter, J. M., Castle, J., Bartel, D. P., Linsley, P. S., and Johnson, J. M. (2005). Microarray analysis shows that some microRNAs downregulate large numbers of target mRNAs. *Nature*, Vol.433, No.7027, (Feburary 2005), pp. 769–773, ISSN 0028-0836

Liu, C.-G., Spizzo, R., Calin, G. A., and Croce, C. M. (2008). Expression profiling of microRNA using oligo DNA arrays. *Methods*, Vol.44, No.1, (January 2008), pp. 22–30, ISSN 1046-2023

Liu, X., Chen, Z., Yu, J., Xia, J., and Zhou, X. (2009). MicroRNA profiling and head and neck cancer. *Comparative and Functional Genomics*, Vol.2009, No.837514, (June 2009), pp. 1-11, ISSN 1531-6912

Liu, X., Jiang, L., Wang, A., Yu, J., Shi, F., and Zhou, X. (2009). MicroRNA-138 suppresses invasion and promotes apoptosis in head and neck squamous cell carcinoma cell lines. *Cancer Letter*, Vol.286, No.2, (December 2009), pp. 217–222, ISSN 0304-3835

Liu, X., Yu, J., Jiang, L., Wang, A., Shi, F., Ye, H., and Zhou, X. (2009b). MicroRNA-222 regulates cell invasion by targeting matrix metalloproteinase 1 (MMP1) and manganese superoxide dismutase 2 (SOD2) in tongue squamous cell carcinoma cell lines. *Cancer Genomics & Proteomics*, Vol.6, No.3, (April 2009), pp. 131-139, ISSN 1109-6535

Liu, Z., Li, G., Wei, S., Niu, J., El-Naggar, A. K., Sturgis, E. M., and Wei, Q. (2010). Genetic variants in selected pre-microRNA genes and the risk of squamous cell carcinoma of the head and neck. Cancer, Vol.116, No.20, (October 2010), pp. 4753–4760, ISSN 0008-543X

Lo, A. K. F., To, K.-F., Lo, K. W., Lung, R. W.-M., Hui, J. W. Y., Liao, G., and Hayward, S. D. (2007). Modulation of LMP1 protein expression by EBV-encoded microRNAs. Proceedings of the National Academy of Sciences of the United States of America, Vol.104, No.41, (October 2007), pp. 16164–16169, ISSN 0027-8424

Lo, E. J., Bell, D., Woo, J., Li, G., Hanna, E. Y., El-Naggar, A. K., and Sturgis, E. M. (2010). Human papillomavirus & WHO type I nasopharyngeal carcinoma. Laryngoscope, Vol.120, No. Suppl 4, pp. S185, ISSN 0023-852X

Lodish, H. F., Zhou, B., Liu, G., and Chen, C.-Z. (2008). Micromanagement of the immune system by microRNAs. Nature Reviews. Immunology, Vol.8, No.2, (Feburary 2008), pp. 120–130. ISSN 1474-1733

Long, X.-B., Sun, G.-B., Hu, S., Liang, G.-T., Wang, N., Zhang, X.-H., Cao, P.-P., Zhen, H.-T., Cui, Y.-H., and Liu, Z. (2009). Let-7a microRNA functions as a potential tumor suppressor in human laryngeal cancer. Oncology Reports, Vol.22, No.5, (November 2009), pp. 1189–1195, ISSN 1021-335X

Lu, J., Getz, G., Miska, E. A., Alvarez-Saavedra, E., Lamb, J., Peck, D., Sweet-Cordero, A., Ebert, B. L., Mak, R. H., Ferrando, A. A., et al. (2005). MicroRNA expression profiles classify human cancers. Nature, Vol.435, No.7043, (June 2005), pp. 834–838, ISSN 0028-0836

Lung, R. W.-M., Tong, J. H.-M., Sung, Y.-M., Leung, P.-S., Ng, D. C.-H., Chau, S.-L., Chan, A. W.-H., Ng, E. K.-A., Lo, K.-W., and To K.-F. (2009). Modulation of LMP2A expression by a newly identified Epstein-Barr virus-encoded microRNA miR-BART22. Neoplasia (New York, NY), Vol.11, No.11, pp. 1174–1184, ISSN 1476-5586

Melo, S. A., and Esteller, M. (2011). Dysregulation of microRNAs in cancer: Playing with fire. FEBS Letters, Vol.585, No.13, (July 2011), pp. 2087–2099, ISSN 0014-5793

Mitchell, P. S., Parkin, R. K., Kroh, E. M., Fritz, B. R., Wyman, S. K., Pogosova-Agadjanyan, E. L., Peterson, A.,

Motsch, N., Pfuhl, T., Mrazek, J., Barth, S., and Grässer, F. A. (2007). Epstein-Barr virus-encoded latent membrane protein 1 (LMP1) induces the expression of the cellular microRNA miR-146a. RNA Biology, Vol.4, No.3, (November 2007), pp. 131–137, ISSN 1547-6286

Muñoz, N., Bosch, F. X., de Sanjosé, S., Herrero, R., Castellsagué, X., Shah, K. V., Snijders, P. J. F., Meijer, C. J. L. M., International Agency for Research on Cancer Multicenter Cervical Cancer Study Group (2003). Epidemiologic classification of human papillomavirus types associated with cervical cancer. The New England Journal of Medicine, Vol.348, No.6, (February 2003), pp. 518–527, ISSN 0028-4793

Muralidhar, B., Winder, D., Murray, M., Palmer, R., Barbosa-Morais, N., Saini, H., Roberts, I., Pett, M., and Coleman, N. (2011). Functional evidence that Drosha overexpression in cervical squamous cell carcinoma affects cell phenotype and microRNA profiles. The Journal of Pathology, Vol.224, No.4, pp. 496–507, ISSN 0022-3417

No, J. H., Kim, M.-K., Jeon, Y.-T., Kim, Y.-B., and Song, Y.-S. (2011). Human papillomavirus vaccine: widening the scope for cancer prevention. Molecular Carcinogenesis, Vol.50, No.4, (April 2011), pp. 244–253, ISSN 0899-1987

Noteboom, J., O'Briant, K. C., Allen, A., et al. (2008). Circulating microRNAs as stable blood-based markers for cancer detection. Proceedings of the National Academy of Sciences of the United States of America, Vol.105, No.30, (July 2008), pp. 10513–10518, ISSN 0027-8424

Näsman, A., Attner, P., Hammarstedt, L., Du, J., Eriksson, M., Giraud, G., Ahrlund-Richter, S., Marklund, L., Romanitan, M., Lindquist, D., et al. (2009). Incidence of human papillomavirus (HPV) positive tonsillar carcinoma in Stockholm, Sweden: an epidemic of viral-induced carcinoma? International Journal of Cancer, Vol.125, No.2, (July 2009), pp. 362–366, ISSN 0020-7136

Nurul-Syakima, A. M., Yoke-Kqueen, C., Sabariah, A. R., Shiran, M. S., Singh, A., and Learn-Han, L. (2011). Differential microRNA expression and identification of putative microRNA targets and pathways in head and neck cancers. Int Journal of Molecular Mediocine, Vol.28, No.3, (September 2011), pp. 327–336, ISSN 1078-0432

Papagiannakopoulos, T., Shapiro, A., and Kosik, K. S. (2008). MicroRNA-21 targets a network of key tumor-suppressive pathways in glioblastoma cells. Cancer Research, Vol.68, No.19, (October 2008), pp. 8164-8172, ISSN 0008-5472

Park, N. J., Zhou, H., Elashoff, D., Henson, B. S., Kastratovic, D. A., Abemayor, E., and Wong, D. T. (2009). Salivary microRNA: discovery, characterization, and clinical utility for oral cancer detection. Clinical Cancer Research, Vol.15, No.17, (September 2009), pp 5473–5477, ISSN 1078-0432

Parkin DM, Bray F. Chapter 2: The burden of HPV-related cancers. Vaccine 2006; 24 (Suppl 3):S/11–S25.

Parkin, D. M., Bray, F., Ferlay, J., and Pisani, P. (2005). Global cancer statistics, 2002. CA: A Cancer Journal for Clinicans, Vol.55, No.2, (Feburary 2005), pp. 74–108, ISSN 0007-9235

Persson, M., Andrén, Y., Mark, J., Horlings, H. M., Persson, F., and Stenman, G. (2009). Recurrent fusion of MYB and NFIB transcription factor genes in carcinomas of the breast and head and neck. Proceedings of the National Academy of Sciences of the United States of America, Vol.106, No.44, (November 2009), pp. 18740–18744. ISSN 0027-8424

Pfeffer, S., Zavolan, M., Grässer, A.-F., Russo, J.-J, Ju J., John, B., Enright, J.-A., Marks, D., Sander, C., and Tuschi, T. (2004) Identification of virus-encoded microRNAs. Science (New York, NY), Vol.304, No.5671 (April 2004), pp 734–736, ISSN 0036-8075

Place, R. F., Li, L.-C., Pookot, D., Noonan, E. J., and Dahiya, R. (2008). MicroRNA-373 induces expression of genes with complementary promoter sequences. Proceedings of the National Academy of Sciences of the United States of America, Vol.105, No.5, (Feburary 2008), pp. 1608–1613, ISSN 0027-8424

Posner, M. R. (2010). Integrating systemic agents into multimodality treatment of locally advanced head and neck cancer. Annals of Oncology, Vol.21, No. Suppl 7, (October 2010), pp. vii246-vii251, ISSN 0923-7534

Rentoft, M., Fahlén, J., Coates, P. J., Laurell, G., Sjöström, B., Rydén, P., and Nylander, K. (2011). miRNA analysis of formalin-fixed squamous cell carcinomas of the tongue is affected by age of the samples. International Journal of Oncology, Vol.38, No.1, (January 2011), pp. 61–69, ISSN 1019-6439

Ribeiro, K. B., Levi, J. E., Pawlita, M., Koifman, S., Matos, E., Eluf-Neto, J., Wunsch-Filho, V., Curado, M. P., Shangina, O., Zaridze, D., et al. (2011). Low human papillomavirus prevalence in head and neck cancer: results from two large case-control studies in high-incidence regions. International Journal of Epidemiology, Vol.40, No.2, (April 2011), pp. 489–502, ISSN 0300-5771

Robbins, K. T., Kumar, P., Harris, J., McCulloch, T., Cmelak, A., Sofferman, R., Levine, P., Weisman, R., Wilson, W., Weymuller, E., et al. (2005). Supradose intra-arterial cisplatin and concurrent radiation therapy for the treatment of stage IV head and neck squamous cell carcinoma is feasible and efficacious in a multi-institutional setting: results of Radiation Therapy Oncology Group Trial 9615. Journal of Clinical Oncology, Vol.23, No.7, (March 2005), pp. 1447–1454, ISSN 0732-183X

Scapoli, L., Palmieri, A., Muzio, Lo, L., Pezzetti, F., Rubini, C., Girardi, A., Farinella, F., Mazzotta, M., and Carinci, F. (2010). MicroRNA expression profiling of oral carcinoma identifies new markers of tumor progression. International Journal of Immunopathology and Pharmacology, Vol.23, No.4, (September 2010), pp. 1229–1234, ISSN 0394-6320

Sengupta, S., den Boon, J. A., Chen, I. H., Newton, M. A., Stanhope, S. A., Cheng, Y. J., Chen, C. J., Hildesheim, A., Sugden, B., and Ahlquist, P. (2008). MicroRNA 29c is down-regulated in nasopharyngeal carcinomas, up-regulating mRNAs encoding extracellular matrix proteins. Proceedings of the National Academy of Sciences of the United States of America, Vol.105, No.15, (April 2008), pp. 5874-5878, ISSN 0027-8424

Skog, J., Würdinger, T., van Rijn, S., Meijer, D. H., Gainche, L., Sena-Esteves, M., Curry, W. T., Carter, B. S., Krichevsky, A. M., and Breakefield, X. O. (2008). Glioblastoma microvesicles transport RNA and proteins that promote tumour growth and provide diagnostic biomarkers. Nature Cell Biology, Vol.10, No.12, (December 2008), pp. 1470–1476, ISSN 1465-7392

Slaby, O., Bienertova-Vasku, J., Svoboda, M., and Vyzula, R. (2011). Genetic polymorphisms and MicroRNAs: new direction in molecular epidemiology of solid cancer. Journal of Cellular and Molecular Medicine, (June 2011), ISSN 1582-1838 (Print)

Spafford, M. F., Koch, W. M., Reed, A. L., Califano, J. A., Xu, L. H., Eisenberger, C. F., Yip, L., Leong, P. L., Wu, L., Liu, S. X., et al. (2001). Detection of head and neck squamous cell carcinoma among exfoliated oral mucosal cells by microsatellite analysis. Clinical Cancer Research, Vol.7, No.3, (March 2001), pp. 607–612, ISSN: 1078-0432

Stefani, G., and Slack, F. J. (2008). Small non-coding RNAs in animal development. Nature Review. Molecular Cell Biology Vol.9, No.3, (March 2008), pp. 219–230. ISSN 1471-0072

Stell, P. M. (1989). Survival times in end-stage head and neck cancer. European Journal of Surgical Oncology, Vol.15, No.5, (October 1898), pp. 407–410, ISSN 0748-7983

Suzuki, H. I., Yamagata, K., Sugimoto, K., Iwamoto, T., Kato, S., and Miyazono, K. (2009). Modulation of microRNA processing by p53. Nature, Vol.460, No. 7254, (July 2009), pp. 529–533, ISSN 0028-0836

Syrjänen, S. (2004). HPV infections and tonsillar carcinoma. Journal of Clinical Pathology, Vol.57, No.5, (May 2004), pp. 449–455. ISSN 0021-9746

Théry, C., Zitvogel, L., and Amigorena, S. (2002). Exosomes: composition, biogenesis and function. Nature Review. Immunology Vol.2, No.8, (August 2002), pp. 569–579, ISSN 1474-1733

Tran, N., McLean, T., Zhang, X., Zhao, C. J., Thomson, J. M., O'Brien, C., and Rose, B. (2007). MicroRNA expression profiles in head and neck cancer cell lines. Biochemical and biophysical research communications, Vol.358, No.1, (June 2007), pp. 12-17, ISSN 0006-291X

Tran, N., Rose, B. R., and O'Brien, C. J. (2007). Role of human papillomavirus in the etiology of head and neck cancer. Head & Neck, Vol.29, No.1, (January 2007), pp. 64–70, ISSN 1043-3074

Turchinovich, A., Weiz, L., Langheinz, A., and Burwinkel, B. (2011). Characterization of extracellular circulating microRNA. Nucleic Acids Research, Vol.1, No.11, (May 2011), pp. 1-11, ISSN 0305-1048

Vasudevan, S., Tong, Y., and Steitz, J. A. (2007). Switching from repression to activation: microRNAs can up-regulate translation. Science, Vol.318, No.5858, (December 2007), pp. 1931–1934, ISSN 0036-8075

Volinia, S., Calin, G. A., Liu, C.-G., Ambs, S., Cimmino, A., Petrocca, F., Visone, R., Iorio, M., Roldo, C., Ferracin, M., et al. (2006). A microRNA expression signature of human solid tumors defines cancer gene targets. Proceedings of the National Academy of Sciences of the United States of America, Vol.103, No.7, (February 2006), pp. 2257-2261, ISSN 0027-8424

Wald, A. I., Hoskins, E. E., Wells, S. I., Ferris, R. L., and Khan, S. A. (2011). Alteration of microRNA profiles in squamous cell carcinoma of the head and neck cell lines by human papillomavirus. Head & Neck, Vol.33, No.4, (April 2011), pp. 504–512, ISSN 1043-3074

Wang, X., Tang, S., Le, S.-Y., Lu, R., Rader, J. S., Meyers, C., and Zheng, Z.-M. (2008). Aberrant expression of oncogenic and tumor-suppressive microRNAs in cervical cancer is required for cancer cell growth. PLoS ONE, Vol.3, No.7, (July 2008), pp. e2557, ISSN 1932-6203

Wang, X., Wang, H.-K., McCoy, J. P., Banerjee, N. S., Rader, J. S., Broker, T. R., Meyers, C., Chow, L. T., and Zheng, Z.-M. (2009). Oncogenic HPV infection interrupts the expression of tumor-suppressive miR-34a through viral oncoprotein E6. RNA, Vol.15, No.4, (April 2009), pp. 637–647, ISSN 1355-8382

Wei, W. I., and Sham, J. S. T. (2005). Nasopharyngeal carcinoma. Lancet, Vol.365, No.9476, (May 2005), pp. 2041–2054, ISSN 0140-6736

Wienholds, E., Kloosterman, W. P., Miska, E., Alvarez-Saavedra, E., Berezikov, E., de Bruijn, E., Horvitz, H. R., Kauppinen, S., and Plasterk, R. H. A. (2005). MicroRNA expression in zebrafish embryonic development. Science, Vol.309, No.5732, (July 2005), pp. 310–311, ISSN 0036-8075

Wightman, B., Ha, I., and Ruvkun, G. (1993). Posttranscriptional regulation of the heterochronic gene lin-14 by lin-4 mediates temporal pattern formation in C. elegans. Cell, Vol.75, No.5, (December 1993), pp. 855–862, ISSN 0092-8674

Wong, S. J., Harari, P. M., Garden, A. S., Schwartz, M., Bellm, L., Chen, A., Curran, W. J., Murphy, B. A., and Ang, K. K. (2011). Longitudinal Oncology Registry of Head and Neck Carcinoma (LORHAN): analysis of chemoradiation treatment approaches in the United States. Cancer, Vol.117, No.8, (April 2011), pp. 1679–1686, ISSN 0008-543X

Wong, T.-S., Liu, X.-B., Ho, C.-W., Yuen, A.-P., Ng, W.-M., Wei, W. (2008). Identification of pyruvate kinase type M2 as potential oncoprotein in squamous cell carcinoma of tongue through microRNA profiling. International Journal of Cancer, Vol.123, No.2, (July 2005), pp. 251–257, ISSN 0020-7136

Wong, T.-S., Liu, X.-B., Wong, B. Y.-H., Ng, R. W.-M., Yuen, A. P.-W., and Wei, W. I. (2008). Mature miR-184 as Potential Oncogenic microRNA of Squamous Cell Carcinoma of Tongue. Clinical Cancer Research, Vol.14, No.9, (May 2008), pp. 2588–2592, ISSN 1078-0432

Wong, T.-S., Man, O.-Y., Tsang, C.-M., Tsao, S.-W., Tsang, R. K.-Y., Chan, J. Y.-W., Ho, W.-K., Wei, W. I., and To, V. S.-H. (2011). MicroRNA let-7 suppresses nasopharyngeal carcinoma cells proliferation through downregulating c-Myc expression. Journal of cancer research and clinical oncology, Vol.137, No.3, (March 2011), pp. 415–422, ISSN 0171-5216

Yu, C.-C., Chen, Y.-W., Chiou, G.-Y., Tsai, L.-L., Huang, P.-I., Chang, C.-Y., Tseng, L.-M., Chiou, S.-H., Yen, S.-H., Chou, M.-Y., et al. (2011). MicroRNA let-7a represses chemoresistance and tumourigenicity in head and neck cancer via stem-like properties ablation. Oral Oncology, Vol.47, No.3, (March 2011), pp. 202–210, ISSN 1368-8375

Yu, Z., Li, Z., Jolicoeur, N., Zhang, L., Fortin, Y., Wang, E., Wu, M., and Shen, S.-H. (2007). Aberrant allele frequencies of the SNPs located in microRNA target sites are potentially associated with human cancers. Nucleic Acids Research, Vol.35, No.13, (June 2007), pp. 4535–4541, ISSN 0305-1048

Zhang, L., Deng, T., Li, X., Liu, H., Zhou, H., Ma, J., Wu, M., Zhou, M., Shen, S., Li, X., et al. (2010). microRNA-141 is involved in a nasopharyngeal carcinoma-related genes network. Carcinogenesis, Vol.31, No.4, (April 2010), pp. 559–566, ISSN 0143-3334

Zhang, S., Hao, J., Xie, F., Hu, X., Liu, C., Tong, J., Zhou, J., Wu, J., and Shao, C. (2011). Downregulation of miR-132 by promoter methylation contributes to pancreatic cancer development. Carcinogenesis, Vol., (July 2011), ISSN 0143-3334

Zhang, X., Cairns, M., Rose, B., O'Brien, C., Shannon, K., Clark, J., Gamble, J., and Tran, N. (2009). Alterations in microRNA processing and expression in pleomorphic adenomas of the salivary gland. International Journal of Cancer, Vol.124, No.12, pp. 2855–2863, ISSN 0020-7136

Zhang, X., Yang, H., Lee, J. J., Kim, E., Lippman, S. M., Khuri, F. R., Spitz, M. R., Lotan, R., Hong, W. K., and Wu, X. (2010). MicroRNA-related genetic variations as predictors for risk of second primary tumor and/or recurrence in patients with early-stage head and neck cancer. Carcinogenesis, Vol.31, No.12, (December 2010), pp. 2118–2123, ISSN 0143-3334

Zheng, Z.-M., and Wang, X. (2011). Regulation of cellular microRNA expression by human papillomaviruses. Biochimica et biophysica acta, (2011), ISSN 0006-3002

Zidar, N., Boštjančič, E., Gale, N., Kojc, N., Poljak, M., Glavač, D., and Cardesa, A. (2011). Down-regulation of microRNAs of the miR-200 family and miR-205, and an altered expression of classic and desmosomal cadherins in spindle cell carcinoma of the head and neck--hallmark of epithelial-mesenchymal transition. Hum Pathology, Vol.42, No.4, (April 2011), pp. 482–488, ISSN 0046-8177

Zubakov, D., Boersma, A. W. M., Choi, Y., van Kuijk, P. F., Wiemer, E. A. C., and Kayser, M. (2010). MicroRNA markers for forensic body fluid identification obtained from microarray screening and quantitative RT-PCR confirmation. International Journal of Legal Medicine, Vol.124, No.3, (May 2010), pp. 217–226, ISSN 0937-9827

16

Structural Features, Biological Functions of the Alpha-1 Antitrypsin and Contribution to Esophageal Cancer

Shahla Mohammad Ganji[1],
Ferdous Rastgar Jazii[1] and Abbas Sahebghadam-Lotfi[1,2]
[1]*Department of Biochemistry, National Institute of Genetic Engineering and Biotechnology (NIGEB), Tehran*
[2]*Department of Biochemistry, Tarbiat Modares University, Tehran*
Iran

1. Introduction

Alpha-1 antitrypsin (AAT) is a member of the serine protease inhibitors (serpin) family. Hepatocytes are the major source of synthesis and secretion of AAT into the blood stream, however macrophages of the lungs also take part in this process to a lower extent [1]. AAT is a proteolytic enzyme which plays major role in the normal physiological processes such as angiogenesis, intravascular fibrinolyis, and wound healing. However it may also participate in pathological conditions such as tumor invasion and metastasis which require degradation of the basement membrane, stimulation of angiogenesis, and migration [2, 3].

Following to synthesis AAT diffuses into tissues where it targets neutrophil elastase, a powerful protease capable of cleaving elastic fibers of alveolar walls and other structural proteins [4]. Apart from synthesis in the liver, AAT may also be synthesized and secreted by the epithelial cells of stomach, intestine, pancreas, and respiratory tract. Additionally, it can be produced by certain cancer cells, including cancers of gastric, colon, and lung. Tumor cells synthesize and release not only an intact native form of AAT, but also a variety of cleaved and/or degraded forms of alpha-1 antitrypsin. AAT has multiple effects on tumor cell viability and play diverse roles in tumorigenesis [2].

Being the most abundant human serum protease inhibitor, AAT is encoded by a single gene of 12.2 kb in length, which is located on the long arm of chromosome 14 (14q31-32.2). The protein is highly polymorphic and a number of alleles have so far been identified for it. These alleles are classified into the following four groups; group 1 or normal allele, whose product is AAT with normal function and serum level ranging from 150 up to 350 mg/dL -1. Group 2 or the deficient alleles is associated with serum AAT level less than 35% of normal subjects. In addition group 2 alleles may also not function normally. Group 3 includes the null allele as this group display no detectable serum AAT; and finally group 4 which includes dysfunctional alleles. The last group encodes AAT present at normal level; however, the AAT produced by this group is a non-functional AAT [5, 6]. Mutations in the AAT gene has shown to be associated with a number of diseases including Cirrhosis, COPD, pneumothorax, asthma, wegener's granulomatosis, pancreatitis , gallstones, bronchiectasis, pelvic organ prolapse, primary sclerosing cholangitis, autoimmune hepatitis, emphysema (predominantly involving the lower lobes and causing bullae), renal, and arthritis. In addition in other malignancies such as Hepatocellular carcinoma, Bladder carcinoma, Gallbladder cancer, Lymphoma, and lung cancer defects and mutations of AAT have also been reported [7, 8].

2. Alpha-1 antitrypsin deficiency (AATD), conformational disease

Alpha-1 antitrypsin deficiency (AATD) is an autosomal recessive genetic disorder caused by defective production of AAT, which leads to the decreased AAT activity in blood and lungs, and deposition of excessive abnormal AAT protein in liver cells. Severe AAT deficiency causes panacinar emphysema or COPD in adults with complications, especially if they were exposed to cigarette smoke. It also include subjects with various liver diseases in a minority of children and adults [9].

Symptoms of AATD include short dyspnea, wheezing, rhonchi, and rales (Crackles). The patient's symptoms may resemble recurrent respiratory infections or asthma that doesn't respond to treatment. Individuals with AATD may develop emphysema during their thirties or forties even without a history of significant smoking, though smoking greatly increases the risk for emphysema. AATD also causes impaired liver function in some patients and may lead to cirrhosis and liver failure (15%). It is a leading cause of liver transplantation in newborns.

The conformational diseases [10], which include diverse disorders such as Alzheimer's and Parkinson's, amyloidoses, AAT deficiency and the prion encephalopathies, take place due to conformational rearrangements of a specific protein that endows a tendency to aggregate formation and deposition within tissues or cellular compartments [11]. AAT deficiency serves as an excellent model for conformational disease because it is one of the few members of this class for which detailed structural data are available on both the wild type and mutant proteins [11]. Indeed, familial conformational diseases occur when a mutation alters specific conformation of protein resulting in abnormal intermolecular interactions, protein aggregation, and consequent tissue damage. The molecular mechanisms of conformational disease are best understood for the serine protease inhibitor (serpin) superfamily of proteins. The serpinopathies include alpha-1 antitrypsin (SERPINA1) deficiency and the newly characterized familial encephalopathy with neuroserpin inclusion bodies (FENIB) resulting from mutations in the neuroserpin (SERPINI1) gene [12].

Robin Carrell and Lomas [11] have described structural rearrangements that take place when AAT meets and inactivates its target, the serine proteases. In the case of AAT, this inherent instability allows the proteins to undergo loop-sheet polymerization, creating an abnormal structure in which the loop from the active site of one AAT molecule inserts itself as another β-strand into a pre-existing β-sheet of an adjacent molecule [11], [13, 14]. In the figure 1, the mechanism of inhibition of proteases by serpins and mutations resulting in disease has been shown [14]. This intrinsic tendency of wild-type AAT to undergo structural transformation is markedly enhanced in mutant forms. As such forms are more prone to accommodate the extraneous strand from an adjacent molecule since mutations destabilize the sheet, allowing an increased mobility of its constituent strands. This loop–sheet insertion is an example of conversion of a loop to a beta- strand through interactions

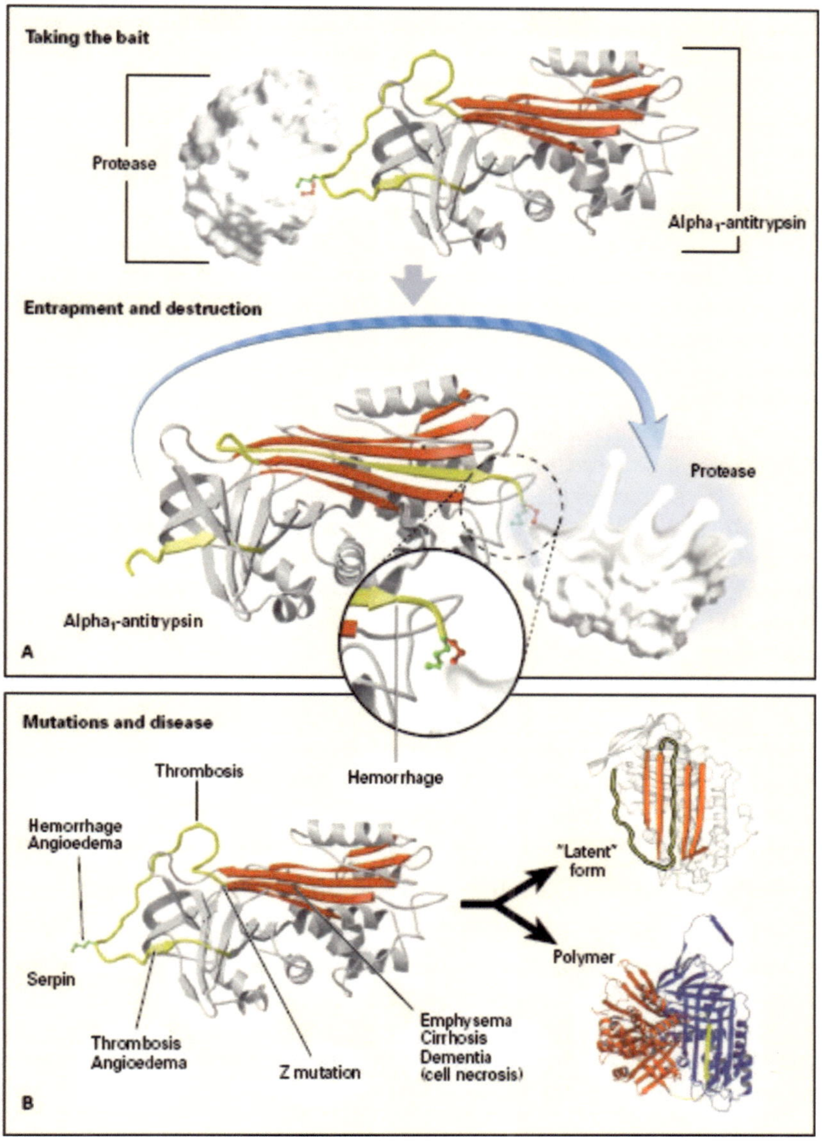

Fig. 1. Mechanism of inhibition of proteases by serpins and mutations resulting in disease.

The mechanism of inhibition of the serpins, represented in Panel A by AAT, is like that of a mousetrap, with a springlike shift from a metastable to a hyperstable state. The protease attacks the reactive center loop (yellow) of alpha1-antitrypsin, with the active serine of the protease (small red side chain) forming a link to the amino acid at the base of the reactive center (small green side chain) of alpha 1-antitrypsin. The resulting cleavage of the reactive loop allows it to snap back into the main *b* sheet (red ribbons with arrows) of the alpha 1 -antitrypsin. This spring-like movement flings the tethered protease to the opposite end of the alpha1 -antitrypsin molecule, distorting its active site (inset) and altering its structure so that it can be destroyed.

A sum 200 different mutations in serpins are known to result in disease (Panel B). In particular, mutations affecting antithrombin confer a predisposition to thrombosis, those affecting C1 inhibitor confer a predisposition to angioedema, and those affecting antiplasmin confer a predisposition to hemorrhage. Mutations at the reactive center result in a loss of function (e.g., causing familial angioedema) or more rarely result in a change in function (e.g., causing hemorrhagic disease). The insertion of an amino acid into the peptide loop containing the reactive center of another serpin, alpha2-antiplasmin, reduces the distortion of the catalytic site (inset) of plasmin, allowing its release, with consequent fibrinolysis and hemorrhage. The most common cause of loss of function of serpin molecules are mutations affecting the critical mobile hinges of the molecule. These lead to spontaneous changes in conformation that allow either the insertion of the intact reactive loop into the main *b* sheet, resulting in the formation of an inactive "latent" form, or the insertion of the loop of one molecule into the *b* sheet of the next, resulting in the formation of polymers. Polymerization occurs in AAT with the common Z variant and with mutations at the opening of the sheet, leading to emphysema and cirrhosis. Mutations at the same site in a neuron-specific serpin result in neurodegeneration and dementia (Carrell R.W. and Lomas D.A. 2002) with pre-existing β-sheet leading to pathological consequence. The tendency to undergo loop–sheet polymerization is not restricted to AAT as other serpins undergo the same transformation. In a rare form of familial encephalopathy where neuronal inclusion bodies (FENIB) form, it was found that inclusion body formation to be the result of a mutant neuroserpin which undergoes loop-sheet polymerization. Structural modeling of the neuroserpin mutants indicate that it may lead to the instability of β-sheet structure, increasing its propensity to gain an extraneous strand. Robin and Carrell [10] have suggested that such β-promiscuity may account not only for the pathologic properties of serpins, but also could explain the 'pathologic property of β-sheets in prion disorder that seems to be caused by the induced transition from α-helix to β-strand [11].

3. AAT, a response to malignancy and inflammation

AAT augments in the serum of gastrointestinal [15], prostate [16], brain [17] as well as biliary tract cancer [18] patients. Also reports indicate increased serum AAT in pancreatic adenocarcinoma [19], breast tumors [20], and esophageal cancer [21]. A significant correlation between serum AAT level and stage of cancer have also been proposed [22, 23]. Several means by which AAT plays role in malignancy and inflammations have been proposed so far as described in the following paragraphs:

a. Equilibrium hypothesis; it is assumed that changes in the ratio of a particular protease to its cognate inhibitor account for the increased potential of tumor formation [23]. Neutrophil elastase and AAT constitute a pair including protease and protease inhibitor counterpart which are in equilibration. Perturbation of this equilibration causes tissue damage and provides a favorable environment for carcinogenesis and tumor progression. Laboratory and clinical findings have indicated that deficiency in AAT is associated with the increased risk of cancers such as liver, bladder, gall bladder, malignant lymphoma, and lung cancer. Conversely elevated concentration of neutrophil elastase may promote development; invasion and metastasis of many types of cancers as a result of tissue damage and air trap which foster longer exposure to the carcinogens and hence promotion of cancer by degradation of extracellular matrix. In this regard tumor-necrosis-factor signaling pathway plays a role [24].

b. The other hypothesis suggests the roles that are played by a protease inhibitor *per se*. While imbalanced equilibration between protease to its cognate inhibitor would affect malignancy (as described above), however the inhibitor by itself seems to play more complicated function. The finding of a high serum concentrations of protease inhibitor even in the advanced stage of cancer at first glance was paradoxical, since inhibitors such as AAT are supposed to counteract the destructive activity of proteolytic enzymes (e.g. trypsin). However, it became clear that the role of protease inhibitors is rather complex and that, in most types of cancers, they play important role in modulating the dynamics of the proteolysis, in which proteases, inhibitors, regulators, cytokines and growth factors interact with each other through unknown mechanisms that have yet to be explored [25]. Tissue dependency of protease inhibitor activity is another phenomenon observed in malignancies. Cancers originated from several tissues often produce tumor associated trypsin inhibitor (TATI), however the strongest expression of which could be seen in mucinous ovarian tumors, both in benign and malignant type of tumors. Thus it appears that expression of TATI is regulated by different mechanisms in different tissues. In the other word expression of TATI is tissue dependent. TATI is a 6 kDa peptide, which is synthesized by several tumors and cell lines and produced by the mucosa of the gastrointestinal tract, where it is thought to protect the mucosal cells from proteolysis. Elevated serum and urine level of TATI occurs in connection with many types of cancer, especially mucinous ovarian cancer, pancreatitis, severe infections and tissue destruction. Thus TATI may behave as an acute phase reactant. While elevation of TATI in cancer and pancreatic disease is associated with expression of trypsin, but such a relationship has not been observed for the inflammatory disease. TATI inhibits trypsin-mediated degradation of extracellular matrix by tumor cells. Therefore it might control activation of tumor-associated trypsinogen [26].

Regarding malignant diseases; increased level of TATI has been observed both in serum and urine. In most cancers the increased secretion is caused by tumors, however in acute-phase reaction which is induced by tissue destruction and advanced disease TATI secretion is associated with cancer invasion. The concentration of TATI in serum and urine correlates strongly with tumor invasion. Howeve there is more variation in urine concentrations of TATI; therefore the serum concentration of TATI is preferred if it is going to be used as an indicator of the degree of invasion [27].

3.1 AAT as an acute phase response

AAT is secreted into circulation and increased level of which is the result of at least three mechanisms: production by tumors, leakage from a diseased pancreas and as a reaction against tissue damage and by impaired renal function [28]. For supporting this proposal, Solakidi, *et al*, have shown that elevated serum tumor associated trypsin inhibitor (TATI) could be due to production of TATI by tumors [28]. They reached to this conclusion because none of patients had any signs or previous history of pancreatic disorders or impaired renal function. Moreover gastric and colorectal neoplasms of patients under study were positive for TATI immunoexpression which could explain the elevated TATI in serum as a result of tumor secretion. To find whether elevation of TATI could be explained in terms of acute-phase reaction, measurement of TATI and CRP (C-reactive protein), a prototype of acute-phase reactant proteins was done; the result of which indicated statistically significant correlation between serum TATI and acute-phase reactant protein level. This finding has indicated regulation of TATI synthesis as an acute-phase reaction. In supporting this notion, Peracaula, *et al*, [29] have suggested that acute-phase proteins might play important role as sensor of diseases. Both level of acute-phase protein and glycosylation have reported to be altered in the inflammation and other diseases including cancer. Factors that promote acute-phase protein synthesis and enhance the expression of specific glycosyltransferases, such as sialyltransferases and fucosyltransferases, may be up-regulated in some tumors which could explain the changes in acute-phase proteins level and specific *N*-glycosylation modifications of some acute-phase proteins in cancer.

4. AAT as a tumor marker and its clinical applicability

Elevation of serum AAT, assessment and association of its phenotype and genotype with regard to specific type of cancer has been subject of many studies on different types of cancers such as gastrointestinal cancers, brain tumors, biliary tract cancer, pancreatic adenocarcinoma, cancers of the prostate, breast, lung and liver [22, 23, 30-32]. Regarding esophageal cancer, there are limited reports available from Japan and Korea as well as our recent repot [21, 33]. These reports have suggested that serum AAT level could be considered as tumor marker. Our results show that the mean range of trypsin inhibitor capacity (TIC) and AAT level are significantly higher in patients than in healthy controls [34]. Hong and colleagues have observed significant increase in serum AAT in malignant esophageal cancer patients compared to benign tumors and healthy controls [35].

Recently Hsu and colleagues identified AAT as a potential biomarker of gastric cancer in gastric juice. They showed gastric juice AAT concentration is markedly higher in gastric cancer patients than in healthy subjects, gastric ulcer patients, and duodenal ulcer patients [2].

Investigating the histological pattern and tumor location of patients, Schena and colleagues [36] showed that AAT represents a diagnostic index of neoplastic diseases, highly sensitive but less specific. Saito and colleagues [37] have investigated severe septic complications as the major cause of post-surgery mortality in esophageal cancer patients. They assessed acute phase proteins in the infection related complications post-surgery in a large number of patients with esophageal cancer and have compared this group of patients with a group of gastric cancer patients and the healthy controls. Elevation of AAT, alpha-1 acidglycoprotein, haptoglobin, and ceruloplasmin was more prominent in patients with esophageal cancer. Stenman and colleagues [27] showed that the TATI level increased in serum of patients with pancreatic, gastric, hepatocellular, biliary tract, and colorectal cancer. They concluded that TATI is a sensitive marker. It increased in 75–95% of pancreatic patients, 40–65% of gastric patients, 60–80% of hepatocellular patients, 75–100% of those with biliary tract, and 34–74% of patients with colorectal cancers [27].

An outstanding study carried out by Varela, and López Sáez [38] indicates that plasma level of A1AP (alpha-1 antiprotease); a member of serpins superfamily increases in clinically active cancer compared to the normal controls and normal range values for clinically defined complete remission. The mean value of A1AP was lower in healthy individuals than individuals with chronic non-malignant diseases. Notably A1AP in both groups was lower than individuals with malignant tumors. They also defined a correlation between plasma A1AP level and the type of malignancy such that increased plasma A1AP follows the following scheme; breast, gastrointestinal, head and neck, and lung cancers. Also the mean range of A1AP has shown to increase in the following clinical order: complete remission, local disease, local-regional disease and metastatic disease. Thus it was concluded that A1AP could be considered as a cancer marker that discriminates cancer from chronic non-tumoral diseases as well as complete clinical remission from relapses[38]. Furthermore Solakidi and colleagues [28] have assessed level of tumor associated trypsin inhibitor (TATI) as well as the carcinoembryonic antigen (CEA), C-reactive protein (CRP), and AAT in association with malignancy or inflammation to demonstrate the role of TATI in gastric and colorectal cancers. Their results showed elevated level of TATI in 50% of patients with gastric cancer and in 41.7% of colorectal cancer patients. Interestingly, elevated level of TATI was observed in only 8% of patients with benign gastrointestinal malignancies. Thus, TATI can be used as a complementary tumor marker in addition to CEA for gastrointestinal cancers. This finding supports our [34] and other reports that elevation of protease inhibitors was observed in the advanced tumor stages. Whether such elevated protease inhibitors, such as TATI and AAT, are functionally effective in the inhibition of proteases or not could be the subject of further investigations. Summarizing our [34] and other reports, it could be concluded that AAT plays role as a biomarker for malignancies including esophageal cancer.

5. AAT and esophageal cancer

Esophageal cancer ranks among the top 10 most frequent cancers, characterized by poor prognosis and 5-years survival rate less than 10%. Despite many efforts and investigations, the mechanism underlying development of esophageal cancer is not well understood [39]. Iran is located in the so-called Asian esophageal cancer belt where reports indicate the highest incidence rate of squamous cell carcinoma of esophagus (SCCE) of the world from certain parts of this country. Although recent reports [40-43] indicate attempts for identifying the molecular etiology of SCCE in addition to achievement of suitable tumor markers for this cancer, such efforts have so far been unconvincing and further efforts are therefore required [34]. Delayed diagnosis is a major problem associated with SCCE that most often results in diagnosis of the disease in the advanced stages of tumorigenesis. In addition, the high invasive phenotype of SCCE together with metastatic potential leads to low curative resection and high frequency of relapses. For developing effective approaches of diagnosis, treatment, and follow-up of SCCE availability of appropriate molecular markers is an asset. In this regard assessing proteases and their inhibitors such as AAT level could be helpful [21, 36, 37].

In a recent study, we investigated the level of AAT in serum of SCCE patients, its trypsin inhibitory capacity (TIC), and association of its phenotype with genotype [21, 36, 37]. AAT deficiency is an inherited disease as it is characterized by the reduced level of AAT in the serum. The two common genotypes of AAT deficiency are type Z (PiZ) and type S (PiS), which are associated with several malignancies. We assessed the AAT phenotype as well as genotypes Z and S in SCCE and their association with malignancy in Azeri patients. Azerbaijan is a region in the north west of Iran composed of at least three provinces where epidemiological studies have indicated a high rate of esophageal cancer from this region in addition to the north eastern region of the country where the highest incidence rate of esophageal cancer in the world has reported from there. AAT phenotype identification was done using isoelectric focusing (IEF) and its genotype was determined by restriction fragment length polymorphism (RFLP). Results indicate that the mean range of trypsin inhibitory capacity (TIC) and AAT nephlometry are significantly different in patients than that of healthy controls. Measurement of AAT indicated higher level of AAT in patients' serum that was in accordance to what previously reported with regard to patho-physiological status and malignancies (as described in detail above). However, and as a significant finding we found that the augmented AAT is non-functional which accounts for further dysfunction as well as reduction of AAT proper protease inhibitor activity in SCCE patients. Moreover, 97.3% of SCCE patients were homozygote for MM (PiMM) (normal genotype), and only 2.7% were MS heterozygous. Neither of the PiZ and PiS genotypes were identified in the patients ($P<0.05$). Thus AAT is among those tumor suppressors whose augmentation doesn't correlate with proper function, though it might be dysfunctional in tumors.

Finding a cogent relationship between stages of SCCE at the time of diagnosis and change in marker serum level is important since it affects survival rate following to surgery as well as helping in choosing proper method of treatment. Assessing the pathology records of patients, we found that most diagnosis were done in the late stages of tumorigenesis when tumors were fully grown and developed into highly invasive and metastatic phenotype. This was unfortunately a shortcoming in some studies [21, 36, 37]. Due to nature of SCCE, disease related complications appear late. As a result, diagnosis by clinical examinations becomes only possible in the advanced stages of tumor development. This has been true for 70.3% of cases in our study. Thus low rates of curative resection and high frequency of relapses was observed post-surgery (67.56% of mortality). This finding is in accordance with Yunping and colleagues[39] who found poor prognosis of esophageal cancer with an overall 5 years survival rate less than 10% [39]. Thus measurement of AAT in the late stages of SCCE raises further challenges for the applicability of which as a tumor marker in order to be applied for early stage diagnosis. We propose that further studies are required regarding to the change in the level of AAT as a marker along with analysis its defective functionality in a large sample size to achieve a definite correlation between serum AAT, tumorigenesis, and stages of tumors. Further study is also required to establish a rational relationship between increased level of ATT as a response to defect in its function or as a response to malignancy and inflammation as suggested by other researchers (above) at cellular and molecular level. It should also be kept in mind that most SCCE are diagnosed in the late stages of tumorigenesis due to late referral of patients to clinics. Thus determining augmented AAT level in the early stages remains to be investigated in future studies. One way for elucidation AAT level in early stages of malignancies would be establishing definite relationship between inflammatory diseases and cancers, though the level of AAT increases in inflammation. In addition most malignancies exhibit increased production of inflammatory cytokines. This is also true for SCCE in which increased cyclooxigenase has been well documented [2, 5, 15, 21, 22, 34, 36, 37, 44].

6. Conclusion

The poor prognosis of malignancies including SCCE in addition to late diagnosis in the advanced stages of tumorigenesis for most cancers demand further efforts for achieving specific and appropriate tumor markers for early stage cancer detection. While we did not have access to the patients at the early stage of SCCE, combining our results with other investigations indicate that AAT is a suitable prognostic rather than early stage diagnostic tumor marker as both we and others found its correlation with the advanced stages of tumors. As a tumor marker, AAT is highly sensitive, however, like most other tumor markers; it lacks tissue specificity which in fact is a drawback for its organ or tissue specific applicability. Increasing the size of the population under study, establishing a rational correlation between malignancies and inflammatory diseases as well as combining AAT with other tumor markers might be helpful for achieving a better picture of AAT applicability for early stage SCCE and other tumors detection as well as specificity for prediction and evaluation of curative treatment.

7. References

[1] Ambiru S, et al., *Effects of perioperative protease inhibitor on inflammatory cytokines and acute-phase proteins in patients with hepatic resection.* Dig Surg, 2000. 17: p. 337-343.
[2] Ping-I Hsu, et al., *Diagnosis of Gastric Malignancy Using Gastric Juice a1-antitrypsin.* Cancer Epidemiol Biomarkers Prev, 2010 AACR. 19(2): p. 405-411.
[3] Pemberton PA., *The role of serpin super-family members in cancer.* Cancer, 1977. 10: p. 24-30.
[4] Carrell R, et al., *Structure and variation of human AAT.* Nature, 1998. 28: p. 3-12.
[5] Crystal RG, et al., *The alpha1-antitrypsin gene and its mutations. Clinical consequences and strategies for therapy.* Chest, 1989. 95: p. 196-208.
[6] Duncan CS., *Natural history of Alpha-1-protease inhibitor deficiency.* Am J Med, 1988. 84(supp6A): p. 3-12.
[7] Topic AS, et al., *Association of moderate alpha-1 antitrypsin deficiency with lung cancer in the Serbian population.* Arch Med Res, 2006. 37: p. 866-870.
[8] Zhou H, et al., *Is heterozygous AAT deficiency type Pi Z a risk factor for primary liver carcinoma?* Cancer, 2000. 88: p. 2668-2676.
[9] http://en.wikipedia.org/wiki/Alpha_1-antitrypsin_deficiency.
[10] Carrell RW. and Lomas DA., *Conformational disease.* Lancet 1997. 350: p. 134-138.
[11] Ron R. Kopito and D. Ron., *Conformational disease*, in *Nature Cell Biology*. 2000. p. 207-209
[12] Crowther DC., *Familial conformational diseases and dementias.* Hum.Mutat, 2002. 20: p. 1-14.
[13] Carrell RW, et al., *Conformational Disease. a1-Antitrypsin Deficiency.* Chest 1996. 110: p. 243S-247S.
[14] Carrell R.W. and Lomas D.A., *Alpha-1-antitrypsin deficiency. A model for conformational diseases.* N Engl J Med, 2002. 346(1).
[15] Bernacka K, Kuryliszyn-Moskal A, and Sierakowski S., *The levels of the alpha 1-antitrypsin and alpha 1-antichymotrypsin in the sera of patients with gastrointestinal cancers during diagnosis.* Cancer, 1988. 62: p. 1188-1193.
[16] Ward MW, Cooper EH, and Houghton AL., *Acute phase reactant proteins in prostatic cancer.* Br J Urol, 1977. 49: p. 411-419.
[17] Sawaya R, Zuccarello M, and Highsmith R., *Alpha-1-antitrypsin in human brain tumors.* J Neurosurg, 1987. 67: p. 258-259.
[18] Hedstrom J, et al., *Time-resolved immunofluorometric assay of trypsin-1 complexed with alpha(1)-antitrypsin in serum: Increased immunoreactivity in patients with biliary tract cancer.* Clin Chem, 1999. 45: p. 1768-1773.
[19] Trachte AL, et al., *Increased expression of alpha-1- antitrypsin, glutathione S-transferase pi and vascular endothelial growth factor in human pancreatic adenocarcinoma.* Am J Surg, 2002. 184: p. 642-648.
[20] Demidov VP, et al., *Alpha 1-proteinase inhibitor in breast cancer.* Vopr Onkol, 1990. 36: p. 23-29.
[21] Shirao K, et al., *Postoperative changes in acute phase protein in patients with esophageal cancer.* Nippon Geka Gakkai zasshi, 1992. 93: p. 675-683.
[22] Yavelow J, et al., *AAT blocks the release of transforming growth factor-a from MCF- 7 human breast cancer cells.* J Clin Endocrinol Metab, 1997. 82: p. 745-752.

[23] El-Akawi ZJ., sawalha DH., and Nusier MK, *Alpha-1 Antitrypsin Genotypes in Breast Cancer Patients.* Journal of Health Science, 2008. 54(4): p. 493-496.

[24] Sun, Z. and Yang P., *Role of imbalance between neutrophil elastase and alpha 1-antitrypsin in cancer development and progression.* Lancet Oncol, 2004. 5: p. 182-190.

[25] Andolfatto S, et al., *Genomic DNA extraction from small amounts of serum to be used for a1-antitrypsin genotype analysis.* Eur Respir J, 2003. 21: p. 215-219.

[26] Stenman UH, Koivunen E, and Itkonen O, *Biology and function of tumorassociated trypsin inhibitor TATI.* Scand J Clin Lab Invest, 1991. 207: p. 5-7.

[27] Stenman UH., *Tumor-associated Trypsin Inhibitor.* Clinical Chemistry 2002. 48(8): p. 1206-1209.

[28] Solakidi S., et al., *Tumour-associated trypsin inhibitor, carcinoembryonic antigen and acute-phase reactant proteins CRP and a1-antitrypsin in patients with gastrointestinal malignancies.* Clinical Biochemistry 2004. 37(1): p. 56-60

[29] Peracaula R., Sarrats A., and Paulin, *Liver proteins as sensor of human malignancies and inflammation.* PROTEOMICS- Clinical Applications, 2010. 4(4): p. 426-431.

[30] Spencer L.T., et al., *Role of human neutrophil peptides in lung inflammation associated with alpha1-antitrypsin deficiency.* Am.J.Physiol Lung Cell Mol.Physiol, 2004. 285: p. 514-520.

[31] Köhnlein T. and Welte T., *Alpha-1 Antitrypsin Deficiency: Pathogenesis, Clinical Presentation, Diagnosis, and Treatment.* The American Journal of Medicine, 2008. 121(1): p. 3-9.

[32] El-Akawi Z J., Al-Hindawi FK., and Bashir NA., *Alpha-1 antitrypsin (alpha1-AT) plasma levels in lung, prostate and breast cancer patients.* Neuro Endocrinol Lett, 2008 Neuro Endocrinol Lett(4): p. 18766166.

[33] Kuramitsu Y and Nakamura K, *Proteomic Analysis in Cancer Patients.* Yamaguchi, Japan: Humana Press, 2008.

[34] Mohammad Ganji S., et al., *Alpha-1 Antitrypsin Deficient Squamous Cell Carcinoma of Esophagus in the Azeri Population of Iran.* LABMEDICINE, 2010. 41(10): p. 21-26.

[35] Hong S-I, Hong E-S, and Choi MS, *Serum alpha-1-antitrypsin in malignant disease.* K J C P, 1991. 11: p. 1-6.

[36] Schena M, et al., *Alpha 1-antitrypsin as a tumor marker.* Quad Sclavo Diagn, 1985. 21: p. 87-96.

[37] Saito T, et al., *Acute phase proteins and infectious complications after surgery for esophageal cancer.* Surgery Today, 1990. 941(1291): p. 1436-2813.

[38] Varela, A.S. and López Sáez J. J. , *Utility of plasmatic levels of alpha-1-antiprotease (A1AP) as a cancer marker.* Cancer Lett, 1995. 89: p. 15-21.

[39] Yunping Z and Ruwen W, *The molecular mechanisms of esophageal cancer.* EXCLI Journal, 2006. 5: p. 79-92.

[40] Rastgar-Jazii F, et al., *Identification of squamous cell carcinoma associated proteins by proteomics and loss of beta tropomyosin expression in eosophageal cancers.* World J Gastroenterol, 2006. 28: p. 7104-7112.

[41] Sepehr A, et al., *Distinct pattern of TP53 mutations in squamous cell carcinoma of the esophagus in Iran.* Oncogene, 2001. 20: p. 7368-7374.

[42] Zare M, et al., *Qualitative analysis of Adenomatous Polyposis Coli promoter: Hypermethylation, engagement and effects on survival of patients with esophageal cancer in a high risk region of the world, a potential molecular marker.* BMC Cancer, 2009. 9: p. 24.

[43] Mohammad Ganji S, et al., *Associations of risk factors obesity and occupational airborne exposures with CDKN2A/p16 aberrant DNA methylation in esophageal cancer patients.* Dis Esophagus, 2010. 23(7): p. 597-602.

[44] Solakidi S., et al., *Tumour-associated trypsin inhibitor, carcinoembryonic antigen and acute-phase reactant proteins CRP and a1-antitrypsin in patients with gastrointestinal malignancies.* Clinical Biochemistry, 2004. 37(1): p. 56-60

Part 7

Miscellaneous

17

Vitamin D3 and Its Role in the Treatment of Head and Neck Squamous Cell Carcinoma

M. Rita I. Young* and David D. Walker
Ralph H. Johnson VA Medical Center, Charleston,
Department of Otolaryngology – Head and Neck Surgery
Medical University of South Carolina, Charleston
USA

1. Introduction

Head and neck squamous cell carcinoma (HNSCC) is the 6th most common type of malignancy worldwide, and represents over 6% of the global cancer burden [1]. Each year, HNSCC accounts for nearly 650,000 new cases of cancer, and over 35,000 deaths worldwide [1, 2]. Historically, HNSCC has been a challenging disease to manage, with locally advanced disease often requiring a multidisciplinary approach of surgery, chemotherapy and radiation. However, despite significant advances among the aforementioned fields, the current 5-year survival rate of approximately 50% has improved very little over the last 30 years [2, 3]. This poor improvement in prognosis is a reflection of the unique treatment challenges presented by HNSCC, which include advanced stages at diagnosis, high recurrence rate after surgical removal and second primary tumor development [4]. Moreover, not only are current treatment options often non-curative, but they are associated with significant morbidity, including substantial physical deformity and functional deficits. Together, these challenges underscore the importance of developing novel anti-neoplastic treatment strategies which may improve survival and quality of life among HNSCC patients.

One of the more intriguing novel anti-neoplastic agents is 1α,25-dihydroxyvitamin D_3 [($1,25(OH)_2D_3$), calcitriol], the hormone first identified as an effective treatment for rickets, which has recently garnered wide-spread support as a possible anti-neoplastic agent in a number of different cancer subtypes [5]. Epidemiological observational studies, performed mainly in the United States, have long postulated a correlation between higher latitude residence and overall cancer incidence and mortality. The first such theory was put forth in 1937 by Peller and Stephenson, who together hypothesized that increased sunlight exposure lowered the risk of cancer [6]. Four years later, observational studies defined the relationship further, demonstrating a significant association between geographic latitude and cancer mortality [7]. Since that time, scientists have continued to hypothesize that inadequate serum vitamin D levels at higher latitudes increases one's risk for a number of different cancers including colon, breast, prostate and ovarian cancers [8-11]. Large cohort studies have

*Corresponding Author

confirmed similar findings among HNSCC patients as well. Such studies have not only demonstrated significantly reduced 25-hydroxyvitamin D [25(OH)D] serum levels among HNSCC patients, but also found disease-free survival time to be significantly associated with 25(OH)D serum levels [12].

However, a definitive causal relationship is perhaps not as clear as it seems. Though these reports have evoked widespread enthusiasm within the scientific community, such zeal has remained tempered. Most of the data regarding an association between 25(OH)D and cancer is derived from retrospective ecological observational studies. To date, no large-scale randomized control trials have ever been done examining serum 25(OH)D levels and a primary outcome of cancer. In fact, smaller randomized control studies are extremely limited and yield conflicting results as to the significance of this relationship [13]. There are several prospective studies examining the relationship, but such studies have offered no consensus findings regarding the association [14, 15].

The continued optimism regarding vitamin D's role as an anti-neoplastic agent is sustained, however, by a number of molecular studies which support the biologic feasibility of the theory. In particular, proponents cite the widely expressed vitamin D receptor (*VDR*), which to date has been found in over 30 different human tissues including lymphocytes, muscle, skin and cancer cells [16, 17]. Furthermore, the terminal enzyme in the synthesis of active Vitamin D, 1-α-hydroxylase, also exhibits widespread expression allowing for synthesis of the hormonally active metabolite in a number of different cell types. Not only is vitamin D capable of ubiquitous synthesis and action, but *in vivo* studies within both human and animal models suggest that the active metabolite of vitamin D (calcitriol) is capable of eliciting a number of non-calcemic downstream effects. Many of these actions can be considered anti-neoplastic in nature, including anti-inflammatory, proapoptotic, and antiangiogenic properties, the promotion of cell differentiation, and the inhibition of cancer-cell proliferation.

In this chapter we describe the relevant molecular and biological mechanisms regarding Vitamin D metabolism. We also describe the basic and inherent anti-cancerous properties of vitamin D metabolites, with a specific emphasis on its role in the management of HNSCC.

2. Overview of vitamin D biological activity

In 1919, Sir Edward Mellanby conducted a series of elegantly designed experiments on rachitic canines. By placing strict restrictions on both diet and sunlight exposure, he was able to establish a causal relationship between the bone disease rickets and a deficiency of an unidentified trace dietary substance. Mellanby concluded, at that time, that the unknown entity was most likely a previously undescribed fat-soluble vitamin. It was not until 1932, however, that Vitamin D's chemical structure was formally characterized, revealing that Vitamin D was not actually a vitamin, but a steroid hormone. In the late 1960s it was discovered that vitamin D was actually a precursor of a new steroid hormone, $1,25(OH)_2D_3$, produced intrarenally. As both the physical structure and physiologic actions of $1,25(OH)_2D_3$ continued to be better characterized, it was soon found to be a critical component of both calcium homeostasis and overall bone health. As research progressed into the 21st century, scientists discovered that the hormone impacted a number of important non-calcemic cell regulatory functions.

Today, what is commonly referred to as "Vitamin D" is actually a combination of ergocalciferol (vitamin D_2) and cholicalciferol (vitamin D_3). Both compounds are readily available in diet form, with vitamin D_2 being found in plant products and vitamin D_3 found predominately in fatty fish, fish liver oil, and eggs with smaller amounts found in cheese and meat products. In either case, the total amount of either vitamin found within food items is relatively small; thus, many developed countries, including the United States, have turned to fortifying numerous food items, such as milk and juices, with both vitamin D_2 and vitamin D_3. Despite food fortification, diet is not the body's primary means for acquiring vitamin D_3 stores. Instead, the majority of the body's cholecalciferol is synthesized *in vivo* through a photosynthic process occurring in the epidermal layer of sun-exposed skin. Upon exposure to ultraviolet radiation, the epidermis is capable of transforming a cholesterol derivative (7-dehydrocholesterol) into vitamin D_3 (cholecalciferol). The catalysis, however, is not uniform among all populations and is subject to significant and intense variations based on skin pigmentation, sunscreen use, age, gender and even obesity [18].

After synthesis, cholecalciferol enters the blood stream and is transported to the liver. There it undergoes intra-hepatic hydroxylation at the 25 position to create 25-hydroxyvitamin D_3 [25(OH)D_3 or calcidiol]. 25(OH)D_3 is the circulating form of the hormone within the plasma as well as the most accurate biomarker of overall Vitamin D3 status [19]. 25(OH)D_3 is next catalyzed into one of two metabolites: the biologically inert 24,25-dihydroxyvitamin D3 [24,25$(OH)_2D_3$] or the biologically active metabolite 1,25-dihydroxyvitamin D3 [1,25$(OH)_2D_3$]. Exactly which metabolite is created depends entirely on what enzyme is expressed within the local tissue. If the tissue expresses 24-hydroxylase (also known as CYP24A1), then 25(OH)D_3 is modified to become 24,25$(OH)_2D_3$. This particular metabolite has poor affinity and avidity toward the VDR and is considered the first step in vitamin D decomposition. Alternatively, if the tissue expresses 1-α hydroxylase (also known as CYP27B1), the biologically active metabolite 1,25$(OH)_2D_3$ is formed. This particular metabolite is most well known for its regulation of calcium homeostasis and is the metabolite capable of exerting anti-neoplastic effects on cancer cells.

3. Vitamin D mechanism of action

The majority of Vitamin D's hormonal action involves direct interaction with a single VDR. An intranuclear regulator of gene transcription, the VDR is a member of the class II steroid hormone receptors and is closely related to the retinoic acid and thyroid hormone receptors [17]. The human receptor is located on chromosome 12q12q14 and consists of nine exons. Fully transcribed, the receptor is a 427-amino acid peptide with relatively simple binding configuration consisting of a DNA-binding domain termed the C-domain, a ligand-binding domain called the E-domain and an activating domain called the F-domain. The receptor acts by interacting with portions of DNA called vitamin D-responsive elements (VDREs). Located in the promoter region of target genes, VDRES are commonly found within 1 kilobase from the gene start sequence. Such areas are composed of hexanucleotide repeats separated by 3 nonspecified nucleotide bases (for example CGACTA-NNN-CGACTA where N represents any nucleotide).

Once 1,25$(OH)_2D_3$ is transported into the cell, it enters the nucleus where it is capable of binding to VDR. After binding, the 1,25$(OH)_2D_3$-VDR complex synergistically heterodimierizes with retinoid-X receptor (RXR). The $1,25(OH)_2D_3$-VDR-RXR complex then binds specifically to a VDRE sequence complex, with the VDR occupying the 3′ region and the RXR positioned at the 5′ end. Conformational changes which occur after $1,25(OH)_2D_3$ binding results in the release of coreppressors and the simultaneous exposure of binding sites for transcriptional coactivators. VDR coactivators are then capable of binding the complex, which results in the acetylation and subsequent release of histones from the DNA strand. Without histones in place, the appropriate transcription factors are capable of binding to the naked DNA strand and transcription of the target gene is able to initiate.

Certain variables that construct this transcriptional machinery apparatus may have a direct role within the formation of cancer. Recent resequencing of *VDR* gene identified 194 single-nucleotide polymorphisms (SNPs). It has been hypothesized that *VDR* SNPs themselves may have a direct impact on formation and prognosis of certain types of cancer, including HNSCC. The two most widely investigated receptors regarding their impact and role within cancer include a *FokI* restriction fragment-length polymorphism (RFLP) in exon 2 and an adjacent *TaqI* RFLP in exon 9. These two polymoprhisms were recently investigated with respect to their association with HNSCC incidence. Such studies yielded mixed results. Findings from one study demonstrated that the heterozygous genotype of *Taq I* (Tt) polymorphism may be associated with an increased susceptibility to HNSCC [20]. In a separate study, however, both homozygous variant genotypes, *TaqI* (tt) and *FokI* (ff), were associated with a reduced risk of HNSCC as compared to the more common *TaqI (TT)* and *FokI (FF)* genotypes. Thus, it remains uncertain as to whether or not specific *VDR* SPNs provide a protective or deleterious effect regarding HNSCC risk [21]. However, demonstrations of both increased and decreased HNSCC risk warrant continued research into how *VDR* SNPs may not only impact cancer incidence, but also mortality and treatment response.

3.1 Biological plausibility within cancer

The general biologic characteristics and mechanisms of action detailed above presented two main molecular hurdles for scientists considering $1,25(OH)_2D_3$ as a plausible anti-neoplastic agent. First, there was the seemingly restricted localization of 1-α hydroxylase. The enzyme responsible for converting vitamin D into its active form is highly expressed in renal proximal tubules and was once thought to be solely expressed intra-renally However, it is now known that many non-renal cells, including bone, placenta, prostate, keratinocytes, macrophages, T-lymphocytes, dendritic cells and several cancer cells all express the converting enzyme capable of producing the hormonally active metabolite $1,25(OH)_2D_3$ [22]. This particular formation of Vitamin D contains a high affinity for the VDR and is capable of eliciting an anti-neoplastic response. It is this formation with which we concern ourselves for the remainder of the discussion.

The second major impasse was the restrictive localization of VDR to skeletal tissues. However, since VDRs were first discovered their localization has been confirmed on a variety of tissues. With respects to SCC, it has been demonstrated that not only do human cancer cell lines (SCL-1, SCL-2) exhibit VDR expression, but in fact they express the receptor in higher amounts than normal human skin cell lines [23]. The discovery of extra-renally expressed 1-α hydroxylase and extra-skeletally expressed VDR was paramount in vitamin D's acceptance as a possible anticancer agent. Such findings sustained the molecular integrity of the theory, paving the way for the initiation of many phase I and phase II clinical trials.

4. Vitamin D and cancer

Thus far, $1,25(OH)_2D_3$has been presented as a secosteroid whose fundamental intra-nuclear action is critical for appropriate regulation of calcium homeostasis and proper bone mineralization. Vitamin D, however, has other non-calcemic regulatory functions, including many which make it an intriguing anti-neoplastic agent. Four separate cellular functions tend to be compromised in order for cancer to thrive within a normal host environment: 1) aberrant regulation of differentiation, 2) dysregulated cellular proliferation, 3) newly acquired ability permitting invasion and metastasis, 4) dysregulated cell destruction of altered self-cells. Numerous published reports have demonstrated that $1,25(OH)_2D_3$ is capable of restoring or repairing each of the aforementioned hallmarks of carcinogenesis. It does so in a number of ways, including inhibition of cellular proliferation, disruption and inhibition of angiogenesis, promoting apoptosis, and improving tumor immunosurveillence.

4.1 Cellular proliferation and differentiation

The processes of cellular proliferation and differentiation are intimately intertwined, and the aberrant regulation of each is critically important to the prosperity of growing cancer cells. The normal cell grows along a continuum of cellular differentiation. As a cell proceeds toward terminal differentiation, its ability to divide and proliferate is decreased. This feature is exploited and utilized by many newer anti-neoplastic agents, including $1,25(OH)_2D_3$. A promising feature of $1,25(OH)_2D_3$ is its ability to manipulate the cell's state of differentiation. *In vitro* studies in human cell lines demonstrated that $1,25(OH)_2D_3$ is capable of reducing cell proliferation by inducing cell cycle arrest in G0/G1 phase while simultaneously promoting cellular differentiation [24, 25].

These results were replicated within murine SCC cell lines which showed that administration of $1,25(OH)_2D_3$to cells induces G0/G1 cell-cycle arrest via the transcriptional activation of *CDKN1B* and subsequent dephosphorylation of pRB [26]. The study demonstrated that in both *in vivo* and *in vitro* studies, the increases seen in CDKN1B were the result of downregulated p21 activity, a potent CDK inhibitor [26]. Human SCC cell lines that positively express VDR showed a potent decrease in cellular proliferation when exposed to $1,25(OH)_2D_3$ and its analogues [27]. Vitamin D's ability to force cells into differentiation may be of critical importance, as such actions can aid in the inhibition of tumor cell proliferation [28].

4.2 Angiogenesis

Cancer cells will often acquire the ability to escape the confines of the original tumor nidus. The tumor cell often relies heavily on its angiogenic properties to spread. In theory, limiting the tumor's ability to aberrantly generate rogue blood supplies may limit its ability to thrive and metastasize, offering a potential avenue to achievement of loco-regional control. Several studies have demonstrated that $1,25(OH)_2D_3$ contains potent antiangiogenic properties capable of reducing the invasiveness of cancer cells. *In vitro* studies demonstrated that

$1,25(OH)_2D_3$ and its analogs directly inhibit tumor-derived endothelial cell proliferation in addition to disrupting angiogenic signaling in cancer cells [29].

Within HNSCC cell-lines, treatment with $1,25(OH)_2D_3$ resulted in a significantly lower production of pro-angiogenic cytokines, VEGF and PDGF [27]. Meanwhile, the pro-inflammatory and proangiogenic cytokine, IL-8, exhibits no change after administration of $1,25(OH)_2D_3$ [27]. The finding of decreasing concentrations of VEGF has prompted considerable interest, as it has not only been cited as a marker for tumor metastasis, but also used as a prognostic factor in HNSCC patients [30, 31].

4.3 Apoptosis

Apart from its actions on the cell cycle, $1,25(OH)_2D_3$ can also suppress cancer growth via induction of apoptosis [32-34]. Results carried out on human HNSCC cell lines demonstrated that exposure to $1,25(OH)_2D_3$ results in the downregulaion of several anti-apoptotic genes. In particular, $1,25(OH)_2D_3$ represses the expression of the anti-apoptotic, pro-survival gene BCL-2 while simultaneously increasing pro-apoptotic gene products of BAX and BAK [35]. Studies completed on mouse SCC tumor cells with $1,25(OH)_2D_3$ revealed a form of caspase-dependent apoptosis involving the growth-promoting/pro-survival signaling molecule, mitogen-activated protein kinase kinase (MEK) [36]. The study was able to demonstrate that exposure to $1,25(OH)_2D_3$ resulted in increased VDR expression and concomitant cleavage of the pro-survival signaling molecule MEK via a caspase-dependent manner.

4.4 Immune escape

Key to the survival of cancer cells is the evasion of destruction, a critically fundamental step of which is the ability to evade the immune system. HNSCC, like all cancers, is capable of evading the host's immune system via a number of different mechanisms. Cancer can evade antigenic recognition via tissue sequestration, improper lymphocytic homing due to improper expression of adhesion molecules, and antigenic shedding and modulation. In certain instances, however, antigenic recognition remains intact, despite a poor immune response. In such cases, cancers continue to thrive by releasing immunosuppressive cytokine, downregulating MHC I complex, or instilling dysregulated or improper costimulation

Numerous studies performed on HNSCC patients have investigated the effects of $1,25(OH)_2D_3$ on the immune profile of patients. Within the past 10 years, it has been shown that not only do monocytes, B-cells, and T-cells express VDR, but also contain the enzyme 1-α-hydroxylase capable of converting $25(OH)D_3$ into $1,25(OH)_2D_3$ [37]. Such findings confirmed long-standing speculation that vitamin D is critical for the appropriate management and integrity of the immune system. Numerous studies have since attempted to understand exactly how vitamin D modulates the host immune profile.

HNSCC itself is associated with profound immunosuppression [38]. This is in part due to tissue infiltration by immunosuppressive immature progenitor cells with surface marker CD34 [39, 40]. In one study, HNSCC patients treated with $1,25(OH)_2D_3$ exhibited decreased levels of intratumoral $CD34^+$ cell populations and diminished the preexisting profound immunoinhibitory effect of the cancer. Such findings suggest that $1,25(OH)_2D_3$ may be helpful in overcoming the profound immunosuppression associated with HNSCC [41].

Tissues of HNSCC patients who received treatment with $1,25(OH)_2D_3$ contained increased levels of $CD4^+$ cells and, more significantly, $CD8^+$T cells. Such findings indicate an increased infiltration of immune effector cells into the tumor microenvironment. Also prominent was an increase in cells expressing the lymphoid activation marker CD69, which represent mainly T cells and monocytes. The same study showed that HNSCC patients who received $1,25(OH)_2D_3$ prior to treatment had a lengthier time to tumor recurrence compared with patients who were not treated before surgery. The treatment arm exhibited a median time to recurrence that was almost 3.5-fold longer than control patients who were untreated before surgery [42]. These findings are complemented by separate studies suggesting that treatment with $1,25(OH)_2D_3$ may be an appropriate method of restarting the immune system [43].

5. Future clinical considerations

One of the most discussed aspects regarding the implementation of vitamin D as an anti-cancer medication is dosing regimen. The Institute of Medicine recently addressed vitamin D dosing regimens in its newly published Dietary Referenced Intakes for Vitamin D. Their review of the literature yielded the suggested dietary intake of 600 IU per day for persons 1 to 70 years of age and 800 IU per day for persons over 70. Such intakes corresponded to serum 25(OH)D levels of at least 20 ng per milliliter (50 nmol per liter) with recommended daily ingestion not to exceed 4000 IU per day [44]. The same review concluded that the prevalence of vitamin D deficiency in North America, which previously published reports had suggested to be as high as 54% in some populations, has been drastically overestimated [45]. The authors concluded that the vast majority of North American individuals have serum 25(OH)D concentrations above 20 ng per milliliter, which is adequate for bone health in at least 97.5% of the population

Another area of debate is the concept of vitamin D screening as a predictor for cancer incidence. Since its inception, many have taken disagreed with such practices. One of the main areas of contention rests in the number of confounding variables associated with low serum 25(OH)D levels. These variables, which include obesity, lack of physical activity, and poor diet or supplementation practices, have the ability to impact cancer risk. Critics also cite reverse-causation bias, noting that in certain individuals poor health reduces one's ability to participate in outdoor activities, resulting in lower vitamin D levels.

6. Conclusion and future perspective

It is the opinion of the authors that the role of $1,25(OH)_2D_3$ as an anti-cancer agent warrants continued clinical and laboratory exploration. Further investigation into the relationship calls for randomized control trials of vitamin D for cancer prevention. As noted by the recently published IRAC review, observational studies themselves are unlikely to "disentangle the complex relationships between vitamin D and known cancer risk factors [46]." Such reports, however, have paved the way for numerous ongoing phase I and II clinical trials which should begin to elucidate what role, if any, $1,25(OH)_2D_3$ may play in the treatment of HNSCC.

7. References

[1] Vokes EE, Weichselbaum RR, Lippman SM, Hong WK. Head and Neck Cancer. New England Journal of Medicine 1993;328:184-94.
[2] Parkin DM, Bray F, Ferlay J, Pisani P. Global Cancer Statistics, 2002. CA Cancer J Clin 2005;55:74-108.
[3] Leemans C, Tiwari R, Nauta J, van der Waal I, Snow G. Recurrence at the primary site in head and neck cancer and the significance of neck lymph node metastases as a prognostic factor. Cancer 1994;73:187-90.
[4] Jones A, Morar P, Phillips D, Field J, Husband D, Helliwell T. Second primary tumors in patients with head and neck squamous cell carcinoma. Cancer 1995;75:1343-53.
[5] Mellanby E. An experimental investigation on rickets. 1919. Nutrition 1989;5:81-7.
[6] Peller S. Skin Irritation and Cancer in the U.S. Navy. American Journal of the Medical Sciences 1937;194:326-33.
[7] Apperly FL. The Relation of Solar Radiation to Cancer Mortality in North America. Cancer Research 1941;1:191-5.
[8] Garland CF, Garland FC. Do Sunlight and Vitamin D Reduce the Likelihood of Colon Cancer? International Journal of Epidemiology 1980;9:227-31.
[9] Garland F, Garland C, Gorham E, Young J. Geographic variation in breast cancer mortality in the United States: a hypothesis involving exposure to solar radiation. Preventive Medicine 1990;19:614-22.
[10] Lefkowitz E, Garland CF. Sunlight, Vitamin D, and Ovarian Cancer Mortality Rates in US Women. International Journal of Epidemiology 1994;23:1133-6.
[11] Hanchette C, Schwartz G. Geographic patterns of prostate cancer mortality. Evidence for a protective effect of ultraviolet radiation. Cancer 1992;70:2861-9.
[12] Gugatschka M, Kiesler K, Obermayer-Pietsch B, Groselj-Strele A, Griesbacher A, Friedrich G. Vitamin D status is associated with disease-free survival and overall survival time in patients with squamous cell carcinoma of the upper aerodigestive tract. European Archives of Oto-Rhino-Laryngology 2011:1-4.
[13] Manson JE, Mayne ST, Clinton SK. Vitamin D and Prevention of Cancer ,Äî Ready for Prime Time? New England Journal of Medicine 2011;364:1385-7.
[14] Freedman DM, Looker AC, Chang S-C, Graubard BI. Prospective Study of Serum Vitamin D and Cancer Mortality in the United States. Journal of the National Cancer Institute 2007;99:1594-602.
[15] Pilz S, Dobnig H, Winklhofer-Roob B, et al. Low Serum Levels of 25-Hydroxyvitamin D Predict Fatal Cancer in Patients Referred to Coronary Angiography. Cancer Epidemiology Biomarkers & Prevention 2008;17:1228-33.
[16] Norman AW. Vitamin D Receptor: New Assignments for an Already Busy Receptor. Endocrinology 2006;147:5542-8.
[17] Jones G, Strugnell SA, DeLuca HF. Current Understanding of the Molecular Actions of Vitamin D. Physiological Reviews 1998;78:1193-231.
[18] Binkley N, Novotny R, Krueger D, et al. Low Vitamin D Status despite Abundant Sun Exposure. Journal of Clinical Endocrinology & Metabolism 2007;92:2130-5.
[19] Hollis BW, Wagner CL, Drezner MK, Binkley NC. Circulating vitamin D3 and 25-hydroxyvitamin D in humans: An important tool to define adequate nutritional vitamin D status. The Journal of Steroid Biochemistry and Molecular Biology 2007;103:631-4.

[20] Bektas-Kayhan K, Unur M, Yaylim-Eraltan I, et al. Association of vitamin D receptor Taq I polymorphism and susceptibility to oral squamous cell carcinoma. In Vivo 2010;24:755-9.
[21] Liu Z, Calderon JI, Zhang Z, Sturgis EM, Spitz MR, Wei Q. Polymorphisms of vitamin D receptor gene protect against the risk of head and neck cancer. Pharmacogenetics and Genomics 2005;15:159-65.
[22] Zehnder D, Bland R, Williams MC, et al. Extrarenal Expression of 25-Hydroxyvitamin D3-Hydroxylase. Journal of Clinical Endocrinology & Metabolism 2001;86:888-94.
[23] Reichrath J, Rafi L, Rech M, et al. Analysis of the vitamin D system in cutaneous squamous cell carcinomas. Journal of Cutaneous Pathology 2004;31:224-31.
[24] Nagpal S, Na S, Rathnachalam R. Noncalcemic Actions of Vitamin D Receptor Ligands. Endocrine Reviews 2005;26:662-87.
[25] DeLuca H. The vitamin D story: a collaborative effort of basic science and clinical medicine. The FASEB Journal 1988;2:224-36.
[26] Hershberger PA, Modzelewski RA, Shurin ZR, Rueger RM, Trump DL, Johnson CS. 1,25-Dihydroxycholecalciferol (1,25-D3) Inhibits the Growth of Squamous Cell Carcinoma and Down-Modulates p21Waf1/Cip1 in Vitro and in Vivo. Cancer Research 1999;59:2644-9.
[27] Satake K, Takagi E, Ishii A, et al. Anti-tumor effect of vitamin A and D on head and neck squamous cell carcinoma. Auris, nasus, larynx 2003;30:403-12.
[28] Stein J, van Wijnen A, Lian J, Stein G. Control of cell cycle regulated histone genes during proliferation and differentiation. International Journal of Obesity and Related Metabolic Disorders 1996;20:S84-90.
[29] Bernardi RJ, Johnson CS, Modzelewski RA, Trump DL. Antiproliferative Effects of 1,25-Dihydroxyvitamin D3 and Vitamin D Analogs on Tumor-Derived Endothelial Cells. Endocrinology 2002;143:2508-14.
[30] Sauter ER, Nesbit M, Watson JC, Klein-Szanto A, Litwin S, Herlyn M. Vascular Endothelial Growth Factor Is a Marker of Tumor Invasion and Metastasis in Squamous Cell Carcinomas of the Head and Neck. Clinical Cancer Research 1999;5:775-82.
[31] Salven P, Heikkila P, Anttonen A, Kajanti M, Joensuu H. Vascular endothelial growth factor in squamous cell head and neck carcinoma: expression and prognostic significance. Modern pathology : an official journal of the United States and Canadian Academy of Pathology, Inc 1997;10:1128-33.
[32] Simboli-Campbell M, Narvaez CJ, Tenniswood M, Welsh J. 1,25-Dihydroxyvitamin D3 induces morphological and biochemical markers of apoptosis in MCF-7 breast cancer cells. The Journal of Steroid Biochemistry and Molecular Biology 1996;58:367-76.
[33] Benassi L, Ottani D, Fantini F, et al. 1,25-dihydroxyvitamin D3, transforming growth factor beta1, calcium, and ultraviolet B radiation induce apoptosis in cultured human keratinocytes. The Journal of Investigative Dermatology 1997;109:276-82.
[34] Vandewalle B, Wattez N, Lefebvre J. Effects of vitamin D3 derivatives on growth, differentiation and apoptosis in tumoral colonic HT 29 cells: possible implication of intracellular calcium. Cancer Letters 1995;97:99-106.
[35] Ylikomi T, Laaski I, Lou Y, et al. Antiproliferative action of vitamin D. Vitamins and Hormones 2002;64:357-406.

[36] McGuire TF, Trump DL, Johnson CS. Vitamin D3-induced Apoptosis of Murine Squamous Cell Carcinoma Cells. Journal of Biological Chemistry 2001;276:26365-73.
[37] van Etten E, Decallonne B, Verlinden L, Verstuyf A, Bouillon R, Mathieu C. Analogs of 1α,25-dihydroxyvitamin D3 as pluripotent immunomodulators. Journal of Cellular Biochemistry 2003;88:223-6.
[38] Heimdal J, Aarstad H, Klemensten B, Olofsson J. Peripheral blood mononuclear cell (PBMC) responsiveness in patients with head and neck cancer in relation to tumour stage and prognosis. Acta oto-laryngologica 1999;119:281-4.
[39] Pandit R, Lathers D, Beal N, Garrity T, Young M. CD34+ immune suppressive cells in the peripheral blood of patients with head and neck cancer. Annals of otology, rhinology, and laryngology 2000;109:749-54.
[40] Young MRI, Lathers DMR. Myeloid progenitor cells mediate immune suppression in patients with head and neck cancers. International Journal of Immunopharmacology 1999;21:241-52.
[41] Kulbersh J, Day T, Gillespie M, Young M. 2009. Otolaryngology Head and Neck Surgery 2009;140:235-40.
[42] Walsh JE, Clark A-M, Day TA, Gillespie MB, Young MRI. Use of [alpha],25-Dihydroxyvitamin D3 treatment to stimulate immune infiltration into head and neck squamous cell carcinoma. Human Immunology 2010;71:659-65.
[43] Fleet JC. Molecular actions of vitamin D contributing to cancer prevention. Molecular Aspects of Medicine 2008;29:388-96.
[44] IOM (Institue of Medicine). 2011. Dietary Reference Intakes for Calcium and Vitamin D. Washington, DC: The National Academies Press.
[45] Bodnar LM, Simhan HN, Powers RW, Frank MP, Cooperstein E, Roberts JM. High Prevalence of Vitamin D Insufficiency in Black and White Pregnant Women Residing in the Northern United States and Their Neonates. The Journal of Nutrition 2007;137:447-52.
[46] IARC. Vitamin D and Cancer. IARC Working Group Reports Vol. 5, International Agency for research on Cancer. Lyon 25 November 2008.